THE
COMPLETE
GUIDE TO
SENSIBLE
EATING

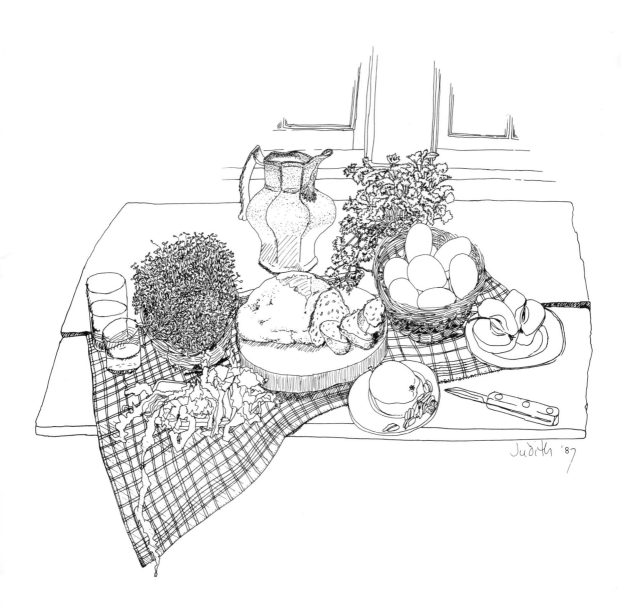

THE COMPLETE GUIDE TO SENSIBLE EATING

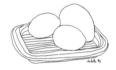

THIRD EDITION

Gary Null

Drawings by Judith Lerner

SEVEN STORIES PRESS
NEW YORK

In the U.K.:
Turnaround Publisher Services Ltd., Unit 3, Olympia Trading Estate, Coburg Road, Wood Green, London N22 6TZ U.K.

In Canada:
Hushion House, 36 Northline Road, Toronto, Ontario M4B 3E2, Canada

Library of Congress Cataloging-in-Publication Data

Null, Gary.
    The complete guide to sensible eating / Gary Null.
      p.   cm.
    ISBN 1-888363-61-4 (cloth)
      1. Nutrition. 2. Food allergy—Diet therapy. 3. Reducing diets.
4. Naturopathy. 5. Menus. I. Title.
RA784.N797 1990
613.2—dc21   97-22206
[B]   CIP

9 8 7 6 5 4 3 2 1

Book design by Hannah Lerner

PUBLISHED BY
Seven Stories Press
140 Watts Street
New York, NY 10013

Printed in the U.S.A.

To Dr. Herbert Shelton

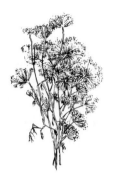

ACKNOWLEDGMENTS

With thanks to some of the men and women whom I have known and communicated with over the years and who inspired me, especially Dr. Herbert Shelton, Adelle Davis, Paavo Airola, Herb Baley, Albert Szent-Gyorgyi, Robert and J.I. Rodale, Bob Hoffman, Broda Barnes, Nathan Pritikin, Linda Clark, John Lust, Lelord Kordel, H.E. Kirschner, John Christopher, Wilfrid Shute, Linus Pauling, Ralph Nader, Irwin Stone, Fred Klenner, Carlton Fredericks, Paul Bragg, Gayelord Hauser and Bernard MacFadden. I would also like to thank Max Friedman, Trudy Gobbic, Adria Eisenmeyer, and Philip J. Hodes, Ph.D. for their invaluable research and editing assistance on the first edition, and Miranda Ottewell for her inspired editing of the second edition.

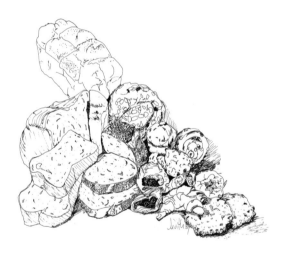

CONTENTS

PART TWO: GETTING TO GROUND ZERO

RECIPES

PROCEDURES AND TESTS

PROGRAMS AND PLANS

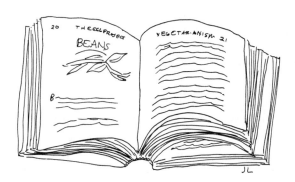

TO THE READER

No one aspect of good nutrition can be applied in isolation; all must be considered together.

What do I mean? Take food combining, for example. The approach has been developed and refined during this century by Dr. Herbert Shelton and many others and forms an essential part of this book. But to try and apply the tenets of food combining without an understanding of your individual nutritional needs is, quite simply, futile. First you must understand what food is, how it works and how it interacts with your body. You must also understand what is wrong with your present diet. If you are American and follow the typical American diet, you may want to know some facts about how food is produced and prepared here, especially animal products and grain foods. Then you must take into consideration the issue of detoxification. In order to pass from an inferior diet to a superior one, you will have to detoxify. Or else you will fail.

Next there is the problem of food allergies. They affect a far greater proportion of the population than is generally acknowledged. Proper testing is important. Low-potency vitamin and mineral supplements may also be appropriate for people seeking proper nutrition, especially in an urban environment. And we cannot ignore the importance of combining enhanced nutrition with regular exercise; the two are inseparable aspects of good health. Finally, you must know how to integrate these changes into your daily life and also how to find an alternative health practitioner for help if and when you need it.

The Complete Guide to Sensible Eating is the shape of things to come, first in this book and then in your life. The various points raised here all come together and form a circle. Other books may attempt to inform you of one or another of them. But only when you bring them all together will you be in a position to really apply them in your life. Food combining alone is of no value, unless joined with a basic understanding of nutrition and health, an appreciation of the importance of regular exercise, and an acute awareness of the environment in which we now find ourselves, late in the 20th century. With access to the right information and the right health professionals, it can be the start of something new.

The Complete Guide to Sensible Eating is the realization that complete well-being is not beyond our grasp, but does not depend on fads or simple answers either. And it may be the only complete, well-rounded, clear, readable guide there is.

Gary Null
June 1990

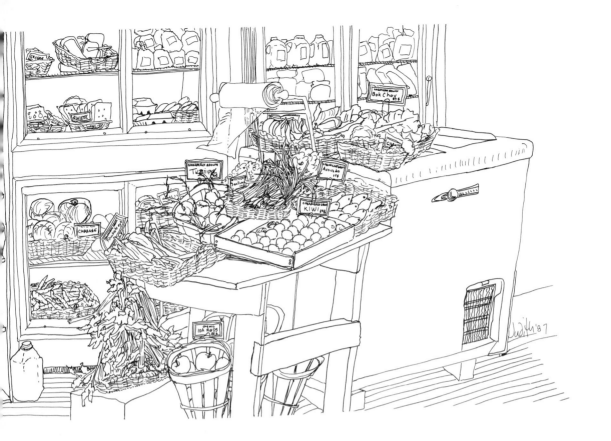

INTRODUCTION

FORTY YEARS AGO, roughly a third of the grocery store was devoted to natural fresh produce. Today, it is a small fraction of that, and even what appears to be natural has been altered. Fruits and vegetables are routinely grown with artificial fertilizers, sprayed with pesticides, treated with hormones and chemicals to control the time of ripening to facilitate mechanical harvesting, dyed, sprayed with chemicals to prevent them from ripening during shipping or to induce ripening after shipping, and coated with waxes to give a glossy appearance.

Modern bread fares no better. The Western world is built on wheat, which, for thousands of years, has been prepared as bread and known as the staff of life. Wheat (and other whole grains) provides a rich source of nutrients: complex carbohydrates, protein, oils, roughage, and an excellent balance of dozens of vitamins and minerals. Grinding wheat with stone rollers blends these ingredients together, providing a product so nutritionally rich that it is prone to spoilage and attacks by vermin and fungi if not immediately used. In order to make a product that could be transported over long distances and stored indefinitely, a product incapable of sustaining life was necessary. White flour was born.

White flour begins with steel rather than stone rollers, thereby flattening and separating the bran and germ, which carry most of wheat's nutrients and are sold as animal feeds, from a chalklike dust. Chlorine gases are used to bleach out any remaining sustenance. The product is then "enriched" with synthetic versions of some of the vitamins removed earlier in the processing. The vitamins considered necessary for this "enrichment" are, not coincidentally, those which are most easily synthesized. These are the ingredients commonly listed on loaves of bread made from enriched flour: barley malt, ferrous sulfate, niacin, thiamine mononitrate, riboflavin, corn syrup, partially hydrogenated vegetable shortening, yeast, salt, calcium sulfate, sodium stearoyl lactylate, mono- and diglycerides, whey dicalcium phosphate, calcium propionate, and potassium bromate.

Some of the flour additives and processing chemicals that need not, according to the Code of Federal Regulations, be listed on the package include: oxides of nitrogen, chlorine, nitrosyl chloride, chlorine dioxide, benzoyl peroxide, acetone peroxide, azodicarbonamide, and plaster of Paris.

One of the most common additives in processed foods is sugar. The average American eats 120 pounds of sugar a year. After processing, many foods are so lacking in taste that there would be no taste at all without adding large quantities of sugar or salt.

Sugar is ideal for the processed food industry because many people like its taste and it is cheap, but primarily because it is addictive. Sugar in large quantities is concealed in many foods; not only in candy, cake, and soft drinks, but in bread, breakfast cereals, cheeses, condiments, and canned or packaged foods. Most processed foods have large amounts of sugar, and those that do not have large amounts of salt. It is not easy to eliminate sugar from your diet.

Americans have grown accustomed to the excellence of their water supplies. Since the turn of the century, treatment of municipal water with chlorine disinfectants has provided protection against disease-causing microorganisms, and private wells are usually tested periodically to assure quality standards. Massive programs to build sewage treatment plants are in effect throughout the country, and standard operating procedures maintain the strict control of disease-causing microorganisms, since much of the water we drink is someone else's sewage. However, even as the problem of human wastes is being controlled, a larger problem is looming: the industrial pollution of drinking-water supplies. Hundreds of thousands of industrial plants discharge grit, asbestos, phosphates, nitrates, mercury, lead, caustic soda, sulfur, sulfuric acid, oils and petrochemicals into many of the waterways from which we eventually drink. Treatment plants designed to handle human wastes are unable to handle many of these more toxic, chemically complex and sometimes unstable substances. Ironically, one of the carcinogens identified as occurring in water results when chlorine mixes with organic matter.

Nationwide, over 700 chemical pollutants have been identified in public water supplies. Most of these are carcinogenic, cause birth defects, or are otherwise toxic. Over 20 scientific studies have documented a consistent link between consumption of trace organic chemical contaminants in drinking water and elevated cancer mortality rates. In spite of mounting evidence, existing United States public health standards reflect virtually no acknowledgement of toxic and carcinogenic substances in drinking water. As a result, no concerted effort has been made to remove them from public water supplies. Parallel failures to protect drinking water quality and to regulate massive discharges of non-biodegradable industrial wastes forecast a grim future for the American public. Toxic contamination has already forced many communities to find alternative sources of water supply. Still, the overwhelming majority of the nation's drinking water systems have never been tested for the presence of toxic pollutants. The response to this dual environmental and health dilemma has been woefully inadequate.

Most of us picture farms as being like those we remember from childhood, or those we have seen in pictures or on television. We imagine farm animals in their pens, or even roaming around a farmyard. Such farms may exist, but they are not the source of the meat we buy and eat today. Chickens are raised by the tens of thousands in giant buildings where they never see the light of day. They are kept in cages in which they cannot move, with conveyor belts bringing them food and water and carrying away their waste. When they do move about, they often slide around on their breasts, as some modern breeds grow too fast for their legs to support them. They are constantly sprayed and their food doused with chemicals, hormones, and medicines. Attempts also are being made to breed featherless chickens.

Many pigs are also raised in cages, without ever seeing daylight. Such conditions are particularly cruel for pigs, which are close to dogs in intelligence and sensitivity. Steers spend most of their lives out of doors, but are no less exposed to chemicals in their upbringing. Today, a steer is born, taken from its mother and put on a diet of powdered milk, synthetic vitamins, minerals and antibiotics. Drugs in its food reduce its activities to save on feed. Next, it is actually allowed to eat some pasture grass, but this is supplemented with processed feed premixed with antibiotics and growth-promoting drugs. At six months, it weighs 500 pounds and is ready for the feed lot. Here it is doused with pesticides and then placed in a pen that is lit around the clock to change natural sleep rhythms and encourage continuous feeding. Food consists of grains, urea, carbohydrates, ground-up newspaper, molasses, plastic pellets, and, most recently, reprocessed manure, a high protein source. After four months in the feed lot, the steer weighs 1,200 pounds. A few more doses of pesticides, antibiotics and hormones to pretenderize it while it is still alive, and it is ready for slaughter. Nearly all poultry, pigs, and veal calves and 60 percent of cattle get antibiotics added to their feed. Seventy-five percent of pigs eat feed laced with sulfa drugs. Cattle feeders use a variety of hormones and other additives to promote rapid weight gain in their animals.

While farmers rely more and more on chemistry to shore up animal health under factory conditions, dangerous residues are showing up in meat and poultry products. Fourteen percent of meat and poultry sampled by the Agriculture Department in the mid and late 1970s contained illegally high levels of drugs and pesticides. According to a recent General Accounting Office report, "of the 143 drugs and pesticides G.A.O. identified as likely to leave residues in raw meat and poultry, 42 are known to cause or are suspected of causing cancer, 20 of causing birth defects and six of causing mutations."

The average American ate two pounds of chemical additives in food in 1960 and ten pounds in 1978, a fivefold increase in less than 20 years. Most of these additives were not put in foods to preserve shelf life or retard spoilage, as is usually claimed; instead, more than 90 percent of the additives (both by weight and by value) were there to deceive—that is, to make the agribusiness product look, taste, feel and nourish more like the real thing.

No one questions the fact that there are a lot of chemicals in our food. Manufacturers contend, however, that these chemicals are safe, that they have been tested and approved by the Food and Drug Administration. Are all these chemicals really safe? The answer is no.

If food additives can be dangerous, why are we told otherwise? The answer lies in the complex interrelations of the food industry, media, government and medical research. The food industry is very big business, with annual sales well over $200 billion. Each year, well over $500 million worth of chemicals are added to foods. The food industry is a major advertiser in consumer magazines and on television, so magazines and television too often are careful of being critical. Food industries are major sources of grants for university research departments. Government agencies have close relationships with the industries they are supposed to regulate. Many research scientists and government management personnel eventually enter the industry they previously regulated—and at much higher paying jobs.

There are literally thousands of chemicals added to food. Few of these have been adequately tested, and none have been tested in combination with others. Many that have been tested have been known to be dangerous for 30 years or more. DES, a synthetic hormone used to fatten cattle, has been known for decades to cause cancer. Industry fights attempts to ban such chemicals every step of the way. When, as in the case of DES, a ban is finally achieved, some producers continue to use it anyway. And by the time the ban is obtained, there are a dozen similar chemicals to replace the one banned, some of which may be worse.

Agribusiness encourages a way of eating that disrupts our physical health and erodes the sense of fulfillment that comes from preparing and eating real food. A fast-food rationale enters the community and the home, with deleterious effects. Agribusiness also undermines small local farmers, who lend economic and ecological stability to the country. And industrialized foods simply do not taste as good as food should. They are dependent on salt, sugar, chemicals, and billions of dollars in advertising. The fact is, most of us simply have forgotten what real food tastes like.

This book talks about real food and how to make the most of it in living a more healthful life.

Part One

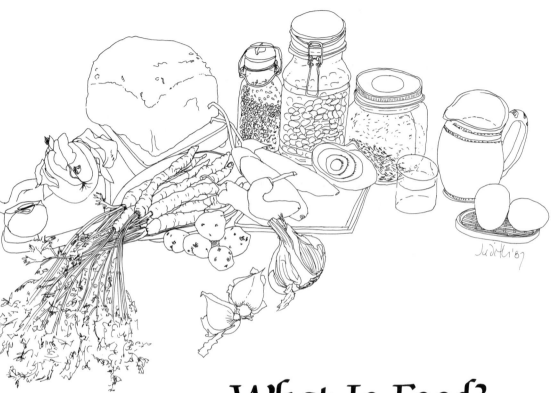

What Is Food?

BASIC NUTRITION BEGINS WITH six major nutrients: carbohydrates, proteins, fats, vitamins, minerals, and water. Along with an understanding of these basic nutrients, for good health you also need to be aware of the air you breathe, the balance of enzymes in your body, and the function of antioxidants in helping your body to combat disease and degenerative processes. Your body needs all of these nutrients every day. How much you need of each depends on your health as well as your energy needs.

Energy may be why we need food, but it isn't necessarily why we eat—sometimes a great deal, sometimes too little, all too often the wrong things in the wrong amounts. When it comes to nourishing our bodies, many of us follow the dictates of myths, fads or bizarre and exotic diets. We all know the proper kind of gas for a car and the best kind of food for our cat or dog. We may know our carburetors and our Siamese, but we don't know ourselves.

Information about good nutrition abounds. Yet many people don't bother to find out more about good nutrition. Some simply don't know where to look or what to trust. These chapters—on our six basic nutrients—should help point the way and begin that journey.

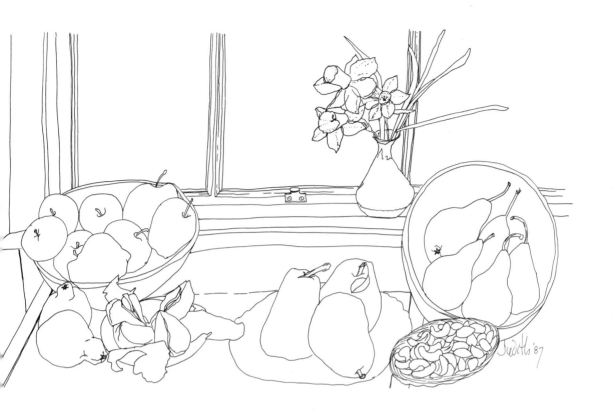

1 · CARBOHYDRATES

*"Buy produce in season, buy it fresh,
and eat it raw when possible."*

UNTIL RECENTLY, CARBOHYDRATES HAVE gotten a bad press. Highly sugared and refined carbohydrates such as candy, soft drinks, pastries, sugared cereals, as well as refined breads and pastas, have been lumped together with complex carbohydrates such as fruit, nutritious starchy vegetables, whole grains, and tubers. When we have thought—carbohydrates—we have tended to think "calories and fattening."

Most people don't understand that there is a distinction between two forms of carbohydrates: the refined starches and sugars that have given carbohydrates their reputation as food for fat, and the complex carbohydrates whose health benefits are finally beginning to be appreciated. Carbohydrates are vital in a proper diet.

3

WHY YOU NEED CARBOHYDRATES

Carbohydrates are everywhere. In fact, they are one of the most abundant compounds in living things. The nutrient group includes nondigestible cellulose (the fibrous material that helps give plants their shape) as well as starches and sugars, two of the storable fuels that supply living things with immediate energy. Each gram of carbohydrates supplies the body with four calories of energy when it is burnt up in our cells. In the U.S., half the calories we get—half of our energy—come from these carbohydrate foods. Many carbohydrate-rich foods also contain substantial amounts of amino acids—the building blocks of protein.

We need carbohydrates. They are the most important source of energy for all our activities. The foods in which they are found—fruits, cereals, seeds and nuts, vegetables, and tubers—also are important sources of the vitamins, minerals, and other nutrients we need to live.

COMPLEX AND REFINED CARBOHYDRATES

Carbohydrate foods come in two forms: complex or refined. *Complex carbohydrates* are starches and fibers in foods like cereals, legumes, seeds, nuts, vegetables, and tubers. They exist in these foods just as they are found in nature, having undergone minimal or no processing.

Refined carbohydrates, on the other hand, have been substantially tampered with. "Refined" may in fact be an overly refined way of putting it. Having been processed by machinery and industry, they are merely skeletons of the complex carbohydrates found in nature.

While the starches and sugars of all carbohydrates supply energy, complex carbohydrates also offer the fiber necessary for good digestive functioning, to supply B and C complex and other vitamins, and/or protein, the building blocks of our bodies. In addition, our bodies tolerate and absorb complex carbohydrates best and most effectively.

Refinement, on the other hand, is a recent innovation in our long history of evolution, food consumption, and food delivery.

When carbohydrates are refined, they are stripped of both their outer shell (the bran layer that contains most of the fiber) and their oil and B vitamin-rich germ (found at their cores). Refined carbohydrates may also be bleached, milled, baked (bread), puffed (some cereals), or otherwise processed (sugar).

Unfortunately, these refined carbohydrates predominate in our diet. Breakfast cereals generally are made from wheat, corn, oats, or rice. But they (with the exception of real oatmeal and a few hot whole wheat cereals) are rarely served in their natural forms. Instead they are dried, refined, bleached, steamed, puffed, flaked, or sugared; occasionally a small percentage of the recommended daily allowance of certain minerals and (usually synthetic) vitamins are added. The cereals can then be labeled "enriched."

But most of the nutrients available from such breakfasts come from the milk that people add rather than from the cereal itself. Our breads (even "rye" and "whole wheat") are usually produced from refined flour and are often loaded with chemical additives. The white rice that graces our plates may look pretty, but it lacks the fiber, vitamins, and minerals found in whole brown rice. Even the potato chips we crunch are a far cry from the vitamin- and fiber-rich whole potatoes from which they are made. Refined carbohydrates may not be good for you. What's worse, they may harm you. They contain little or no fiber, so overreliance on them as a source of energy can lead to poor intestinal health and a myriad of digestive disorders. Also, overconsumption of refined sugar is linked to obesity, hypoglycemia, diabetes, and other blood-sugar disorders.

Complex carbohydrates are closer to their natural state.

Refined carbohydrates are highly processed foods, depleted of nutrients and fiber, and contain little more than pure starch or sugar, which are energy sources of no practical use to anyone.

DANGER: SWEETS CAN QUICKLY SOUR

As we said, you need carbohydrates for energy, especially to fuel your brain. But you don't really need refined sugar. Too much glucose in your bloodstream, an aftereffect of a typical high-sugar coffee and doughnut break, for example, may actually worsen fatigue and overburden your vital organs rather than picking you up. If you have a well-balanced diet, you should be relying on your liver to send forth new energy from its reserves to your working muscles, not on candy bars or doughnuts. Sugar also has been implicated in cardiovascular problems and diabetes.

We know that anyone with hypertension (or high blood pressure) should avoid salt. They should also avoid refined sugar. Animal studies suggest that high blood pressure may even lead to blood-sugar disorders.

Another bonus you receive when you aviod refined sugars is improved resistance to infections. The protective functions of your cells are depressed by all forms of sugar, but especially by sucrose. Also, sugar seems to provoke and worsen skin conditions such as acne. Withdrawing it often results in visible healing. Omitting refined sugar from your meals will also keep the various acids and other digestive juices in your stomach at normal levels.

Your brain must have a constant supply of glucose (blood sugar) in order for its "circuits" to communicate and function properly. Hypoglycemia or low blood sugar, often caused by overconsumption of refined sugars and flour, can distort perception and alter behavior.

If you suspect you are one of America's hypoglycemia victims, don't take this blood sugar disorder lightly. Consult your doctor for the necessary lab tests. Hypoglycemia not only may lead you to snack too often or to nap too often because of the fatigue and hunger it causes, it could also lead to diabetes or obesity. Remember, if you follow a poor diet high in refined carbohydrates—especially sugars—you are inviting hypoglycemia's damage to your brain and nervous system. But at the same time you need a constant supply of glucous in your bloodstream. A proper diet can help.

Too much refined sugar could be a contributing factor in causing children to become hyperkinetic or learning-disabled. It may also cause young adults to be learning-disabled or delinquent. Some studies even suggest that too much sugar is a causative factor in adults who behave criminally or antisocially.

Even naturally occurring sugars can pose problems. Gastrointestinal complaints, for example, can be caused by a sensitivity to the milk sugar lactose in dairy products. Cultured dairy products, including yogurt, which are more easily digested, can provide a substitute for this as well as providing the vitamins and minerals you would miss if you avoided milk.

Fructose (the form of sugar predominant in fruits and honey) has been much praised recently as being superior to sucrose (cane sugar) or glucose (corn sugar). Not always true. It may be sweeter, so you may use less of it—but a simple sugar is sugar to your body. Watch out for any simple or concentrated sugar!

HOW MANY CARBOHYDRATES DO YOU NEED?

Half the calories Americans consume come from carbohydrates. Unfortunately, most of these are refined carbohydrates. The breads most people eat are 55 percent carbohydrate, since the refined flour from which they are made is 75 percent refined carbohydrate. Most flour cereals are 80 percent refined carbohydrate; our spaghettis and pastas are 75 percent refined carbohydrate. Jams, candies, and some pastries may be 90 percent refined carbohydrate.

In contrast, fresh fruit is only 15 percent carbohydrate; dry legumes, even before being doubled in size by the addition of water in cooking, are just 60 percent carbohydrate; and uncooked whole grains, before the absorption of water, are 70 percent carbohydrate. Green leafy vegetables average 8 percent carbohydrate or less; starchy vegetables such as potatoes or corn, 20 percent or less. The point is, by eating vegetables, grains, legumes, seeds and some fruits, with moderate to low carbohydrate content, we are actually reducing calories and sugars in our diet.

The ideal diet gets most (85 to 90 percent) of its calories and protein from complex carbohydrates, and 10 to 15 percent from fats found in nuts, seeds and oils. This ratio allows complex carbohydrates to be the mainstay of the diet, with fewer calories from fats and fewer from complete protein foods. But, in most cases, that is not what happens.

Our bodies are factories—processing foods, making chemicals , storing materials, and producing energy. Just as plants do, your body factory stores much of its energy in the form of simple sugars and starches. Our backup energy reserve is stored as fat. The form of stored energy immediately available and most easily converted into action comes from carbohydrates. The sugars we absorb from our food may be converted into energy, starch, or fat, by the body. At any given time, we usually have available about a 13-hour supply of glycogen (starch) and glucose (a simple sugar). Our blood levels of glucose are supposed to remain stable, with about 15 grams circulating at all times. Each gram of glycogen or glucose, when oxidized by the cells, provides four calories of energy for all the body's needs.

Despite what our backgrounds, palates, or emotions may tell us, supplying energy remains the number one purpose of food. Carbohydrates yield immediately available energy; if they are oversupplied, the body builds up its muscle and liver glycogen reserves or converts the extra amount into fat. High-protein diets, on the other hand, can be dangerous. Protein is mainly a building material—not a primary energy source. It can be burnt up as fuel, but this is an inefficient way to provide energy to our systems; it requires extra energy, and it results in a waste product called urea, which must be disposed of through the kidneys. Over the long term, eating too much protein and burning protein as fuel can overstress and even weaken the kidneys.

Tip: To keep our bodies in balance and get proper supplies of complex carbohydrate, try to have three or four servings a day of fruits or vegetables, and three servings daily of whole grains or legumes. In later chapters you'll see how to combine those foods to get the best possible kinds of proteins from them.

SOURCES OF COMPLEX CARBOHYDRATES

Complex carbohydrates are not hard to find. You just have to know where to look. Basic whole grains, for example, include whole wheat (to which, unfortunately, too many people have became allergic because they have consumed so much refined wheat flour in breads, cakes, pastas, and packaged, processed foods), rye, triticale (a cross between rye and wheat you may be able to tolerate if you are allergic to real whole wheat), corn, barley, brown rice, oats, millet, and buckwheat. All these can be served whole, as cereals or side dishes, mixed in soups and casseroles, ground into whole grain flour and baked into bread, or rolled into whole grain pastas.

Legumes, an excellent source of complex carbohydrates, are also more varied then most people realize. Among the common varieties are soy-beans and soy products such as tofu, tempeh, and miso, mung beans, lentils, aduki beans, split peas, black-eyed peas, kidney beans, navy beans, red beans, pink beans, pinto beans, black beans, turtle beans, fava beans, chick-peas (garbanzos), and peanuts.

Seeds such as sunflower, pumpkin, chia, and sesame are high in both protein and carbohydrates; alfalfa, chia and flax seeds (those grown organically for food, not for fabrics, to avoid pesticide contamination) are highly nutritious when sprouted. Most nuts are mainly fat, but almonds, cashews, pistachios, and pine nuts are high in carbohydrates as well.

The entire vegetable family is a rich source of carbohydrates. Those lowest in calories, such as celery, broccoli, and mushrooms, contain mostly water and fiber; the starchier, root vegetables like carrots, beets, potatoes, and yams, tend to be higher in unrefined starches and sugars as well as in fiber.

Fruits are excellent sources of complex carbohydrates, natural sugars, minerals, vitamins, and fiber. Choose from apples, pears, peaches, nectarines, plums, grapes or citrus fruits. Although the sugar content of these fruits is fairly high, it is diluted with water and released relatively slowly into your system as you chew and digest the cellulose-encased cells of the pulp. Your body doesn't get the kind of sudden jolt it receives from refined, pure sugar. Bananas and other tropical fruits should be eaten in moderation by those sensitive to sugar, since their sugar content is higher. Similarly, dried fruits, including figs, prunes, raisins, dates, apricots, pears, and apples contain three times the sugar dose of fresh fruit; like refined sugar, they are highly concentrated carbohydrates, which should only be eaten occasionally. *Hypoglycemics and diabetics should take special note of this precaution.*

Eating too much fruit can add extra calories, but as long as you don't eat fatty foods as well, fruit will not make you fat. An apple indeed may contain the equivalent of three teaspoons of sugar and the calories that go with that. But it is much harder to down three whole apples than nine teaspoons of sugar. Some people consume as much sugar in one cup of coffee, one mug of cocoa, or one doughnut—without getting all the beneficial vitamins, minerals, fiber, and enzymes of the apple.

PREPARING COMPLEX CARBOHYDRATE FOODS

Grains should be rinsed before use, and the larger legumes—such as beans—should be soaked overnight before cooking. Cooking time can be shortened by using pressure cookers.

People who eat meat and wish to switch to a more complex-carbohydrate-oriented, vegetarian diet often worry that eating will become a boring, asensual experience, limited in variety and taste. Pilgrims, seek no more. There are vegetarian recipes and menus to satisfy every palate and taste. The vegetarian recipes included in later chapters will provide a sampling of their variety and set you on the right nutritional track.

For those who must restrict their sodium intake, a variety of other herbs and spices are available that are even livelier than salt. They include leeks, dill, oregano, cumin, curry, and chili peppers. Vegetables may be mixed with legumes for stews and casseroles as well as soups; seasoned grains, such as millet (perhaps combined with soy granules or lentils for protein enhancement), are delicious stuffed into peppers, tomatoes, or hollowed-out zucchinis.

FACILITATING DIGESTION OF CARBOHYDRATES

Cooked starches are easier to digest than uncooked ones, since heat ruptures the cell walls of plants and allows certain chemicals, called enzymes, to convert the starches to sugars more easily in the mouth and the intestines. These sugars are then used by the body for energy.

Normally, carbohydrates are digested quickly. The carbohydrates in fruit juice may be digested in as little as 40 minutes; starchy foods, such as beans or grains, may take up to 1 1/2 hours. Cooked and eaten properly, the digestion time of a carbohydrate meal may be only 80 to 90 minutes. The more fiber you consume with your meals, the faster the digestion process, since fiber absorbs water and stimulates the actions of the digestive tract.

Animal proteins and fats take much longer to digest, and if sweet or starchy foods are eaten at the same time as meat and fish, they can remain in the stomach for much of the time the protein foods take to digest (up to six hours). This can cause gas and indigestion, since the sugar from the carbohydrates may begin to ferment in the warm acid environment of the digestive tract. For this reason, it's a good idea if you eat meat, fish, or fowl to serve your meal with only a salad and vegetables, saving primary carbohydrate foods for other meals. Also, as we age we may lose some of our digestive capacities, which increases digestion time. This may vary widely, depending on the size of the animal protein portion, how long it was cooked, how thoroughly the food was chewed, and the age as well as the mental and physical condition of the individual.

If you begin your meal with a beverage, you can briefly dilute the acid in your stomach and slow digestion. Cold beverages can suspend initial digestion for a short time, since the acids and enzymes of your digestive system usually operate at body temperature.

Some people complain that they have trouble digesting beans, and that flatulence is a problem. Partly, this is because these products may ferment in the large intestines, producing gas. Beans should be soaked for at least 15 hours before cooking. Cook them slowly to avoid altering the protein, and thoroughly so that their fiber is completely softened. Digestion will then be easier.

Bean sprouts also may be easier to digest than cooked dried beans. Sprouting increases the nutrient content as well as the digestibility of beans, grains, and seeds. Alfalfa and mung beans are two of the most popular types. Alfalfa sprouts are a nutrition powerhouse, containing five times the amount of vitamin C of alfalfa seeds. Two ounces of sprouts a day will supply you with vitamins and live, raw enzymes you might not otherwise obtain from your diet, as well as chlorophyll, which is considered an intestine and blood cleanser. Always steam soy bean sprouts briefly before serving them, since the raw beans contain digestion inhibitors, trypsin, and other natural toxins that can only be neutralized by heating.

The typical American dinner, consisting of meat, potatoes, vegetables, and perhaps a salad, with dessert afterwards, mixes up all four digestive processes at once, weakening them all. The acid from the meat's protein neutralizes the enzyme in your mouth that breaks down starches into sugars, so starch digestion is limited and extended. When a sugary dessert is added, its simple refined sugars start fermenting, resulting in too much acid in the stomach. If you then take an antacid, this plays additional havoc with the digestive process. Such habits eventually can lead to chronic indigestion and too much stress for the gastrointestinal tract.

It would be best to eat complex carbohydrates at one meal, protein at another, and fruits as snacks between meals. Protein meals take a long time to digest, and can leave you with less energy for several hours after eating them, since, ironically, much of your energy is used just to digest the protein, with blood channeled from other parts of the body to the digestive organs to help with the work.

If you eat some fruit 10 to 15 minutes before such a meal, you can also prevent your blood-glucose levels from declining during the time you are digesting your meal. The glucose in the blood has also been diverted to help in the digestive process. Someone who eats complete protein at every meal may spend the whole day with part of his or her energy involved in digestion—a strange way to spend a day!

If, on the other hand, you eat three or four small meals that include complex carbohydrates, your energy levels are likely to be higher and more constant throughout the day. What's more, your intestines will be spared the somewhat exhausting, though necessary, process of prolonged digestion.

There are some people who are allergic to one or more grains, legumes, seeds, or nuts; however, most people who in the past have been diagnoised as "carbohydrate intolerant" can actually benefit from complex instead of refined carbohydrates. (For fuller discussion of allergies, see Chapter 8, "Food Allergies.")

A WORD OR A FEW ABOUT FIBER

Fiber, quite simply, is made up of carbohydrates that the human body cannot digest. But just because they are nondigestible does not mean they serve no useful purpose. Fiber substances such as cellulose are in the cell walls, giving plants the power to grow structurally strong. Fiber does a great deal for us, too.

In the late 1980s, fiber has been rediscovered both by the physician and the nutritionist. More and more researchers—at the National Cancer Institute, the America Cancer Society and elsewhere—are jumping on the fiber bandwagon of digestive health. They have pinpointed the value of fiber in our food to act as a kind of super janitorial service for our intestines, keeping them free of hazardous substances, including some powerful cancer-causing chemicals, that may enter our bodies.

Fiber is not found in meats, cheeses, refined carbohydrates or highly processed foods—that is, in the typical American diet, already too high in fatty meats, bleached breads, and sugary desserts.

Fibrous foods stimulate and exercise your mouth and gums, oral membranes and facial muscles. Fiber also scrubs the cell walls of your colon and bowels, cleaning and hastening transit time though the digestive system for the foods you eat, reducing the possibility that your body will harbor toxins longer than it should. Fiber also fills you up, so you don't have to snack so often.

When adequate amounts are missing from your diet, you may develop constipation, and are at risk of colorectal cancer, or one of the other common diseases that attack the gastrointestinal system. This risk becomes greater when your diet is low in fresh, nutritious whole foods and instead is high in fats and sugars.

By contrast, a diet emphasizing moderate amounts of protein, high intake of natural fiber foods, and low fat intake results in better health of the bowels and the whole body and provides protection against certain types of cancer. Fiber, for the most part, does not even contribute calories.

Fiber should be eaten in its natural form. Our bodies have evolved according to the foods our ancestors ate, and are adapted to derive the toal value of a food: protein, fats, carbohydrates, water, vitamins, minerals, trace minerals, and enzymes, along with the bulk necessary for good bowel movements. The processing of most supermarket cereals originally was based on several not necessarily healthful factors. One of these was profit, which continues to play a major role. Another was the erroneous belief that fiber serves no useful purpose. Now that we know better, processing and food industry methods and beliefs are changing. For example, whole-fiber breakfast cereals have begun to be distributed through supermarkets. Read the labels of "natural" cereals carefully to avoid sugar. Some are genuine whole foods, others contain large quantities of sugar in various forms, or are packaged with preservatives.

If you are in fairly good health, 20 to 30 grams, or about an ounce a day of fiber from natural souces should be adequate. If occasional periods of irregularity are a problem, a few extra tablespoons of untreated, unheated oat germ, wheat bran, or even a tasty variation such as rice or corn bran can be sprinkled over your morning cereal or evening salad and will provide extra benefits.

If you prefer to use fruits and salad foods to meet your roughage requirements, a raw salad for lunch and a partially cooked grain salad such as tabouli for dinner, plus a big puree of fresh fruit in season, would fill the bill nicely. Some researchers believe these absorb the most water in your intestines. Oat fiber will absorb up to six times its weight in water, and vegetables generally hold roughly half as much.

All vegetables weren't created equal in terms of fiber. Root vegetables such as carrots are at the top of the list: their crunchy quality and hardness indicate a high fiber yield. They also require beneficial exercise of your jaws and teeth. Buy produce in season, buy it fresh, and eat it raw when possible. Vegetables can be grated for uncooked salads. But do not neglect the less common tubers: yams, kohlrabi, parsnips, even eggplant can be eaten whole. Never peel away any vegetable skin if it isn't essential to your recipe to do so, since in and near the skin is stored much of the plant's roughage and nutrients.

The whole legume family deserves special attention. A good way to eat these and profit by the skins is to sprout your peas, chick-peas, mung beans, and lentils rather than cook them. Thus you are rewarded with the full value of the live food, including minerals, amino acids and carbohydrate energy. Remember to steam bean sprouts briefly before serving.

A little bran every day will improve your health and regularity, but there's no substitute for a well-balanced diet. And no two fibers are the same. Fiber in fruits and vegetables is different from that in grains. Include them all.

Take, for instance, the fiber in citrus fruits. If you've had a grapefruit or orange for breakfast, you've already had a beneficial two-carbohydrate food factor—protopectin. The pulp of all citrus fruits contains this combination of cellulose plus pectin.

The cellulose in the citrus fruit absorbs fluid from your intestines. So as it enlarges, it quickly pushes along any contents in the intestinal tract. Meanwhile, the pectin becomes gelatinous, and in counterpoint to the cellulose, it provides lubrication and ensures smooth passage for the food.

In addition, protopectin helps you get maximum value out of the other nutritious foods you eat, and enhances your system's use of dietary fats. This, in turn, helps provides some protection against the cardiovascular dangers that high cholesterol levels pose.

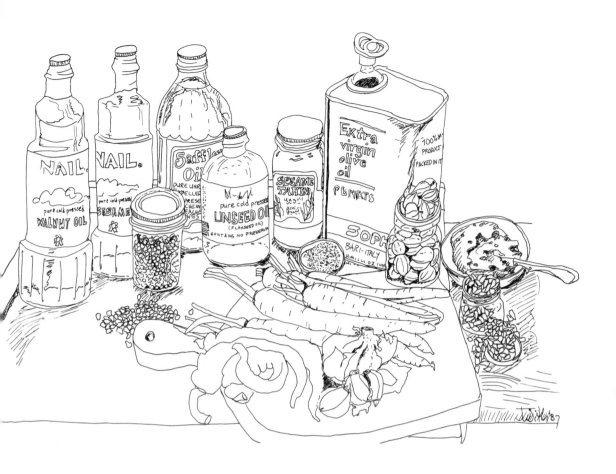

2 · FATS

"Fat is fine for fitness—in limited amounts."

AMERICANS RECEIVE NEARLY HALF (45 percent) of their total calories from fats. Our overindulgence in fatty foods has taken its toll by contributing to a high proportion of overweight Americans as well as to the degeneration of our heart and blood vessels, with fats reducing blood flow through our arteries and increasing blood pressure. The American Heart Association has declared that we should reduce the amount of saturated fat and cholesterol in our diet to help prevent heart disease. In 1984, the government's National Heart, Blood and Lung Institute concluded a 10-year study and issued a report conclusively implicating cholesterol in individuals with an increased risk of heart attack. Several other studies have confirmed the 1984 finding. We should not avoid fat completely. Reducing the fat in your diet doesn't mean eliminating it. People need not overreact, just act.

WHY YOU NEED FAT

Fat provides one of the body's primary nutrients. We need it in small amounts because it allows us to use the fat-soluable vitamins A, D, E, and K, which are essential for the health of our immune system. These vitamins only work when in the presence of fatty molecules or tissue. Fat helps prevent viral infections, protects our heart, blood vessels, and internal organs, slows down the aging process, and helps keep skin healthy. Most importantly, fats, like carbohydrates, are a usable and essential source of energy. They serve as a reserve supply of energy deposited in various parts of the body called adipose tissue.

Fat is a concentrated source of energy. It yields nine calories per gram when it is burned up or oxidized. Proteins and carbohydrates each yield only four calories per gram. Therefore, a little bit of fat goes a long way in carrying out normal body functions.

Body fat acts as an insulator and prevents excessive heat loss. It also acts as a shock absorber. You need some fat around your internal organs to prevent bruising, hemorrhage or rupture. It also is essential for the utilization of nutrients and the production of hormones. In fact, much of your body's chemistry revolves around the proper utilization of fat. Fat is fine for fitness—in limited amounts. But you don't want too much fat, because it may not only surround the organs but can also penetrate them. In excess it can lace itself through the organs, and through the muscle tissue, so your risk of disease (such as heart disease and diabetes) increases.

SATURATED AND UNSATURATED FATS

Not all fats are equal. They may be equal in calories, as the fat in margarine is no different in terms of its caloric count than the fat in olive oil or butter. But fats have unique properties. The omega 3 fatty acids, which are found in fish, for example, have been shown to be healthful to the heart. They also allow the body to use energy more efficiently. The essential fatty acids found in the oil from sesame seeds, sunflower seeds, safflower seeds, and soy beans are vital for the maintenance of health, growth, maturation, hormone production, and other functions. It is important, therefore, to have a variety of fats in the diet in small amounts. It is not necessary to add tablespoons of fat in the form of oil when grains, legumes, fish, seeds and nuts are plentiful sources, with a combination of long and short chain fatty acids found in each food.

There are two kinds of fats—saturated and unsaturated. *Saturated fats* are found in animal food sources such as meat and dairy products, constituting half of the USDA's dietary recommendations for the "basic four food groups." Technically speaking, fat is saturated if the carbon atom chain that makes it up is also saturated with hydrogen atoms. You can tell if fat is saturated if it turns solid at room temperature. Examples of saturated fats include butter, the fatty part of chicken, fish, veal, lamb, pork, and beef (the actual marbled fat that you can see), lard, and coconut oil.

Unsaturated fats are primarily found in grains, legumes, seeds, nuts, and the oils derived from them, including corn oil, safflower oil, sunflower oil, and soy oil—all of which are liquid at room temperature. These unsaturated oils should represent the majority of your fat intake. Unsaturated fats should be used because they provide us with certain essential fatty acids. These have several functions: controlling high blood pressure; helping form prostaglandins (important chemicals for a host of bodily functions); and regulating the ability of substances to enter and leave cells. The body can manufacture those fatty acids not considered "essential" if your diet doesn't provide them.

There are a variety of types of unsaturated fats. Most common are polyunsaturates—such as those found in corn or safflower oil. There are also monounsaturates—such as those in olive oil. There is new evidence suggesting that the latter type actually helps protect your heart by raising levels of certain types of cholesterols (high density lipoproteins), a blood fat in your body. The omega 3 fish fat mentioned above, for example, is also a monunsaturate.

All fats, however, are combinations of saturated and unsaturated, and we need both each day. But, primarily, the fats in our diet should be of an unsaturated quality. Not more than 25 percent should be saturated.

HOW MUCH FAT DO YOU NEED?

There is considerable disagreement regarding how much fat is necessary and appropriate in the diet. Estimates range from 10 to 30 percent of total caloric intake. To be safe, your consumption of calories from fat probably should be limited to 15 percent of your total calories. A quarter of these could be saturated. The rest should come from the unsaturated fats found in cooking and salad oils or, more beneficially, from those naturally occurring oils in vegetables, grains, legumes, nuts, and seeds. In their natural state, if they are unbleached, unadulterated, and have not been clarified or chemically altered to destroy their nutritional benefits, oils not only provide you with fat that the body can utilize, but also supply vitamin E, a substance that has powerful antioxidant properties, preventing the destruction of essential fatty acids and helping your body heal itself. Vitamin E promotes nerve growth and keeps our cells functioning normally.

HYDROGENATION

Once a vegetable oil has been hydrogenated (a process in which hydrogen is added to it to give it a longer shelf life) it becomes solid. It is therefore no longer a polyunstaurated fat (or liquid). It is now saturated.

Be wary of food labels that declare a product is made from polyunsaturates, including certain salad oils and margarines, as well as egg and cream substitutes. One part of the statement is true. What the labels may fail to mention is that now you are eating a saturated fat. The verdict on hydrogenated or partially hydrogenated oils, like margarines, is not yet conclusive concerning their harmful or beneficial effects.

FATS AND DIETING

One of the reasons doctors may prescribe high-fat, high-protein, low-carbohydrate diets is because of the ability of fat and protein to keep you feeling full after a meal, allaying between-meal hunger pangs. If, on the other hand, you eat a complex carbohydrate in the form of a grain or vegetable, it is digested and goes through your system in a matter of 30 to 80 minutes. You benefit from the energy and you're not taxing your digestive system. But it also means there will be a tendency to get hungry sooner.

After all, we tend to gain weight in large part because we get hungry and have in-between meal snacks. A fatty or high-protein food eaten at mealtime will require four to six hours of digestion just to empty out the stomach. As long as you have that much food in your stomach, your appetite is suppressed so you do not feel hungry. Snacks usually come in the form of high-sugar, refined carbohydrate foods like jelly rolls, candy bars and soft drinks. Bypassing the midmorning, midafternoon, and late evening snack, can mean eliminating 400 to 900 calories. In a period of a week you would be able to knock off a pound just by modifying your diet to reduce snacks and increase the protein and fat content.

THE DANGERS OF FAT

Many people like deep-fried foods such as french fries, onion rings, fried fish, potato chips, and doughnuts. These are prepared with fatty oils heated to high temperatures that alter the chemical structure of the fat, creating free fatty acids that can have an irritating effect upon the stomach and on the sensitive mucous linings of the intestines. Eating fried foods frequently can set into motion the ultimate dysfunction of your intestine. Colitis, spastic colon, or some other form of irritable intestine condition may be the result. Heated fats also slow down digestive time. The longer fat is cooked, the more difficult it is for the enzymes in the stomach and the intestine to break it down. Liquid fats are easier to digest. Oils (or unsaturated fats) go through the system much more rapidly than saturated fats.

As I've said before, when you have a lot of fat in your stomach after a meal, you will have less energy. Your energy is being diverted to facilitating the proper digestion, utilization, absorption, and elimination of your food—a lengthy process. Blood and oxygen, also, are diverted, to a degree, even from your brain, just for digestion.

Nearly 95 percent of the fat you consume is digested and utilized by the body. It is fine to have some amount of fat as reserve, but in the absence of regular, daily exercise the muscles begin to atrophy and fat infiltration into the muscle occurs. Fat then takes the place of unused, atrophied muscles. We lose our strength, endurance and stamina, and we become more susceptible to body injury, accident, and disease.

Fats are necessary nutrients. We need unsaturated fats from seeds, grains legumes, and nuts. We don't need all of the oils from salad oil to cooking fats that are typically part of our diet now. Try to keep the fats in your diet to 15 percent. And be selective, choosing certain types of fish, like salmon, for their healthful fat content.

POLYUNSATURATES

For man, it is extremely important to know that the *essential* fatty acids—those we need for certain vital functions—are all polyunsaturates. Our systems can manufacture saturated and even some mono-unsaturated fats from carbohydrates, but not the polyunsaturates. So we must supply these substances from our diet.

What are the vital functions that we need polyunsaturated fatty acids for? First, they are an important part of the membranes that interconnect every cell in our body. Almost all of our cells have both inner and outer membranes. Most of the enzymes in the body are strung along the inner cell membranes, which therefore form a physical locus for the performance of our metabolic functions. And how these membranes influence our enzymes depends largely on the fatty acids in them. A membrane with a high proportion of saturated fat will be very stiff. On the other hand, a higher proportion of mono- and polyunsaturates will allow it to function in a more balanced, responsive way.

A second function performed by fatty acids is to make a special class of hormones, the prostaglandins. A classic hormone is made in one gland—the thyroid, for example—and travels throughout the body giving various signals to cells. Prostaglandins, on the other hand, are made throughout the body. Every single cell, with the exception of the red blood cells, makes prostaglandin. These hormones don't travel far, though, and tend to be destroyed after one passage through the circulatory system. They regulate the local responses of the body to other stimuli, including other hormones, brain chemicals, and drugs.

There are about fifty different biologically active prostaglandins, and the balance between these hormones can have a profound effect on our bodies' functions. Since prostaglandins are manufactured from various fatty acids, an imbalance in the intake of fatty acids can disturb the balance between prostaglandins and trigger a wide range of disorders. These include almost all of the degenerative diseases which have largely emerged in the twentieth century. Heart disease, cancer, auto-immune diseases like AIDS, allergies, asthma, and premenstrual syndrome are consistently accompanied by prostaglandin imbalances.

A NATION AT RISK

Almost anyone in the modern United States has a fatty acid problem. We are all at risk, and the reason can be found in the dietary changes we have seen in this country over the past century. We consume no more fat today than our grandparents did a hundred years ago. We consume much more sugar and less fiber, however, and we also consume a lot less of the foods that provide fish oils and their plant oil analogues.

One group of essential fatty acids is found in corn oil, as well as safflower, sunflower, liver, and kidney oils. These fatty acids are present to some extent in almost all whole foods, but they are by far most concentrated in these oils. Americans do generally consume a substantial amount of these oils, largely because of publicity from the medical community about the need for their fatty acids and about the desirability of avoiding saturated fats.

Another group of essential fatty acids, however, is found in foods and oils which Americans seldom use—most typically in fish oils, particularly those from oily, cold water fish like salmon, tuna, mackerel and herring. These fatty acids are also found in some plants; flax seed—which is used to make linseed oil—is the richest plant source. Other northern-climate plants also have seeds which are rich in these fatty acids—the germ of winter wheat, walnuts, and soybean oil, for instance.

One reason for our deficiency in "fish-oil" type essential fatty acids is that we now mostly use oils that contain less of these fatty acid groups. Another is that we process the oils we do use for convenience. Almost all the oils we buy have been at least partially hydrogenated. This is done to prolong shelf life—but it is a nutritional disaster.

A century ago, people living near water ate a lot of fish, of the kind they could catch. In England, for example, herring, a good source of this group of fatty acids, was a staple food. But over the years the great schools of herring in the North Sea were wiped out, although efforts have begun to revitalize these food sources. Salmon was another staple—reportedly, workers in one plant in England petitioned not to be served salmon at lunch more than five times in a week! Until World War II, food-grade linseed oil was used widely and frequently in the mountains of northern Europe. Today, salmon is a rare luxury, and linseed oil is something to treat furniture with.

Codliver oil is another casualty of changing customs. Not all that long ago codliver oil was a common supplement in the winter; we need more of its unsaturated fatty acids when it's cold, and the vitamin A and D it supplied was an additional benefit. The dying away of the popularity of codliver oil has also deprived us of a valuable arthritis treatment. The fatty acids found in this oil decrease production of some of the prostaglandin hormones that cause arthritic inflammation.

How can you tell if you are at risk? One sign of essential fatty acid deficiency is dry skin, which tends to get worse in the winter. Another is the rough skin that can appear on the backs of our arms or on our thighs, sometimes called "chicken-skin." Brittle or weak fingernails, especially those that tend to split, and dry, unmanageable hair are also warning signs, as is excessive thirst, which usually is not accompanied by a corresponding increase in urination. These are not surefire guides, though; vitamin A, B_6, or zinc deficiencies can produce similar symptoms.

Intense menstrual cramps are signs of an excess production of certain prostaglandins, as well as asthma, eczema, and arthritis. Families with a shared tendency to have allergies often have an inherited dysfunction in the way their bodies process essential fatty acids. This is due to a weak enzymatic link, and these people need more essential fatty acids than the average person.

CORRECTING A DEFICIENCY

Americans consume the greatest number of nutritional supplements in the world; we're something of a joke in this regard in Europe. Taking in fatty acids as supplements is no magic formula; they have to be utilized in the body, and that requires a balance of vitamins and minerals. In fact, without using oil supplements, it's possible to increase the efficiency with which your body uses essential fatty acids by taking extra zinc and B vitamins. Many people have a problem absorbing and metabolizing fatty acids, as we noted above. But if the basic levels of these substances aren't provided it is impossible to tell if the problem is metabolic. Many experts state that essential fatty acid deficiencies are rare due to their wide distribution in our diet, but only the corn-oil type is actually widely consumed. The first step, then, is to boost your intake of the fish-oil type of fatty acids. Sometimes this will bring out the other weak links; once they've been exposed, other supplements can be added more judiciously.

Certain kinds of fish which themselves are good sources of these fatty acids have had much of their value in this regard removed by the time they are purchased. For example, sardines are usually canned not in their own oil, but in olive or soybean oil; in fact, due to potential spoilage problems, it's illegal to can sardines in their own oil. Fresh sardines, however, and almost any fresh cold water fish, are a good source.

Nut butters are also rich in these fatty acids, particularly those made from walnuts and chestnuts. So are cold-pressed nut oils—though "cold-pressed" is a misnomer; the process does heat the oil to a degree, and some of the valuable fatty acids are lost. This also happens with the processing of nut butters, when some oils are lost or altered through the exposure to air during chopping and grinding. These losses, however, are far outweighed by the food value that does remain.

As mentioned before, one of the richest sources of fatty acids is food-grade linseed oil. Whole-grain winter wheat is a palatable and practical source. Vegetable leaves have "fish-oil" type fatty acids in high proportion to other types of fat, but have so little total fat that they are not a very efficient way of supplying these oils. Although olive oil is a good oil to use and may play a role in lowering cholesterol, it does not contain fish oil type fatty acids.

One way to ensure that we get enough essential fatty acids for ideal functioning is to remove foods from our diet which can interfere with their processing. Saturated fats and partially or fully hydrogenated vegetable oils should be avoided. Sugar and alcohol also hamper the efficient metabolizing of fatty acids.

Evening primrose oil is more similar to corn oil than to fish oil in its fatty acids. It has an advantage over corn or safflower oil, though; it bypasses a step in the metabolic process required to utilize the other oils. Some people who have a weak enzyme which makes it difficult to metabolize essential fatty acids can utilize evening primrose oil, which doesn't require this enzyme.

CAUTIONS

Oils lose much of their value when they are used for cooking; heat destroys much of their fatty acid content. So if you're going to rely on oils as supplements, they should be taken in an uncooked form. This can be done by using oils as salad dressing, or mixing them into margarine. In addition, the essential fatty acids in oils oxidize easily, and so have a short shelf life. The byproducts of oxidation are dangerous; so as you increase your intake of essential fatty acids it is wise to also take in antioxidants—particularly Vitamin A and selenium—to safeguard yourself against oxidation.

All of the substances which supply concentrated essential fatty acids should be used carefully as supplements, as it is possible to "overdose" on essential fatty acid intake. It is also important to be aware of a competitive relationship between some different types of fatty acids in the body's metabolic processes. For example, the fish oil type competes with the corn oil/primrose oil fatty acids for the enzymes used to metabolize them. Taking too much of either can produce a relative deficiency of the other.

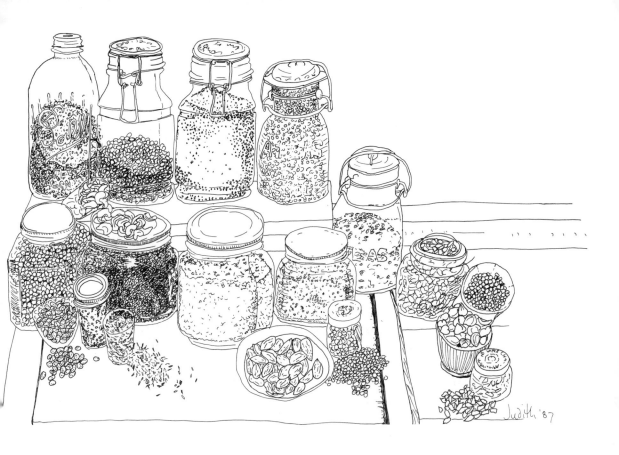

3 · PROTEIN

> *"Sprinkle brewer's yeast on your cereal or blend it with milk, combine tofu with algae in salads, add wheat germ to lentil burgers, and spread peanut butter on whole wheat bread to increase the usability of the protein in these excellent sources."*

A THICK, RARE STEAK, a hamburger, or a platter of fried chicken—the joys of protein? For many of us, protein equals meat equals strength, endurance, growth, health. We have been misled! Meat is only one of several possible dietary sources of protein. Yet it has become the predominant and most expensive source in the average American diet. Our image of protein as the one most important nutrient ("protein" is derived from the Greek "protos," meaning first) has led us to eat so much meat that we often consume more than twice the protein we need each day.

On average, Americans eat nearly 100 grams or 3$^{1}/_{2}$ ounces of protein every day when all most of us actually need is half of that. And despite the legends, even athletes are better off increasing their carbohydrate rather than their protein consumption if they want to increase their endurance and stamina. Eggs, dairy products, grain, legumes, nuts, and seeds are all excellent sources of protein that can supplement meat or replace it in the diet.

WHY YOU NEED PROTEIN

Proteins are the building blocks of life. They are the basic material from which all your cells, tissues, and organs are constructed. Only water represents a larger percentage of your total body weight than protein. Proteins are constantly being replaced, twenty-four hours a day, throughout your entire life, as your body uses and loses cellular materials. The optimal intake of high-quality proteins allows the body to grow and maintain healthy bones, skin, teeth, muscles, and nerves; it keeps the blood count correct; and it allows the metabolism—the body's ability to use food sources—to function at the highest level. Hemoglobin, the part of the red blood cells that provides oxygen to the cells, is made primarily of protein.

When we think of protein, we usually think of it as a body-building substance found in muscles. However, only one-third of our body's protein is concentrated in muscle tissue. Protein is part of every living cell in our body, from the hair on our heads to the nails on our toes. Skin, nails, hair, muscles, cartilage, and tendons all have fibrous protein as their main constituent.

And, with four calories per gram, it is also available as a source of heat and energy. When carbohydrates and fats are in short supply, protein can be converted to glucose, providing necessary energy to the brain and central nervous system.

Protein molecules called *enzymes* start the metabolic process; they must be present for hundreds of necessary chemical reactions and interactions in our body to occur. Enzymes allow energy to be stored and released in each cell; and they allow protein, fats, carbohydrates, and cholesterol to be synthesized by the liver. Protein is responsible for keeping your blood slightly alkaline, and it is the raw material out of which the antibodies that shield you from infection are created. Hormones, which regulate your metabolism, also contain some protein.

HOW MUCH PROTEIN DO YOU NEED?

Generally speaking, adults require .9 grams of protein per kilogram of body weight. (A kilogram is 2.2 pounds.) Thus, a 60-kilogram (132-pound) woman probably needs about 54 grams of protein a day. During spurts of growth, as in infancy, early childhood, and puberty, more protein is needed. Others with higher protein needs include pregnant women and lactating mothers; hypoglycemics; convalescents from surgery and certain types of infection, shock, or fever; and those under any kind of stress. Under certain conditions, such as kidney disease, lower protein intake for a period of time also may be in order.

COMPLETE PROTEINS: THE EIGHT ESSENTIAL AMINO ACIDS

The hundreds of proteins your body synthesizes are all made up of chains of only 23 smaller, basic protein substances, called *amino acids*—composed of nitrogen, carbon, oxygen, hydrogen, and in some cases, sulfur. Of these, the body can synthesize 15 on its own, leaving eight that must be present in your food to be used. These eight are called the essential amino acids. A ninth amino acid, histamine, is essential for children.

Amino acids, of which proteins are made, are necessary for certain vitamins and minerals to be utilized. The amino acid tryptophan, for example, initiates the production of the B vitamin, niacin. Proteins help transport fats through the bloodstream by combining with them to form lipoproteins. In fact, the only fluids in your body that do not normally contain protein are perspiration, urine and bile. It is possible to live without eating protein, but not for very long.

In order for your cells to make the proteins they need for growth, all the necessary amino acids must be present simultaneously in sufficient amounts. This means that if any one amino acid is not present, the protein cannot be constructed. Since protein cannot be stored (except, perhaps, by lactating mothers), it is necessary to eat complete proteins at each meal, or, if you are eating nonanimal products, to mix your protein sources to form complete proteins. To provide your body with only some of the amino acids it needs is like being a baker who buys 100 pounds of flour, 100 pounds of shortening, but only 1 ounce of yeast. Because of the yeast he still can bake only one or two cakes. What does he do with all that flour and shortening? In your body, unused amino acids might be excreted or broken down and oxidized for energy and other metabolic needs.

Protein deficiencies occur when we don't consume enough protein for our body's needs, or when the proteins we do consume lack one or more of the eight essential amino acids. These eight are threonine, valine, tryptophan, lysine, methionine, histidine, phenylalanine, and isoleucine. Foods that contain all eight of these essential amino acids are called complete protein foods. Eggs, meat, fowl, fish, and dairy products—all animal products—contain complete proteins.

For protein to be absorbed and used by the body, all eight essential amino acids must be present in a certain proportion, actually in about the same proportion in which they occur in eggs, nature's complete food package for chicken embryos. Partially complete proteins may contain all eight, but not in the correct proportions. Thus foods high in partially complete proteins, such as brewer's yeast (also called nutritional yeast), wheat germ, the soy food tofu, peanuts, and certain micro-sea algae, should be eaten in combination with other protein foods.

We have been led to believe that animal products—such as meats, poultry, fish, dairy products and eggs—are the only adequate sources of protein. This is based on misconceptions that originated over 40 years ago. If we can't thoroughly digest something, we can't utilize its protein—no matter how complete it is. In addition to digestibility, our ability to utilize protein may be influenced by the functioning of our digestive tract, the presence of any disease or infection, and age. Plant sources, once disparaged, are now starting to get higher ratings.

PREPARING PROTEIN FOODS

Protein digestion is improved by correct cooking practices. Moderate heating of most protein foods increases their digestibility, particularly in the case of beans, grains, and meat. Beans and other legumes contain several toxins (such as trypsin inhibitors) that can inhibit digestion, but that become harmless when they are cooked or sprouted.

Legumes should never be eaten raw: several of them contain even stronger toxins that must be neutralized by heat. All grains and some legumes contain phytic acid in their outer husks. In the intestines, these can form phytates that bind with zinc, calcium, and other minerals and can cause deficiencies in these minerals. Thus, grains should be sprouted, baked with yeast (unleavened breads contain more phytates than leavened), or cooked thoroughly, and vegetarians should supplement their diet with zinc and calcium or foods containing them. Zinc is present in sea-food, peas, corn, egg yolk, carrots and yeast.

It is also very important to cook meat slowly but thoroughly, because of the microorganisms it contains. Pork harbors a parasite than can cause trichinosis if it is not thoroughly cooked. Other meats should be broiled or roasted. Excessive heating of any protein, whether of animal or plant origin, may cause what are known as cross-linkages (the same mechanisms that cause your hair to stay curled after a permanent wave). Cross-linkages make it difficult for protein-digesting enzymes to break protein down into simple amino acids so they can be absorbed. Therefore, it is best to stay away from deep-fried or overdone protein foods. Milk and milk products are especially sensitive to heat, and should not be heated above the boiling point.

If you have trouble digesting milk, you might try yogurt, buttermilk, or other cultured milk products. These contain live, healthy microorganisms that "pre-digest" lactose, the sugar in milk that many people cannot toler-ate, changing it to more easily absorbed lactic acid.

On the average, about 90 to 93 percent of the amino acids in the foods you eat are absorbed after digestion commences.

Sprinkle brewer's yeast (if you are not allergic to it) on your cereal or blend it with milk, combine tofu with algae in salads, add wheat germ to lentil burgers, and spread peanut butter on whole wheat bread to increase the usability of the protein in these excellent sources.

TOO LITTLE PROTEIN

Eating an inadequate amount of high-quality protein forces our bodies to break down more tissue than it can build up, resulting in overall dete-riorization. Some symptoms of protein deficiency are muscle weakness, loss of endurance, fatigue, growth retardation, loss of weight, irritability, lowered immune response, poor healing, and anemia. Pregnant women must be extra careful to avoid this deficiency, since it will not only affect their health but that of their unborn baby. A protein deficiency can pro-mote a miscarriage, premature delivery, or toxemia. Its effects on the baby's development may set the stage for chronic diseases later in life.

The amino acids in grains are high quality and will maintain life and growth, but when supplemented with foods containing other amino acids, they may yield even higher quality protein in greater quantities. For exam-ple, wheat is a fairly good protein. It can maintain life, and millions of poor people have subsisted on bread or cereal alone for long periods of time. However, wheat alone cannot promote optimal growth, and even adults who restrict their protein to one or two food groups or types of foods (a mono-diet) run the very real risk of lowering their body's immune response. Remember, proteins also are needed for the body's natural disease fighters—the antibodies that combat infection. The poor quality of the hair and skin of those on mono-diets reflects their nutritional deficiencies. Their body functions much as a car does that runs on four cylinders when it was built for six or eight.

On the other hand, Americans have been led to think of meat, eggs, fish and milk as the only real suppliers of protein. They have been led to believe that any meat is a good protein source. Wrong! Cured ham has only 16 percent protein; hot dogs, only 7 percent, less than dried skim milk, which has over 34 percent, or sunflower seeds with 27 percent; lentils have more than 23 percent protein. And while all we need to satisfy our protein needs is a few ounces of complete high-quality protein a day, we are getting far more than that.

It is true that incomplete proteins alone do not provide an adequate diet. But one can create complete, or high-quality, proteins by combining foods so that those that are low in some amino acids are eaten together with ones that are high in those same acids. These complementary proteins—all from plant sources—are in this way completed and so can supply protein needs quite nicely. You just have to know how.

Soybeans, for example, are low in the amino acid tryptophan, but high in lysine. To enhance their biological values to you, combine them with complementary proteins like nuts, grains, and seeds, low in lysine but high in tryptophan. In countless combinations, they can make satisfying, delicious dishes.

Tofu, for example, made by curdling soybean milk and packing the solids in layers of cloth, has a protein value—in terms of completeness, digestibility and other factors—only slightly less than animal flesh. It can be made even higher in quality by combining it with grains such as brown rice. Soybean sprouts and soy flour, can also be used in cooking to enhance the complementary values of other foods.

Other legumes, like chick-peas, lentils, and various kinds of beans are low in certain amino acids, but high in others. They also can be combined with grains, nuts, and seeds to form complementary proteins of high nutritional values. Consider, after all, how the rest of the world, which has not had the luxury of high meat diets, subsists. Central American and Caribbean nations use beans and rice as staples. Middle Eastern countries combine sesame paste with chick-peas, while Italians mix lentils, chick-peas, and other beans with pasta.

Grains and cereals make ideal complements to legumes because they are generally high in tryptophan and low in isoleucine and lysine. Grains and cereals supply half the world's protein and are great sources of fiber, too. They do not need to be complemented with meat products to raise the protein values. The myth has been that cereals, grains, and seeds are incomplete, poor sources of protein even when combined. This is false. When you combine grains, seeds, and legumes, you can easily exceed animal protein quality. Consider breakfast cereals with soy milk, or macaroni and cheese, or tofu eggs—or real eggs if you prefer—served with whole grain breads. These sorts of combinations work well because they complement each other.

Why bother switching from what is easy, the protein found in animal products, to what may take some slight effort or change of habit, creating complementary proteins? Simply because health disadvantages of meats and other animal products should outweigh any slight discomfort in seeking new or improved sources of protein. And because our typical diet is based on an unhealthy protein excess.

TOO MUCH PROTEIN

Researchers now agree that American meat eaters and vegetarians alike are generally getting more protein than they need. A study done by the United States Department of Agriculture found that the average consumer of animal products gets over 165 percent of their Recommended Daily Allowance for protein. Children fed by their overcautious—and sometimes protein-fanatical—parents, get a whopping 209 percent. Surprisingly, vegetarians were getting only 15 percent less protein than their nonvegetarian counterparts, still 50 percent more than the Recommended Daily Allowance. Children had identical results in both categories. And in the two groups, women over age 65 consumed the least amount, yet still more than the recommended allotments.

Studies done in the mid-1960s concluded that both vegans (who eat no animal products) and lacto-ovo-vegetarians (who include dairy foods and eggs in their diet) both received protein in excess of the established requirements. The plant-eating vegan men ate an average of 128 percent of their requirements and the women 111 percent; the egg- and dairy-eating, lacto-ovo vegetarians all ate 150 percent; and the nonvegetarian men ate 192 percent. The nonvegetarian women consumed slightly less than 171 percent of their required protein requirements. It is not difficult to obtain your protein. One researcher at Harvard, whose studies showed that only one ounce, or 30 grams, of protein met daily amino acid requirements, has stated that "it is most unlikely that protein deficiencies will develop in healthy adults on a diet in which cereals and vegetables supply adequate calories."

When it comes to certain nutrients, the more the merrier. For example, research indicates that water-soluble vitamin C helps fortify our immune system, and in high doses it may even prevent or reverse certain forms of cancer. In the case of protein, however, more does not mean better. Depending on your age, sex, and the number of calories your require, the total amount of protein needed will average between 30 and 40 grams a day.

PROTEIN AND DIETING

It is estimated that nearly 80 million Americans in any given year are following some dietary program to lose weight. Regretably, many will be going on one version or another of a high-protein, low-carbohydrate diet, with the misconception that protein is low in calories. In fact, the protein foods, such as beef or pork, recommended on most of these diets, are very high in calories.

One gram of protein yields nine calories per gram. Filet mignon, for example, is nearly 40 to 50 percent fat; a single 10-ounce portion can contain up to 1,400 calories. But a certain nutritional sleight of hand makes those diets work for some people. Meats require six to eight hours to digest. You will probably not be very hungry during digestion. To really control overeating, exercise remains more important than limiting calorie intake, since exercise increases your metabolic efficiency. Like carbohydrates, proteins also contain four calories per gram. Four calories remain four calories.

Many diet doctors claim high-protein diets melt away fat. When we want to lose weight, they say, we should limit our diets to beef, hard-boiled eggs, chicken, and cottage cheese. But these foods contain substantial amounts of saturated fats and lack carbohydrates. Such low-carbohydrate, high-protein diets create an abnormal biochemical state within the body, resulting in weight loss.

But it is not a healthy weight loss. In effect, these diets prevent proteins from being stored as fat, leading to a buildup of high-calorie compounds called ketones in the blood stream or ketosis. Many dieters experience anorexia due to the toxic effects of ketones, eliminating large amounts of water and salt, which contributes to weight reduction. Under normal conditions, our bodies would not excrete this unburned high energy compound. Ketosis, therefore, can lead to dehydration, burning of essential body proteins, kidney infection, kidney stones, renal damage, and in several cases, it has lead to coma and death. These more dangerous conditions usually occur only during starvation or as a metabolic side effect of diabetes.

So before embarking on the new monthly best-seller's advice, consider the potential long-term health hazards. It is not uncommon for participants in fad diets to experience bleeding gums, depression, lowered resistance to infection, fatigue, weakness, irritability, and dizziness. A high-protein diet has been shown to encourage the onset of degenerative diseases such as arteriosclerosis (hardening of the arteries). Excesses of the amino acid methionine, can break down into the nonessential amino acid hymocycsteine, which can irritate the walls of the arteries, generating fat deposits in these vessels. And if we omit foods with carbohydrates or with fiber, like fruits, grains and vegetables, we may be inducing vitamin and mineral deficiencies and hurting our digestive system.

PROTEIN AND DISEASE

In the short run, your body can cope with an excess of protein by burning it for energy. This may be inefficient, since protein takes more energy than carbohydrates or fat to metabolize, but it is not harmful. However, over the long run, too much protein can hurt. Ammonium is released when protein is burned in the cell. The ammonium is turned into urea and excreted through the kidneys. Along with the excess of sodium that generally characterizes the animal protein diet, this stepped-up excretion process taxes the kidneys. Too much animal protein can also lead to localized edema and generalized dehydration, as people on high-protein diets require more water than others. To process a high-protein diet the body may require up to four times as much water as for a high-carbohydrate diet.

There are numerous other side effects of eating too much protein. Too much protein causes you to lose calcium through the urine, sometimes resulting in a deficiency in that important mineral. High-protein intake has even been linked to osteoporosis, a degenerative disease that causes the demineralization and loss of calcium from our bones by increasing urinary excretion of calcium. Older women suffer most from this condition.

High-protein diets can be dangerous. For example, eight ounces of beef supplies more than 500 calories, while it is only 22 percent protein. But it also contains lots of fat and water. High-protein diets provide too much saturated fats, cholesterol and sodium, all implicated in heart diseases.

If you eat more protein than you need, your body will have to dispose of extra urea, the nitrogen-containing waste product of protein metabolism. Urea is formed in the liver and excreted through the kidneys. This extra work for your liver and kidneys can be stressful, can make you tired or cause other problems if you don't drink lots of extra water to flush out the kidneys.

Older people and infants are specially vulnerable if they have to use too much water to flush out this excess urea. They can become dangerously dehydrated. Infants are particularly at risk for such conditions. Protein deficiency is very uncommon in the United States. If anything, as we've said before, we eat too much protein compared to our other food nutrients.

Statistics show that on average, individuals in the United States annually eat approximately 200 pounds of red meat, 50 pounds of chicken and turkey, 10 pounds of assorted fish, 300 eggs and 250 pounds of various dairy products.

In this country animal sources of protein often contain large amounts of synthetic hormones, saturated fats, antibiotics, pesticide residues, nitrates, and a host of other potentially harmful ingredients. Although we've heard warnings about the nasty ingredients in those plump "butterball" turkeys, about the carcinogenic (or cancer-causing) effects of charcoal broiling or frying fatty beef, the residues in milk and the mercury and toxic wastes in fish, we're still buying them.

Animal foods are much higher in saturated fats and cholesterol than vegetable protein foods. Especially when combined with the refined carbohydrates of the typical American diet, animal foods have been implicated in increasing our risk of heart disease and arteriosclerosis.

Studies indicate that animal sources contribute to arteriosclerosis much more than vegetable sources. The incidence of arteriosclerosis is substantially higher in those getting their protein from animals than with vegetarians whose protein comes primarily from plant sources.

PROTEIN AND ATHLETICS

One of the most enduring myths in the protein story is in the field of athletic prowess. Despite scientific evidence to the contrary, many athletes and trainers alike still equate protein with strength. This false notion is based upon the premise that protein, especially animal protein, is turned into muscle when ingested. But what is really needed during a strenuous workout or competition is a quality source of energy. For this, protein is actually a less efficient source than complex carbohydrates, since carbohydrates have more deliverable calories.

Depending on the athletic training schedule a person follows, some extra protein may be advisable. This can amount to about ten more grams of high-quality protein, which will be used to replace the nitrogen lost by perspiration and to provide the extra protein needed during periods of accelerated muscle growth. However, after the training period, the athlete only needs more calories than the average person, not more protein. Such misconceptions get many a hungry athlete into trouble each year.

Many trainers are well aware of the scientific void behind the "steak and egg" fortification diets, yet they continue high-protein diets because their athletes believe in them, a tradition that has a strong psychological hold and may, in fact, have an effect on their performance.

Yet these athletes are hurting themselves in many ways. As we work, play, or sleep, our systems are maintaining a biochemical balance of amino acids. If we make a habit of consuming more than we need, our bodies may start abnormally increasing the rate of amino acid replacement in our cells. This rapid turnover of cells is believed to accelerate the aging process. A high-protein diet, therefore, may be counterproductive to longevity. Athletes on high-protein diets also run the risk of dehydration. Protein does not give us that extra edge. Complex carbohydrates, if anything, may.

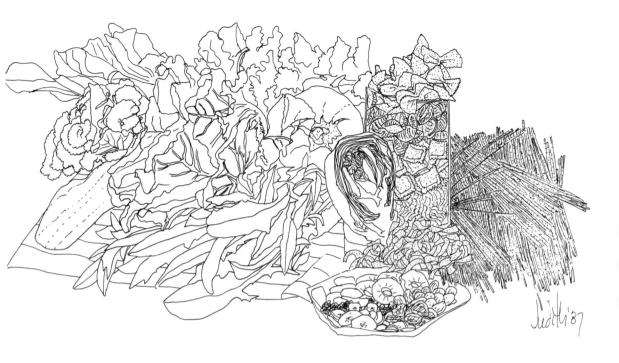

4 · VITAMINS

"People who have had surgery need more vitamin C; those with certain chronic infections or cancers require more folic acid; alcoholics require a full range of vitamin supplements because drinking results in poor absorption of all vitamins from foods; and heavy smokers need more vitamin C to repair cells damaged by the toxins in cigarette smoke and tars."

VITAMINS ARE ORGANIC COMPOUNDS necessary for life. They have no caloric value, but are important parts of enzymes, which help our bodies use food to supply energy. They also help regulate metabolism, assist in forming bones and tissue and build major body structures.

There are two categories of vitamins, the oil-soluble and the water soluble. *Oil-soluble vitamins* (A, D, E, and K) require oil to be absorbed and are stored in the body. When too much of an oil-soluble vitamin builds up in your tissues, it can be dangerous. The *water-soluble vitamins* (B complex, C, and the bioflavonoids) are not stored by the body and need to be replenished daily.

VITAMIN A

Vitamin A, an oil-soluble vitamin, is necessary for growth and repair of your body's tissues. It is essential in the maintenance of your body's immune response, which helps the body fight infections. It helps maintain healthy skin and protects the mucous membranes of the lungs, throat, mouth, and nose. It also helps the body secrete the gastric juices necessary for protein digestion, and it protects the linings of the digestive tract, kidneys, and bladder. Vitamin A is essential in the formation of blood, strong bones, and teeth and in the maintenance of good eyesight.

While abundant in carrots, especially in the form of fresh carrot juice, vitamin A is present in even higher concentrations in green leafy vegetables such as beet greens, spinach, and broccoli. Yellow or orange vegetables are also good sources. Eggs contain vitamin A, as do whole milk and milk products. And while animal livers are concentrated sources of vitamin A, livers also are waste-filtering organs, so one most take care when obtaining nutrients from them. Any hormone or chemical to which the animal was exposed will be concentrated in the liver. It is therefore a problematical food to eat.

One of the first symptoms of vitamin A deficiency is night blindness, an inability of the eyes to adjust to darkness. Other signs include fatigue, unhealthy skin, loss of appetite, loss of sense of smell, and diarrhea. The recommended daily intake of vitamin A, as established by the National Research Council, is 5,000 IU for adults. It is not difficult to obtain this amount from the foods mentioned above in moderate quantities. During times of disease, trauma, pregnancy, or lactation, supplements may be advisable, but should be administered under a physician's or nutritionist's direction, since megadoses of vitamin A can be harmful.

THE B VITAMIN COMPLEX

This family of water-soluble vitamins works together to unlock the nutrients in fats, carbohydrates, and protein, making them available as energy. When each component of the B vitamin group is present in the proper ratio, the entire complex will work harmoniously in every cell of the body. B vitamins are found in nutritional yeast, seed germs, eggs, liver, meat, and vegetables. Whenever muscular work increases, when you run or participate in other endurance sports, the need for B vitamin complex increases.

VITAMIN B₁ (THIAMINE)

Vitamin B_1 is essential to normal metabolism and normal nerve function. It converts carbohydrates into glucose, which is the sole source of energy for the brain and nervous system. B_1 helps your heart by keeping it firm and resilient. It is found in a variety of foods, including whole grains, legumes, poultry, and fish.

A deficiency of vitamin B_1 may result in the degeneration of the insulating protective sheath (myelin) that covers certain nerve fibers. Your nerves can then become hypersensitive, causing irritability, sluggishness, forgetfulness and apathy. If such nerve destruction continues, nerves in the legs may become weakened, and pain may develop in the legs and feet. Paralysis may result. A deficiency may also result in constipation, indigestion, anorexia, swelling, and heart trouble caused by increased blood circulation.

Adult males need a daily minimum of 1.4 mg. of vitamin B_1, and adult females need at least 1.0 mg. If you drink tea or coffee, perspire a great deal, or if you are under heavy stress, are taking antibiotics, or have a fever, your intake of vitamin B_1 should increase. Some nutritionists suggest that athletes should increase their intake to between 10 and 20 mg. daily. Such quantities are not easily obtained from food alone. Therefore, a low-potency, all-natural vitamin may be good insurance.

VITAMIN B₂ (RIBOFLAVIN)

Vitamin B_2 helps promote proper growth and repair of tissues, and enhances a cell's ability to exchange gases such as oxygen and carbon dioxide in the blood. It helps release energy from the foods you eat, and it also is essential for good digestion, steady nerves, assimilation of iron and normal vision. It is vital to the health of your entire glandular system, most particularly to the adrenal glands, those involved in stress control.

Dairy products, meat, poultry, fish, nutritional yeast, whole grains, leafy green vegetables, and the nutrient-rich soybean can provide ample supplies of vitamin B_2.

Lack of vitamin B_2 is one deficiency that can be seen readily. If your tongue is purplish red, inflamed, or shiny, you may need more B_2. Other symptoms are cracking at the corners of the lips; greasy skin; vision problems such as hypersensitivity to light, itchiness, bloodshot eyes, or blurred sight; headaches; depression; insomnia; or loss of mental alertness. A minimum of 1.6 mg. of vitamin B_2 daily for adult males and 1.2 mg. daily for females is recommended. Two servings of most grains will satisfy this requirement without difficulty.

VITAMIN B_3 (NIACIN)

Vitamin B_3 is essential to every cell in the body. It is the fundamental material of two enzyme systems and helps transform sugar and fat into energy.

Many vital functions in our body's food processing plant would stop without an adequate supply of vitamin B_3. Low levels of this vitamin have been linked to mental illness and pellagra, a disease that produces disorders of the skin and intestinal tract.

You can get a reasonable amount of vitamin B_3 from green leafy vegetables, wheat germ, brewer's yeast, beans, peas, dried figs, prunes, and dates. Organ meats, salmon, and tuna are also plentiful sources. Adult males need a minimum of 18 mg. of vitamin B_3 daily, and adult females need 13 mg. daily. Studies have shown that excessive amounts of B_3 can cause glycogen (a starch that helps the body utilize the energy of sugars like glucose) to be consumed hyperactively by the muscles, resulting in the early onset of fatigue. Again, a low-potency vitamin is a worthwhile investment to be sure you are getting sufficient amounts of niacin.

VITAMIN B_5 (PANTOTHENIC ACID)

Vitamin B_5 also works in all our cells. It converts carbohydrates, fats, and protein to energy, acts as an antistress agent, and manufactures antibodies that fight germs in the blood. B_5 is found in many foods including eggs, peanuts, whole grains, beans, and organ meats.

The signs of deficiency include high susceptibility to illness and infection; digestive malfunctions such as abdominal pains and vomiting; muscular and nerve disturbances like leg cramps; insomnia and mental depression. Although the requirement for pantothenic acid is not yet known, 5 to 10 mg. daily for adults is suggested. A low-potency vitamin supplement is suggested.

VITAMIN B$_6$ (PYRIDOXINE)

Vitamin B$_6$ nourishes the central nervous system, controls sodium/potassium levels in the blood, and assists in the production of red blood cells and hemoglobin. It helps protect against infection, and assists in manufacturing DNA and RNA, the acids that contain the genetic code for cell growth, repair and multiplication. It is valuable for those involved in endurance sports.

The best sources of B$_6$ are brewer's yeast, brown rice, bananas, and pears. It is also found in beef, pork liver, and fish such as salmon and herring. Deficiency signs are similar to those of vitamin B$_2$: irritability, nervousness, weakness, dermatitis and other skin changes and insomnia. The official recommended daily amount for adults is 2 mg. of vitamin B$_6$ per 100 grams of protein consumed. This amount is easily obtained from the food sources listed above.

VITAMIN B$_{12}$ (CYANOCOBALAMIN)

Vitamin B$_{12}$ is the most complex of the B vitamins. Every cell in the body depends on it to function properly. It is especially vital to cells in your bone marrow, gastrointestinal tract, and nervous system. It helps prevent fatty deposits from accumulating in your liver, and helps maintain normal weight. All B$_{12}$ in its natural state is manufactured by microorganisms, so it is not normally found in fruits and vegetables. Fermented soybean products such as tempeh, nonfat dry milk, poultry, and meat all contain B$_{12}$.

Common symptoms of B$_{12}$ deficiency are motor and mental abnormalities, rapid heartbeat or cardiac pain, facial swelling, jaundice, weakness and fatigue, loss of hair or weight, depression, and impaired memory. Adults need a daily minimum of 30 mcg. of vitamin B$_{12}$. If you are a vegetarian, you should include a low-potency vitamin supplement with your diet.

FOLIC ACID

Folic acid works mostly in the brain and nervous system. It is a vital component of spinal and extracellular fluid, is necessary for the manufacture of DNA and RNA, and helps covert amino acids.

Brewer's yeast, dark green leafy vegetables, wheat germ, oysters, salmon, and chicken all contain folic acid.

Your body needs comparatively miniscule amounts of folic acid; 400 micrograms daily are recommended. This is easily obtained from the food sources listed above. If you are pregnant, elderly, or suffer from any nervous disorder, you may benefit from additional amounts.

PARA-AMINOBENZOIC ACID (PABA)

Para-aminobenzoic acid is a component of folic acid, and acts as a coenzyme in the body's metabolism of proteins. It helps manufacture healthy blood cells and can help heal skin disorders. In addition, it protects your skin against sunburn by absorbing the portions of those ultraviolet rays of the sun known to cause burns and even skin cancer.

Eggs, brewer's yeast, molasses, wheat germ, and whole grains are good sources of PABA. Signs of deficiency include digestive trouble, nervous tension, emotional instability, and blotchy skin. No official daily requirements have been established for PABA.

CHOLINE

Choline is present in all your cellular membranes and works to remove fat. It also helps regulate your cholesterol levels and is vital to the liver's functions. It aids in building and maintaining a healthy nervous system.

If choline is not present in your system, your liver is unable to process any sort of fat. Fatty deposits in the liver interfere with its normal filtering function. A deficiency can also lead to muscle weakness and excessive muscle scarring. Choline is found in a variety of foods, including: wheat germ and bran, beans, egg yolks, brewer's yeast, whole grains, nuts, lecithin, meat, and fish.

Your body also produces its own supply of choline, using protein and other B vitamins. Daily requirements are not yet known, but the average daily intake has been estimated to be between 500 and 900 mg. In addition to the foods listed above, two tablespoons of lecithin granules may be taken as a supplement to help meet these requirements.

INOSITOL

Inositol carries the responsibility for breaking down fats, and thus plays an important role in preventing cholesterol buildup and normalizing fat metabolism. Studies indicate that inositol has an anxiety-reducing effect similar to some tranquilizers.

A good supply of inositol can be found in wheat germ, brewer's yeast, whole grains, oranges, nuts and molasses. Keeping your intestinal tract healthy may be the best way to make sure you are getting enough inositol. The bacteria or intestinal flora found there are indispensable for making inositol in the body. If you suffer from insomnia, hair loss, high cholesterol levels, or cirrhosis of the liver, you may have a deficiency of inositol. A minimum daily requirement for inositol has not yet been established.

BIOTIN

Biotin helps keep your hair, skin, bone marrow, and glands healthy and growing. It helps produce, and then change into energy, fatty acids, carbohydrates, and amino acids. It is vital to the production of glycogen. Your body manufactures biotin in the intestinal tract. You can also get it from eggs, cheese, nuts, and many other common foods.

Deficiencies are rare. However, when they occur, symptoms include fatigue, depression, skin disorders, slow healing of wounds, muscular pain, anorexia, sensitivity to cold temperatures and elevated blood cholesterol levels. Between 150 and 300 mcg. of biotin will meet your body's daily needs. This is best obtained from your low-potency vitamin supplement.

VITAMIN C

Vitamin C strengthens the immune system, keeps cholesterol levels down, combats stress, promotes fertility, protects against cardiovascular disease and various forms of cancer, maintains mental health, and ultimately may prolong life. Its presence is necessary to build collagen, the "cement" that holds together the connective tissue throughout the body. Athletes, for example, need more vitamin C for collagen synthesis and tissue repair. Vitamin C combats toxic substances in our food, air, and water, and is a natural laxative.

Whole oranges and other citrus fruits, sprouts, berries, tomatoes, sweet potatoes, and green leafy vegetables are important sources of vitamin C. Symptoms of vitamin C deficiency include bleeding gums, a tendency to bruise easily, shortness of breath, impaired digestion, nosebleeds, swollen or painful joints, anemia, lowered resistance to infection, and slow healing of fractures and wounds.

The daily recommended allowance of vitamin C is 45 mg., according to the Food and Nutrition Board. This amount is easily obtained from the fresh fruits and vegetables in your diet, including oranges, sweet peppers, and potatoes. Some nutritionists believe that much higher doses (up to 10 grams daily) can help heal serious illnesses and reduce the risk of cancer (see "The Megadose Controversy" below). Hence, supplements may be beneficial. Those with elevated needs for vitamin C are the elderly, dieters, smokers, heavy drinkers, users of certain medications including oral contraceptives, pregnant and nursing women, and those under any type of stress.

VITAMIN D

Vitamin D helps your body utilize calcium and phosphorus to help form strong bones and teeth and healthy skin. Its action also is vital to your nervous system and kidneys.

A prime source of vitamin D is sunshine, but it may be necessary to get this vitamin from food sources and supplements if sunlight is inaccessible, or if sunshine is to be avoided for other health reasons. Food sources include fortified milk and butter, egg yolks, fish liver oils, and seafood such as sardines, salmon, tuna, and herring.

The symptoms of deficiency include brittle and fragile bones, pale skin, some forms of arthritis, insomnia, sensitivity to pain, irregular hearbeat, soft bones and teeth, and injuries that take an abnormally long time to heal. At least 400 I. U. of vitamin D are needed daily. Greater amounts may be necessary to build strong resistance against bone disease. However, megadoses of this oil-soluble vitamin are not recommended. One-half hour of good sunlight per day is the best supplement.

VITAMIN E

Vitamin E is basically an antioxidant; that is, it protects your fatty acids from destruction and maintains the health and integrity of every cell. It is especially important for promoting the health of your muscles, cells, blood, and skin. It is a primary defense against respiratory infection and disease. Vitamin E also is an excellent first aid tonic for burns. It is believed that vitamin E's antioxidant effects make available larger amounts of fats for metabolism, providing the body with extra energy for muscle contractions, and so is useful in exercise as well.

Ideal sources of vitamin E are wheat germ and wheat germ oil. Leafy plant foods eaten with cold-pressed oils, whole grains, seeds, nuts, and fertile eggs are also good sources. Some common symptoms of low vitamin E levels are swelling of the face, ankles, or legs, poor skin condition, muscle cramps, abnormal heartbeat, and respiratory difficulties.

Nutritionists and doctors recommend a daily dosage for adults of between 30 and 400 I. U., unless a condition requiring higher amounts is present. It's best to supplement.

VITAMIN K

Vitamin K is an oil-soluble substance that helps your blood clot properly, and aids in proper bone development and function.

The microorganisms and bacteria that naturally live in your large intestine produce vitamin K. You can help them work by eating yogurt and other fermented dairy and soy products. Other good sources include green leaves of plants like kale and spinach, cauliflower, broccoli, and cabbage. A tendency to bruise easily is a symptom of vitamin K deficiency . It can be the symptom of other nutritional deficiencies as well. Little is known about the precise daily minimum need for humans, and supplements are not available over-the-counter.

BIOFLAVONOIDS

Bioflavonoids are a group of water-soluble substances that ensure the strength and proper function of your capillaries. Along with vitamin C, with which they are almost always found in food, the bioflavonoids help manufacture collagen. They also protect your cells against attack and invasion by viruses and bacteria.

Excellent sources of bioflavonoids are grapes, rose hips, prunes, oranges, lemon juice, cherries, black currants, plums, parsley, cabbage, apricots, peppers, papaya, cantaloupe, tomatoes, broccoli, and blackberries. The white pulp of the inside of a grapefruit is also an rich source.

Symptoms of bioflavonoid deficiency include bleeding gums and easily bruised skin. There is no established minimum daily requirement for bioflavonoids, but most nutritionists agree that 900 mgs. may be an optimum amount. This amount is obtainable from the foods listed above.

VITAMIN SUPPLEMENTS

Vitamin supplements may be necessary. The world has changed since our ancestors lived on diets without one-a-day vitamins with iron, special mixtures of stress vitamins, or supplemental vitamins for infants or children. For a variety of reasons, individuals often overlook foods that contain essential vitamins or nutrients. They may just be eating less regularly because of the hectic pace of their lives, they may be unable to eat certain foods for health reasons, or they may be dieting. For many of these people, supplements in controlled, recommended doses, could help.

Others who may benefit from vitamin supplements include:

• Infants—particularly those who are not breastfed and therefore may be getting uncertain amounts of various vitamins and minerals.

• Pregnant or lactating women—pregnant women often have reduced levels of a number of vitamins, even though their caloric intake is usually greater than normal, and therefore, they are getting more foods with more vitamins in them. Vitamin supplements are often prescribed. Iron, as a mineral supplement, is almost always prescribed as well.

• Women on oral contraceptives—studies indicate that birth control pills cause shortages of a number of water-soluble vitamins, including thiamin, riboflavin, B_6, B_{12}, folic acid and vitamin C. Diet changes may not be sufficient and supplements are often suggested.

• The elderly—older people tend to absorb less vitamin C and less of the B vitamins than the rest of the population. Also, many older people eat a limited choice of foods. Multivitamin supplements may be in order.

• Those with other special problems—people who have had surgery would need more vitamin C. Those with certain chronic infections or cancers require more folic acid. Alcoholics require a full range of vitamin supplements because drinking results in poor absorption of all vitamins from foods. Heavy smokers need more vitamin C to repair cells damaged by the toxins in cigarette smoke and tars.

THE MEGADOSE CONTROVERSY

Dr. Linus Pauling, the Nobel Prize winner, has engaged in an ongoing controversy in the media and the scientific press, and with other medical and biochemical researchers, about the possible values of megadoses of vitamin C to help fight the common cold and for use in a number of other health situations. While conflicting research studies support both positions, it would seem logical that Dr. Pauling has hit on something substantial. Vitamin C is known to increase the body's ability to ward off infection, to repair tissue damage, and in general to help the body's natural immune system to function properly.

Whether vitamin C is most effective in fighting the common cold or other more serious disorders is debatable. What is clear is that vitamin C plays a role in helping the body fend off diseases—common colds and others.

Vitamin C in large doses seems to have some efficacy in helping treat cancer of the colon, and while not curing the disease, it might slow its development. Research is still minimal in this area.

However, vitamins alone do not work miracles. Megadoses of vitamins should not be used in place of a balanced diet, or to replace days, weeks, or more of neglect of important natural vitamin sources in natural foods. It is important to remember that megadoses as well as vitamin supplements also cannot and should not replace a healthful regular regimen of exercise. Some research does indicate that megadoses of specific vitamins or nutrients can aid in certain specific conditions.

It is possible, for example, that depression can be relieved by taking typtophan (one of the eight essential amino acids) in elevated doses. However, more than one gram, should not be exceeded. Vitamin B_6 may also find some use in larger doses to help women taking the Pill fight depression, a possible side effect, and to help women relieve premenstrual syndrome (PMS) effects.

Megadoses of vitamin A for both acne and for deafness has received some experimental attention in recent years. However, large doses of vitamin A can be toxic to the system. Also women who are trying to conceive, or those already pregnant, should avoid taking any excessive doses of vitamin A, under any circumstances.

All in all, the case for megadoses of vitamins is yet to be made to the general population. Megadoses of, for example, vitamins A or D can be toxic to the body under certain circumstances. As for vitamin C, researchers are still studying effects of megadoses and the verdict is not yet in. However, there are indications that substantial healthful effects can sometimes be realized.

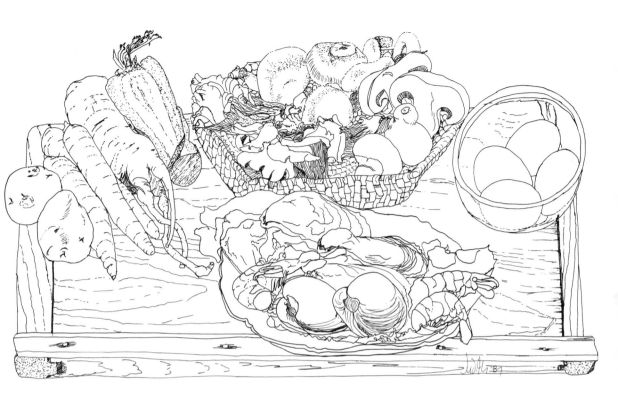

5 · MINERALS

"Your body needs between 55 and 440 mg. of sodium daily to perform its functions. Many of us consume between 7,000 and 20,000 mg. daily. Too much sodium can result in serious health problems, including hypertension, stress, liver damage, muscle weakness, and pancreas disease."

MINERALS SERVE AS BUILDING materials for bones, teeth, tissue, muscle, blood and nerve cells. They help spur many biologic reactions in the body and maintain the body's fragile balance of fluids.

You need minute amounts of minerals. They constitute only 4 or 5 percent of your total body weight. Although we will examine them individually here, understand that the actions of minerals within your body are interrelated. No one mineral can function in isolation.

CALCIUM

Calcium is the body's chief mineral. It is the principal component of your bones and teeth, and a vital component of the liquid that bathes your cells. Calcium is one of the raw materials used in the bloodstream. You need it to help you cope with stress. An active ingredient of some enzymes, calcium is also an enzyme stimulator, that is, it must be supplied before you can store the sugar (glucose) as glycogen in your muscles. Along with several other minerals, calcium also helps maintain the delicate acid/alkaline balance in your blood, protecting it against overacidity.

Without a steady supply of calcium, your bones and teeth would not remain hard and durable. Your brain would not function properly, nor would your muscles be able to store energy. Without enough calcium in your diet, the digestive, circulatory, and immune systems would suffer. Adequate amounts are necessary to avoid the many complications that can come from calcium deposits, which are caused by calcium that has been removed from the body's reserves and lodges in soft tissue. Warnings of calcium deficiency include nervousness, depression, headaches, and insomnia.

Milk is one of the best sources of calcium, as are other, more easily absorbed dairy products such as buttermilk, yogurt, acidophilus milk (a healthful bacteria-rich fermented milk product), and kefir (also a milk product). Most cheeses are good sources. Oatmeal, collard greens, and tempeh are also rich in calcium. Sesame seeds, torula yeast, carob flour, and sea vegetables all contain calcium in smaller quantities.

However, the body will not always properly absorb or utilize calcium. For example, if there aren't enough complete proteins in your diet, the necessary substances that allow calcium to be absorbed by your bones won't be available. Also, protein is needed for your body to make collagen. If you eat high protein foods, you will absorb 15–20 percent of the calcium in your food, as opposed to 5 percent if you don't. However, an excessively high protein diet will cause you to lose calcium thorough the urine. Sugar in the diet (except for lactose or milk sugar) will also antagonize the absorption of calcium.

For a healthy adult, 800 to 1,200 mg. of calcium daily is sufficient. This is usually obtainable from foods in the diet such as those listed above. For women who are pregnant or breast feeding, 1,200 mg. is required. As women age, calcium supplements, ideally in forms like amino acid chelate, might be necessary to fight the onset or severity of osteoporosis.

CHROMIUM

Chromium is important to your heart, liver, brain, and glucose metabolism system. It is vital to the production of protein and to white blood cells, where it helps fight bacteria, viruses, toxins, arthritis, cancer, and premature aging. To counteract stress, your adrenal glands must have an adequate supply of chromium.

The best food sources of chromium are whole wheat flour, brewer's yeast, nuts, black pepper, all whole grain cereals except rye and corn, fresh fruit juices, dairy products, root vegetables, legumes, leafy vegetables, and mushrooms.

Without chromium, insulin cannot transport glucose from your bloodstream to your cells, nor can your liver properly remove excess fats from your blood. A deficiency can result in rapid premature aging, since protein production will be seriously impaired. Symptoms of chromium deficiency include fatigue, dizziness, anxiety, insomnia, a craving for alcohol, blurred vision, depression, and panic.

No definitive guidelines have been established by the government on the amount of chromium necessary on a daily basis, but trace mineral experts suggest that 200 mcg. will provide an adequate daily supply. This is usually obtainable from the diet.

IODINE

Iodine is essential to the manufacture of thyroxin, the hormone that controls the speed at which your blood takes the food from your intestines to the cells, where it is used for energy. It is particularly important to your heart, your immune system and your system of protein synthesis.

Fresh seafood is a good source of iodine, as is garlic. You can enhance the iodine content of your diet by using sea vegetables such as hiziki, wakame, kelp, or dulse. Dried mushrooms, leafy greens, celery, tomatoes, radishes, carrots, and onions also supply iodine.

Without adequate amounts of iodine, the way your cells use energy would be seriously impaired. Proper growth in childhood could not take place, and maintenance of healthy adult tissue could not occur. An iodine deficiency can lower your resistance to infection and impair metabolism of fat in the bloodstream. Thyroid malfunctions are a direct result of iodine deficiency. Symptoms of inadequate iodine consumption include sluggishness, bad complexion, and unhealthy-looking hair, teeth, and nails. You need 150 mcg. of iodine. Some nutritionists believe that 3 mg. a day of this trace mineral is necessary to prevent serious thyroid disorders. Sufficient amounts of iodine are generally available in the foods we eat without supplements.

IRON

Without the oxygen-carrier iron, you could not live. The hemoglobin in your red blood cells, the myoglobin in your muscles, and the enzymes tied in with energy release, all depend on iron.

The most concentrated sources of iron are animal livers, but as we have mentioned, the liver is a waste-filtering organ, and any hormone or chemical—like pesticides or antibiotics fed to animals—to which the animal was exposed will be concentrated there. Egg yolks contain more iron than muscle meats. Other good sources include leafy green vegetables, dried beans, peaches, apricots, dates, prunes, cherries, figs, raisins, and blackstrap molasses.

A deficiency of iron can cause certain types of anemia. Deficiency symptoms include chronic fatigue, shortness of breath, headache, pale skin, and opaque or brittle nails. The daily requirements for iron are 10 mg. for adult males and 18 mg. for women. For pregnant women, 30–60 mg. are required. Starting the day with a hot cereal on which you've sprinkled two tablespoons of rice bran, torula yeast, or pumpkin seed meal will go a long way toward satisfying your iron needs. Daily iron supplements are also recommended.

MAGNESIUM

Magnesium is a versatile, tireless worker in your body's protein production process. In addition, it is one of your body's most important coenzymes. It works with calcium to turn it into something the body can use. It is necessary for the production of hormones, and it works in your muscles, cells, nervous system, digestive system, reproductive system, blood, and immune system.

Green leafy vegetables are one of the best sources for magnesium. Nuts, seeds, avocados, and turnips also contain significant amounts. Whole grains, legumes, organic eggs, and raw milk are excellent sources. Many fruits and natural sweets such as carob, honey, and blackstrap molasses also contain magnesium.

Magnesium deficiency can result in lowered immunity, improper muscle function, and impaired digestion. Without adequate magnesium, your nerves can become ragged and supersensitive to pain. Your bones would be too soft to support you, and production of new protein would be impaired. Without it you would be unable to store energy, synthesize sex hormones, or prevent your blood from clotting. Signs of magnesium deficiency are an irregular heartbeat, hair loss, and easily broken nails.

The recommended daily intake of magnesium is 350 mg., but 450–650 mg. may be a more realistic figure for maintaining optimal health. Sufficient amounts of magnesium can be obtained in the diet from some of the foods listed above.

MANGANESE

Manganese is a trace mineral that is active in protein production and essential to the correct structure of your bones, teeth, cartilage, and tendons. Vital in the formation of new blood cells in your bone marrow, it is also necessary for transmitting nerve impulses in your brain. Manganese plays an important role in the metabolism of blood sugar and fats, and is necessary for the production of sex hormones.

Nuts, seeds, and whole grains are excellent sources of manganese. Green leafy vegetables, if grown organically in mineral-rich soil, can supply you with manganese. So can rhubarb, broccoli, carrots, potatoes, peas, and beans. Pineapples, blueberries and raisins, cloves and ginger are also good sources.

Without manganese, a slow deterioration of muscle health—myasthenia gravis—can develop. Protein production and carbohydrate/fat metabolism would be inhibited. Manganese deficiencies can be related to blood sugar disorders and sexual dysfunction There is no official recommended daily requirement for manganese, but trace mineral experts suggest up to 7 mg. daily. It is worthwhile to supplement here.

PHOSPHOROUS

Phosphorous works in your bones, teeth, collagen, nerves, muscles, metabolic and cellular systems, brain, liver, digestive and circulatory systems, and eyes. It is an important part of your genetic materials, RNA and DNA, and helps maintain your body fluids in the right balance. It is indispensible to the runner since it plays a vital role in supplying energy to muscles by burning carbohydrates.

Phosphorus is available in nearly every food you eat. Eat a lot of refined foods, though, and you are in danger of getting too much. Protein foods like meat, poultry, fish, eggs, dairy products, whole grains, nuts, and seeds supply phosphorus in abundance. Vegetables that contain phosphorus include legumes, whole grains, celery, cabbage, carrots, cauliflower, string beans, cucumber, chard, and pumpkin. Fruits also contain a healthy supply. Too little phosphorus, although rarely seen, is responsible for certain anemias. It might also affect your white blood cells, and immunity to bacteria and viruses would be hampered. The recommended daily intake of phosphorus is 800 mg. for adults. Pregnant or lactating women need 1,200 mg. A well-balanced meal plan should provide you with all of this requirement.

POTASSIUM

Potassium, in conjunction with sodium, helps form an electrical pump that speeds nutrients into every cell of your body, while speeding wastes out. It is vital to the function of all cells, helping maintain the proper acid/alkaline balance of your body fluids. Potassium is particularly vital to the workings of your digestive and endocrine systems, your muscles, brain, and nerves.

In general, vegetables, fruits, and other plant foods are far richer sources of potassium than animal foods. Green leafy vegetables are an excellent source. High potassium fruits include bananas, cantaloupes, avocados, dates, prunes, dried apricots, and raisins. Whole grains, beans, legumes, nuts, and seeds are also good sources.

If you find that injuries take a long time to heal, or your skin and other tissues seem "worn out," you may be suffering from a potassium deficiency. Lethargy and insomnia typically are other early signs of deficiency, along with intestinal spasms, severe constipation, swelling of tissues, thinning of hair, and malfunctioning muscles.

If you eat correctly, you needn't worry about your potassium intake, although studies show that runners can lose extraordinary amounts of potassium through sweating. You can easily consume the 2 to 4 grams needed each day to replace the amount normally lost in your urine. A variety of grains and legumes will meet this requirement easily. Runners can eat extra amounts of potassium-rich foods during times of heavy training. I suggest four medium soy pancakes or two potato fritters as a potassium-rich treat.

Those on certain medications, like diuretics to combat hypertension, also require extra amounts of potassium to replace the mineral that is lost by the diuretic's actions. However, potassium supplements should not be taken without a doctor's advice.

SELENIUM

Selenium's primary function in your body is as an antioxidant, protecting your cells from being destroyed. It plays a vital role in your enzyme system, and is necessary for the manufacture of prostaglandins, which control blood pressure and clotting. Selenium is needed to protect your eyes against cataracts, contributes to protein production, and protects the artery walls from plaque.

Animal foods tend to have more selenium than plants. Whole grains, mushrooms, asparagus, broccoli, onions, and tomatoes are the best vegetable sources. Eggs are excellent sources of selenium; they also contain sulphur, which helps your body absorb and utilize selenium.

Signs of selenium deficiency include lack of energy, accelerated angina, and the development of degenerative diseases. Deficiencies have been implicated in blood sugar disorders, liver necrosis, arthritis, anemia, heavy metal poisoning, muscular dystrophy, and cancer. There are no official recommended daily amounts for selenium, but the Food and Nutrition Board suggests an intake of 150 mcg. daily. It is best to supplement with a 50 mcg. vitamin and mineral tablet.

SODIUM (SALT)

Sodium, along with potassium, pumps nutrients into cells and waste products out. It also regulates fluid pressure in the cells, thus affecting your blood pressure. With other nutrients, it helps control the acid/alkaline blood levels in the body. Sodium is vital to the ability of nerves to transmit impulses to muscles and to the muscles' ability to contract. It also helps pump glucose into the bloodstream, produces hydrochloric acid for digestion, and keeps calcium suspended in the bloodstream ready for use. Sodium is available in almost every food we eat, including water. Refined foods contain enormous quantities of sodium.

Sodium deficiency is uncommon. But, when it occurs, it is usually caused by stressful situations such as exposure to toxic chemicals, infections, digestive difficulties, allergies, and injuries. Symptoms of deficiency include wrinkles, sunken eyes, flatulence, diarrhea, nausea, vomiting, confusion, fatigue, low blood pressure, irritability, difficulty in breathing, and heightened allergies.

Your body needs between 55 and 440 mg. of sodium daily to perform its functions. Under normal conditions, obtaining sufficient quantities is not the problem. Many of us consume between 7,000 and 20,000 mg. daily. Too much sodium can result in serious health problems, including hypertension, stress, liver damage, muscle weakness, and pancreas disease.

ZINC

Zinc plays an important role in the body's production of growth and sex hormones, and in its utilization of insulin. As a coenzyme, zinc helps start many important activities and sparks energy sources. It is an important element in the body's ability to remain in a state of balance, keeping your blood at a proper acidity, producing necessary histamines, removing excess toxic metals, and helping your kidneys maintain a healthy equilibrium of minerals. Zinc works in the protein production system, in blood cells, the circulatory system, liver, kidneys, muscles, bones, joints, eyes, the immune system, and the nerves.

Eggs, poultry, and seafood contain sizeable amounts of zinc, as do organ meats. Excellent vegetable sources include peas, soybeans, mushrooms, whole grains, most nuts, and seeds, especially pumpkin.

Lack of taste or smell is a sign of zinc deficiency. Skin problems also may indicate zinc deficienices. Stretch marks are an indication that elastin, the fibers that make your skin springy and smooth, are not incorporating enough zinc to keep your skin healthy. Acne and psoriasis can result from zinc deficiency, as can an abnormal wearing away of tooth enamel. Other signs of zinc deficiency include opaque fingernails, brittle hair, and bleeding gums The daily zinc requirement for adults is 20 to 25 mg. By including sesame, sunflower, and pumpkin seeds, we can supply a good portion of this daily.

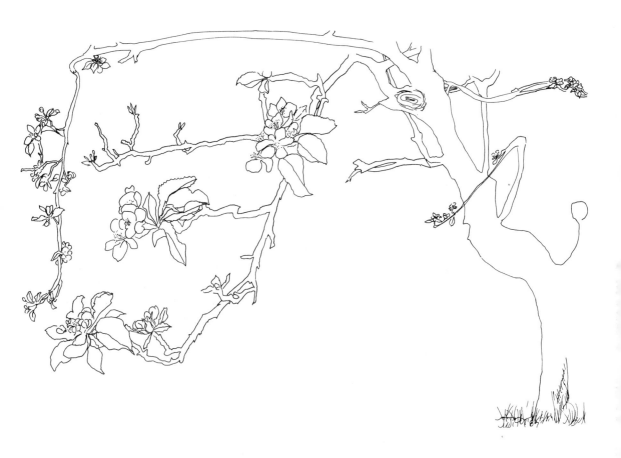

6 · WATER, AIR, ENZYMES, AND ANTIOXIDANTS

"The urban or suburban dweller faced with these challenges should stock up on vitamin E."

THE ENVIRONMENT FROM WHICH we gain sustenance can also have an adverse effect on us. Consider these life-giving and life-supporting elements and aspects of the world around us. Although it comprises 50 to 70 percent of our body weight, water is too often overlooked or taken for granted when we consider amounts of water needed and proper balance of nutrients necessary for good health. Similarly, we too often pay little attention to the quality of air we breathe and the very activity of breathing itself. By not taking seriously the impact of our environment on the enzymes and antioxidants in our bodies, we place our health in danger. We must be as aware of the air we breathe and the water we drink as we are of the food we eat.

▷ WATER

You can go 60 days without food, but only about 18 days without water, the sixth of the major nutrients. Water is second only to oxygen in importance, of all the components necessary for life. It is present in all tissues, including teeth, fat, bone, and muscle. It is the medium of all body fluids, such as blood, digestive juices, lymph, urine, and perspiration. It is a lubricant for the saliva, the mucous membranes, and the fluid that bathes the joints. And it regulates body temperature. Water also prevents dehydration, flushes out toxins and wastes, supplies the body with oxygen and nutrients, and aids muscle cells in producing energy.

The average body contains 40 to 50 quarts of water, with 40 percent of that water inside your cells. Lean persons have a higher percentage of body water than fat persons; men have a higher percentage than women, and children have a higher percentage than adults. Water is your life's blood. Indeed, 83 percent of your blood is water. With a loss of 5 percent of your body water, your skin shrinks and muscles become weak. The loss of less than a fifth of your body water is fatal.

How Much Water Do You Need?

Although water occurs naturally in most foods, it must be consciously included in our daily diets. Include 8 glasses, 8 to 10 ounces each ,every day. To rehydrate after exercise, drink one glass of water every 20 minutes for the first hour, then one glass for several hours afterward. Your body will determine how much it needs; it will absorb water at a particular rate and eliminate whatever is excess.

Eating a high-protein diet results in the body eliminating water. If you are not a vegetarian, it's especially crucial for you to keep careful track of water consumption to replenish the water lost in the excretion of animal protein wastes. If you are concerned or uncertain about pollutants in your tap water, buy pure spring water, not distilled water. Be sure to read the label, even on spring water jugs.

Despite popular theories and practices to the contrary, fruit juice, soda pop, and Gatorade-type drinks—ones that mix sugar and water—will not aid in athletic performance. A Rube Goldberg-type series of reactions occur instead. The sugar in these drinks triggers insulin to be released into the blood. The insulin inhibits epinephrine, which is needed to release free fatty acids, substances you will need for fuel. The insulin also lowers blood sugar levels, which causes glycogen stored in the muscles to leave the muscles and enter the blood. This reduces the store of energy you need to exercise. Drinking such sugar drinks 30 to 60 minutes before exercise, therefore, has a negative effect on athletic performance. Also, concentrations of too much sugar force the body to tap water from other cells to help dilute and digest the sugar. This activity will lead toward dehydration.

It's best to avoid beer, wine, and other alcoholic beverages, although some recent studies support extremely moderate amounts (one glass per day) for cardiovascular health. In general, though, they cause fatigue and dehydration through their diuretic actions. Avoid caffeine drinks like coffee and iced tea. They also act as diuretics, resulting in dehydration.

Drinking during meals, in a sense, can "drown" your enzymes, reducing their strength. When foods are dry, it is better to allow extra salivation prior to swallowing, to moisten them, rather than washing them down with liquids. Eating green and succulent vegetables with a meal also will help provide natural water to lubricate dry foods.

BREATHING

The first and last thing we do on this planet is breathe. But too often we go through life almost ignoring this vital process. Oxygen enters the body through the food we eat and the water we drink as well as the air we breathe. Our bodies have elaborately designed mechanisms for taking in, absorbing, distributing, and utilizing this oxygen.

Disciplined breathing exercises such as those performed in yoga are designed to control the vital energy represented by our breath. Some people believe you can tune into the larger energies of the universe by working on proper breathing techniques. Breath and thought are integrally related: calm one and you calm the other. It is known that deep breathing can reduce stress and tension and regularize body rhythms.

It is not within the scope of this book to provide a comprehensive discussion of proper breathing—a subject worthy of several volumes. But it is important to note here that attention should and must be paid to proper breathing in everyday life, even as we eat. This is an important key to success, as we try to relieve stress and relax.

ENZYMES

Enzymes are natural substances that stimulate some of the internal reactions necessary for life. Your body contains more than 700 types of enzymes, each one responsible for a different task. A shortage of even one type can dramatically affect health. Enzymes are found throughout the body, with the most vital ones in the salivary glands, pancreas, stomach walls, intestines, and liver.

Without enzymes, food could not be digested. Enzymes help transform food products into muscles, nerves, bones and glands. They assist in storing excess nutrients in the muscles and liver for future access, help create urea to be excreted in the urine, and facilitate the departure of carbon dioxide from the lungs. Enzymes also help stop bleeding and serve to decompose poisonous hydrogen peroxide to liberate needed oxygen. They help you breathe and attack poisons in the blood.

Enzymes are abundant in fresh, raw foods. However, they cannot survive at temperatures higher than 122°F., which means that they won't exist in cooked foods. The best sources of enzymes are fresh fruits and vegetables, which should be eaten in season and fresh. When cooking vegetables, use as little water as possible to conserve the enzyme content as well as the vitamin content. Cook vegetables only until tender, in a tightly covered pot. Do not soak most fresh foods; the water can destroy enzymes.

The enzyme that begins the entire digestive process is found in the saliva. Proper chewing is necessary to make that enzyme best perform its work. Food that is not chewed well enters the digestive canal only partially prepared; digestion is therefore less nutritious.

Mental strain or worry also has a deleterious effect on enzyme actions. It is better to avoid large meals during such times, since stressful situations tend to inhibit the flow of enzymes and interfere with the actions of the digestive tract.

In order to perform their life-sustaining tasks, enzymes must be continually replaced. Unnatural components of our environment, such as pollution, artificial additives in foods, and stress, all negatively affect the makeup of your cells and increase your need for health-promoting enzymes. To get enough of these fragile chemicals, it would be better to avoid processed, refined foods as much as possible, looking to natural foods for nourishment instead.

ANTIOXIDANTS

Antioxidants, which oppose oxidation or the burning of substances within the body, have been identified as important factors in helping make us live longer, helping fight heart disease and lung problems, and combating carcinogen formation. They accomplish these, in part, by battling the degenerative processes associated with *free radicals*.

Free radicals are substances released by your body when certain fats are broken down in specific ways. Radiation exposure—either accidental or intended—can cause the release of free radicals. They are also released by a variety of other inopportune circumstances—from the presence of chemical pollutants found in water, air, food, tobacco smoke, and in many cancer-causing agents.

Antioxidants can save us from these free radicals, trapping them and preventing the degenerative processes associated with their reactions with unsaturated fatty acids to form the molecules that ultimately cause harmful disruptions in our cells.

Free radicals also have been linked to certain symptoms of aging. It is with some degree of logic then that scientists believe antioxidants, which can slow down the destructive processes of free radicals, can also help reduce some of the effects of the aging process. Vitamin E is the most common antioxidant. It is known to have some effect, for example, on preventing or delaying the brown pigmentation of skin caused by the aging process—so-called liver spots. Vitamins A, C, and D are less powerful antioxidants, as are selenium and sulfur-containing amino acids.

Pollution can have a serious effect on a variety of body processes. Environmental pollution, for example, seems to defeat or otherwise interfere with the beneficial effects of antioxidants. It is therefore necessary to take nutrients that will contribute to their formation—in the face of such environmental obstacles.

Pollution poses a variety of challenges for those seeking healthful nutrition. Much of our fish comes from rivers, lakes, and waterways poisoned by sewage, chemicals, and a host of other pollutants. Shellfish, particularly, are prone to feed on this sewage and absorb them into their bodies. Fatty fish, as well, are more prone to absorb chemical pollutants and then pass them on to the humans who eat them.

In addition to all the obvious stresses environmental pollution causes, it also depletes our vitamin E supplies. Vitamin E, you'll recall, is a potent antioxidant, and therefore serves to help our bodies by blocking the actions of dangerous free radicals. A deficiency in vitamin E can put the urban or suburban dweller at even greater risk from pollution in the air we breathe, the water we drink, the food we eat. Vitamin E is our major hedge against environmental stress. It helps dilute the harmful effects of drinking water that may have lead in it, an excess of minerals like sodium in it, or an otherwise unbalanced mineral content. Vitamin E as an antioxidant protects us from many types of contaminants simply by impeding the formation of compounds that lead to cellular destruction.

The urban or suburban dweller faced with these challenges should stock up on vitamin E. Wheat germ and wheat germ oil are superior sources of vitamin E. All whole grains, unrefined cereals, whole grain baked goods, seeds, nuts, bran, and organic eggs are also excellent sources. Vegetable oils like safflower oil are likely to have vitamin E if they have been refined only minimally. The best source for such scarcely refined oils—so-called cold-pressed oils—are to be found in natural foods from health food stores.

The active chemical ingredient in vitamin E is pure alphatocopherol. If you're seeking a supplement, get natural vitamin E. There is some indication that the natural form is more active and therefore more useful than the synthetic variety.

Since environmental pollution and other factors seem to have a negative effect on antioxidants, it may be necessary to supplement your intake of nutrients to help you make more antioxidants for possible use.

For a more detailed discussion of the detrimental effects of our environment and suggestions on combating those effects, see Chapter 7, "Detoxification."

Part Two

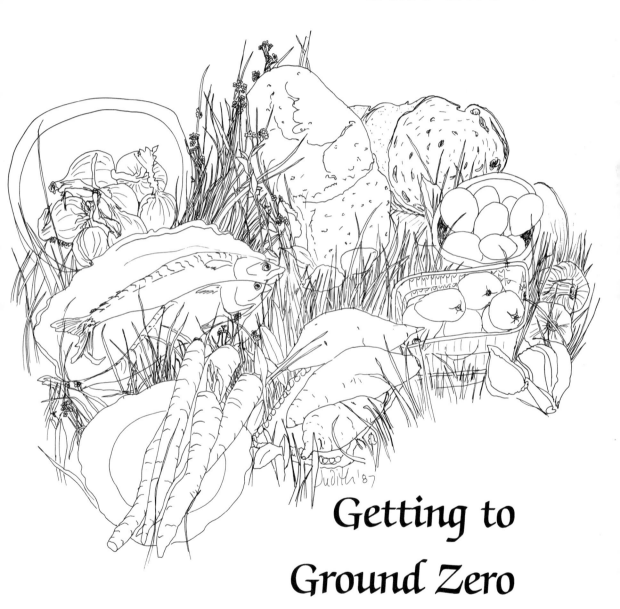

Getting to
Ground Zero

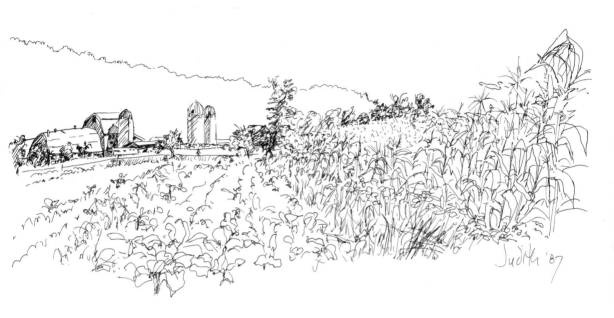

7 · DETOXIFICATION

"*Offer the body the right nutrients. Allow the body to open up the eliminative processes, in which the liver and digestive tract play key roles. Start to detoxify by getting used to natural juices, natural mineral sources, and other organic substances, sometimes supplemented by enemas or medically supervised short-duration fasts. The process may be a slow one at the start. When toxins have had so long to build up, their breakdown also will take time.*"

WE ARE SURROUNDED IN our world by toxic substances in the air, water, soil, and food. Food that is manufactured or processed is also usually treated with chemical preservatives, dyes, and food additives. A healthy body can usually eliminate these potentially toxic or harmful substances through the liver and other organs. But a diet that is too high in fats, processed proteins, sodium, refined sugars, and other refined foods, reduces this natural capacity to rid the body of these toxins. When that happens, the toxins in the body can accumulate.

▷ THE PROBLEM

Toxins in food may not all be poisons in the classic sense. They often do their damage more insidiously, inhibiting the actions of enzymes in our bodies. Many things can go wrong if enzymes don't properly do their work. Since enzymes are important activators of almost every digestive or energy-producing activity in the body, our digestive systems can become sluggish and slow down if they are adversely affected by toxins, with the result that fat digestion can become difficult and protein digestion inefficient. Our kidneys and liver then become overloaded and fat may be deposited in arteries. Cardiovascular illness and other degenerative diseases can result.

Foods that are commercially fertilized may also be denuded of their proper mineral levels. Potassium, for example—our most important activator or catalyst of enzyme actions in the body—is one of the most vital minerals to be lost in this way. Without the right amounts of this mineral, the natural chemicals and enzymes that make our digestion efficient could not function. Yet potassium is reduced—and sodium added—in many of our processed foods and toxins will often deplete potassium supplies. This changes our basic metabolic balance, opening the door for a host of potential problems. The detoxification process will often depend on rebuilding potassium supplies in the body by including fresh fruits and vegetables in our daily diet.

Toxic substances may severely depress the immune system. It is only in the past half century, with the increase in environmental pollution and dependence on processed foods, that we have seen a rapid increase in diseases like cancer, heart disease, arthritis, Legionnaires disease—maladies, unknown not too long ago, that a healthy, normal immune system would be able to fight off.

While those who live in polluted urban or suburban areas may say they have little control over many toxic substances—like air pollution—there *are* things we all can do. People can stop smoking, drinking liquor, using drugs, and eating processed foods. These are all toxic substances. What we need to do instead is to start using fresh untreated foods, raw foods, and fresh juices, whose actual nutrients are more easily available to the body than packaged foods. They can help restore and reactivate our depressed immune systems and eliminate many toxins.

THE SOLUTION

Offer the body the right nutrients. Allow the body to open up the eliminative processes, in which the liver and digestive tract play key roles. Start to detoxify by getting used to natural juices, natural mineral sources, and other organic substances, sometimes supplemented by enemas or medically supervised, short-duration fasts. The process may be a slow one at the start. When toxins have had so long to build up, their breakdown also will take time.

FINDING OUT WHAT'S WRONG THROUGH PROPER TESTING

Once you have decided to make a change in your diet and life-style, you may want to undergo some simple inexpensive tests to ascertain whether there are specific aspects of your health that should be taken into consideration in your diet. According to Dr. Martin Feldman, a preventive medicine physician practicing in New York City, some of the most useful standard testing options include: the glucose tolerance test (also called the GTT or blood-sugar test), hair analysis, the SMA-24 blood test (Sequential Multiple Analyzer, a multiple blood-chemistry screening test), the complete blood count (CBC), and tests of the red blood cell sedimentation rate (also called the ESR or sed rate), and thyroid function. The tests are particularly appropriate if your decision is prompted by health problems or health complaints, such as generalized fatigue, that you already have. But very often a state of imbalance may be present long before symptoms appear. The best care is prevention, correcting the imbalance nutritionally before it has developed into a symptomatic disease state.

Personal Medical History

Every individual is biologically unique. This should be reflected in the health profile. Testing should always be preceded by a proper medical history, taken by a physician. If you ever go to a medical facility and they don't take your medical history—thoroughly—then there is something wrong with that group of physicians. By taking a history, symptoms begin to stand out. Some of these symptoms are early warning signals of what later may become a toxic or imbalanced state.

Some types of symptoms that will appear during a personal history have not always been duly appreciated by physicians as indicators of an imbalanced or toxic state. For example, problems on the surface of the skin may signify underlying toxic states requiring attention and treatments. The skin, after all, is not just a covering on the body like a coat. It is a living, breathing part of our bodies. It is, in fact, our largest organ and has a great deal to do with our internal health. If the body is in a toxic state, one of the routes to eliminate poisons, besides the kidney, the liver, and the lungs, is the skin. Many early warnings of toxicities often appear as minor skin problems, even as simple blemishes on the face. Acne, for example, is a manifestation of an internal hormonal toxicity. Red, blotchy skin, may provide an early warning that the liver, kidneys, or lungs are malfunctioning by not eliminating toxins. Headaches also can provide clues. Many headaches are responses to stress or tension. But other headaches may instead signal a toxic condition. Generalized fatigue may also be caused by a toxic state. Premenstrual syndrome (PMS) in women may reflect a state of hormonal toxicity; cystic breasts may also reflect an imbalance; osteoarthritis may reflect a calcium imbalance associated with toxicity. These are a small sampling of conditions that may come up during the personal history taking. While many physicians will accept these conditions as being without a specific, treatable cause, these symptomatic states may in fact stem from correctable toxic states.

The Glucose Tolerance Test

The glucose tolerance test (also called the GTT, blood-sugar, or glucose test) measures the blood level of glucose, the most important sugar in the body. Glucose is usually maintained at a constant level by means of insulin and other hormones so that, for example, when a person fasts, the body produces glucose from its stores of fat and protein. Normally, blood glucose is obtained from the digestion of carbohydrates in the diet.

There are certain imbalanced states, however, where the glucose level is either too high or too low. Symptoms of lethargy, dizziness, or irritability may be caused by an abnormally low blood-sugar level, or hypoglycemia.

It can occur without a clearly identifiable cause, or as the result of excessive use of alcohol or strenuous exercise. At the other extreme, an abnormally high glucose level may cause frequent urination and chronic infections.

The glucose tolerance test requires that you eat adequate carbohydrates for several days prior to being tested, and then fast 12 hours immediately beforehand. Blood and urine samples are taken prior, during, and at the termination of the test, during which glucose is administered, either orally as a syrup or intravenously. The test should cost well under $50.

Other tests to measure glucose in the blood include the hemoglobin, A1C test, also called the glyco-sloated hemoglobin test. This measures the glucose in the red blood cells and may be performed during routine blood tests. It will measure average glucose levels over many weeks, rather than the minute-to-minute glucose levels measured by the glucose tolerance test.

Tests of pancreatic function, adrenal gland fuction, and liver function may also be used to measure the glucose levels since, ultimately, glucose is controlled by those three parts of the body. The pancreas, for example, is in charge of insulin production. If the pancreas does not create enough insulin, high glucose levels result. If insulin is excessive, low glucose levels appear. Chromium levels are also important in any glucose test since they control how cells actually absorb or use glucose. The chromium can be determined via hair analysis or blood analysis methods, which are inexpensive.

Hair Analysis

Hair analysis as a valid scientific measurement is often criticized and maligned. Yet, there is a specific advantage of hair analysis: When you examine just three inches of hair, you're observing growth over a period of three to four months. You therefore can obtain the average level of the body's status over a several-month period. As the hair grows each day, the mineral status of the body is reflected in the growth of the hair on that day. When examining hair, you're looking at a relatively stable part of the body—almost like examining a fossil—as opposed to the blood, which is constantly in flux.

In the case of exposure to mercury through a silver amalgam mercury filling that you received from your dentist, for example, the blood level of the mercury may rise for about 12 to 24 hours after you were exposed. After a day or so, the mercury leaves the blood stream. But hair analysis will show mercury's impact over days, weeks, or months. This is true of other minerals as well. Lead is another good example. In the case of exposure to lead in a work environment, blood levels rise during the exposure, but 12 to 24 hours afterward, the lead level in the blood will be nondetectable. Hair analysis will continue to show evidence of the change.

The cost of hair analysis is relatively modest compared to other tests (between $25 and $60). The most problematic aspect is in the proper interpretation of the results. Many labs overinterpret by overemphasizing data of minor importance. The hair has two major strengths in analysis. First, it is useful in showing when the body is not absorbing particular minerals efficiently and an imbalance has occurred due to this malabsorption, particularly of minerals like calcium, magnesium, zinc, manganese, and chromium. Second, the hair shows toxic metals very well, including lead, mercury, cadmium, arsenic, and aluminum.

The Classic Blood Test— SMA-24

The standard blood test gives us a lot of data, some of which can serve as an early warning, and some of which, unfortunately, is already a late warning. Commonly called the SMA-24, or the SMA-12 when abridged, the test is relatively complete, reasonably inexpensive, and provides a lot of data for the money. It should be performed as part of the six-month or yearly examination.

A patient should always be tested on an empty stomach, that is after not having eaten for six to eight hours. No food, no juice, no coffee, no tea. Water only. If you've eaten within four hours before the test, this makes it very difficult to interpret the glucose and triglyceride levels on the blood specimen that is drawn.

The first item on an SMA-24 is the *glucose level*. Glucose, if a body has been fasting, should be roughly between 75 and 100. A glucose below 75 is evidence of a possible hypoglycemic (low blood sugar) tendency.

Above 100 is too high. Does that mean you have diabetes? No. Does that mean that the body may get diabetes? The answer is maybe in time. A high glucose level serves as an early warning sign. The next step is to look into whether the cause is the glucose "thermostat" imbalance or a malfunctioning of the pancreas, the adrenal glands, or the liver. Chromium levels should be considered as a related aspect. A glucose imbalance may mean that something is going to go *more* wrong in the future and is deserving of more attention now.

Next on the SMA-24 are the *sodium levels*. Occasionally sodium is too low. An important aspect rarely appreciated by traditional physicians is that low sodium may indicate an adrenal malfunction. The adrenal gland may be sluggish, not making enough aldosterone, which is the sodium-retaining hormone.

Potassium is a potential problem if it is too low. This may happen when people take blood pressure medicines, and the body is asked to remove salt. One can remove too much potassium.

Carbon dioxide is usually tested on the SMA-24. An elevation of the carbon dioxide is a reflection of an alkaline state. The most comon cause of an excessively alkaline state is a diminished flow or amount of stomach acids.

Next is *blood urea/nitrogen*. If the urea/nitrogen levels are elevated, the body is experiencing urea toxicity. One should then look at whether the kidneys are working properly, or whether one is protein toxic. Too much protein can eventually lead to excessive urea.

Creatinine is a kidney-related enzyme. Its elevation is kidney related, so one has to go beyond the blood levels themselves.

Blood calcium may be normal and appear normal on the test, even if our true calcium status is not. Here's an example where one has to intelligently analyze the blood and not assume that the calcium overall is correcly balanced, just because the blood level is. In about one person in five with a severe calcium imbalance, the blood will show too low calcium levels. On the other hand, in four out of five people, the calcium may be off without the imbalance appearing on the blood test.

Phosphorous. When phosphorous is too high, it can adversely affect calcium levels.

Uric acid. Elevation of uric acid indicates a gout condition. Many people have gout early on. Even then, uric acid may not appear over the upper end of the range. But high uric acid can be a warning of gout that will develop later on, so one has to keep watching the uric acid. In such cases, the physician may also need to take a family history, since parents may have had gout.

Alkaline phosphatase is a complex part of the blood. If elevated, it may reflect a liver imbalance or bone problem.

The *total protein* in the blood may occasionally be low and may indicate a malabsorption of protein.

Albumin in the blood relates to its protein component as do *globulin* levels.

The measurement of *SGOT* and *SGPT* in most SMA-24's are measures of liver-related enzymes. Elevation of either may indicate that the liver is out of balance. If the liver is even slightly off balance, it can cause a variety of health problems. Such an imbalance should be dealt with nutritionally.

Bilirubin levels also are potentially liver related. Elevation of bilirubin may also have other meanings.

The *cholesterol* in the blood should be looked at. One also has to look at the *HDL* (high density lipoproteins, or "good" cholesterol) versus the total serum cholesterol levels. Ratios of four to one (of total cholesterol to HDL) or better are desirable.

In day-to-day practice almost all people with cholesterol levels above 225 provide some indication that the liver is sluggish or out of balance. This problem plays a major role in cholesterol elevation.

One should always also ask for a *triglyceride* level as part of the SMA-24 test results. Triglyceride levels are almost as important as cholesterol levels. An elevated level is usually due to malfunctioning of either the liver or the pancreas. Triglycerides are dangerous because they are blood fats and may play some part in clogging our arteries with harmful plaque.

These are the primary items of importance that can be tested with the SMA-24.

The CBC or
Complete Blood Count

In the CBC, we look both at the white blood cell components and the red blood cell components.

White Blood Cells. You could have a white blood count (WBC) as low as 4.8, or as high as 10.8 and still be within the normal range. It you fall below 4.8 WBC, it probably indicates that your immune system is not working properly. Even just slightly below the 4.8 level is an early warning sign that your immunity is not at 100 percent. The CBC is very inexpensive (roughly $10); at the same time it provides a lot of valuable information.

Occasionally the white blood count may be very high (counts in the range of 9, 10, or 11). This is usually indicative of an internal infection. The elevation of the white blood cells represents the body's attempt to deal with the invasion of a foreign substance or agent. The white blood cells are the soldiers that the body mobilizes to do battle. When the enemy has entered it, the body will, if it can, make many more white blood cells. The elevation that appears on the CBC is an indication that there is some kind of internal battle raging.

Conversely, when the body, even at rest, is not making enough white blood cells (in the case of a low WBC), it means there aren't enough soldiers around to do battle in case the need arises.

It is also important to go beyond the total number of the white cells, to look at the differential, or types, of white blood cells.

While all red blood cells are identical and do the same job, we have different types of white blood cells. The basic types of white blood cells are the neutrophils or the polymorphonuclear white blood cells, something called a segs, the lymphocytes, the monocytes, the eosinophils, and the basophils.

The neutrophils or polys tend to make up between 50 and 70 percent of the total white cells. We have more neutrophils or polys than any other type. That's normal. That's the way the body is set up. The lymphocytes comprise between 20 and 40 percent of our white blood cells. There are only a few eosinophils, monocytes, and basophils.

If there are more lymphocytes than neutrophils, an inversion of the usual ratio, most doctors would not even mention it to the patient. They may not even notice it, or if they notice, they don't mention it. But it should be examined. It's a potential early warning that the body's immune mechanism for making white blood cells is really not up to par. If there were a viral illness, either recently or at the time when the test is taken, that may explain the imbalance. During a viral illness, the body will make more lymphocytes because lymphocytes tend to be the main soldiers against viruses. In the absence of a viral problem or an infection, when lymphocytes still outnumber polys, the possibility of an immune imbalance should be examined further.

Red Blood Cells. There is basically one issue with red blood cells— anemia. Occasionally there's an excess of red blood cells, but that's a rare unusual state. Most of the time the question is are there too few, indicating anemia.

There are two types of anemia, depending on the size of the red blood cells. If the cells are too small, small-cell or iron deficiency anemia may be at cause. This condition is almost always related to an iron deficiency, where the body doesn't have enough iron or isn't properly handling the iron it does have. Since the body can't make enough cells without the necessary quantities of iron, it produces smaller cells and fewer cells.

In the second type of anemia, the cells are too large. The most common reason for this abnormality is a vitamin B_{12} deficient anemia. Treatment is different for each specific type of anemia.

Tests of Sedimentation Rates and Thyroid Function

People should also be tested on a routine basis to determine *sedimentation rates* and *thyroid function*. The sedimentation rate is a very inexpensive test. In women, if the sedimentation rate is above 20, there is an indication that some inflammatory process exists or is developing. If there is no cold, sore throat, or other obvious infection, one has to seek out other possible causes. In men, a sedimentation rate above 15 is considered an abnormal elevation.

Thyroid testing can involve special difficulties. For example, thyroxin is the hormone that allows the thyroid gland to carry out its function. You can have normal thyroxin levels and normal blood iodine levels at the same time as a food sensitivity to the thyroid gland is causing your metabolism to slow down, so that you gain weight at an abnormal rate. Chronic fatigue may also be caused by malfunctioning of the thyroid gland.

A standard blood test for thyroxin would not detect either the food sensitivity or the chronic fatigue.

An expenditure of $150 should cover most of the important tests for the average person to determine the state of their overall health.

DETOXIFICATION TECHNIQUES

There are a variety of detoxification techniques available. Several that can be used in combination to improve your well-being and increase your self-awareness are described below.

Maintaining Intestinal Fortitude

It is estimated that nearly half of all illness originates in the intestinal tract—the receptor of the foods we eat, the water we drink, and the air we breathe. Anything that passes through the intestines will impact, positively or negatively, on your health. Cleansing the intestines will help free the body of some hazardous toxic substances.

According to Heather Muir, an authority on the intestines and their role in maintaining good health, certain organisms proliferate in the colon, depending on what we eat and what foods go through it. One of those organisms is the *Candida albicans* organism, which causes candidiasis or yeast in the intestine. Another is the *E. coli* bacteria. Still other bacterial flora help maintain a healthy balance in the colon. If we eat the right types of food that can be digested quickly, transit time in the colon should also be fast. This helps keep bacteria in balance and diminishes harmful bacteria activity. However, if we eat animal proteins such as meat and hard cheeses, food transit time in the colon slows down. Everything begins to clog up, and the trouble begins.

Another concern in keeping the colon healthy is the sometimes deleterious effect of antibiotics on our digestive system. Most antibiotics destroy the friendly bacterial flora in the colon in a short time. This allows the proliferation of two harmful organisms, the *E. coli* and the *Candida albicans*.

We are exposed to antibiotics in many ways. We may take them as medication to cure infections, but we also get them in the meat we eat. The antibiotics, tranquilizers, and hormones that the animals have been fed before slaughter remain in the meat. Some believe that we also are being flooded by the animal's adrenalin, which it produces just prior to being killed.

In any case, there are a number of nutritional experts who urge people to consult with specialists on ways to cleanse the colon of these harmful substances—either by having a yearly colonic irrigation, where water is used to clean out the colon, or by using a variety of different types of enemas.

Yeast Infection Control

Successfully combating candida or common yeast infections may require changing the diet. But cleansing of the colon will also help. One reason these infections affect large numbers of people is that many of the foods we eat have molds in them. Mushrooms and wheat are prime examples.

To fight candida, people can go on a special diet. For their new diet, they should first go off wheat, breads and cereals, yeast, vinegar, cured or processed meats, and all sugars. They should include Kyolic garlic, Vitamin C, Biotin, B$_6$, caprilic acid, beta carotene pau d'arco, and acidopholis—all as daily supplements. Fresh vegetable juices and some fresh fruit juices also are important in any cleansing program because they provide needed vitamins and minerals, and they help specifically to cleanse the colon.

In particular, papaya and watermelon juices both have useful cleansing and therapeutic properties. Carrot juice, celery juice, and cucumber juice, mixed in a one to one ratio, are sometimes useful for intestinal cleansing.

Adding kelp to a carrot, celery, parsley, and spinach juice combination—quite rich in potassium—may be beneficial for the glandular system. The juice made from Jerusalem artichoke has alkaline mineral elements, particularly potassium and calcium. And small quantities of fresh garlic juice helps us to get rid of some intestinal parasites.

Detoxification with Herbs (See Chapter 17)

Detoxification with herbs can be another key approach to renewed health. Two authorities in this area are Dr. Paul Lee, Director of the Platonic Academy in Santa Cruz, California, and one of America's leading spokespersons on the health properties of herbs, and Jeanne Rose, author of *Herbal Guides to Inner Health* and *The Herbal Body Book*.

Both experts point to specific herbs that are excellent detoxifiers, primarily because they stimulate macrophage activity. Macrophages are parts of our immune system that attack, engulf, and digest toxins and other substances that cause us to be ill.

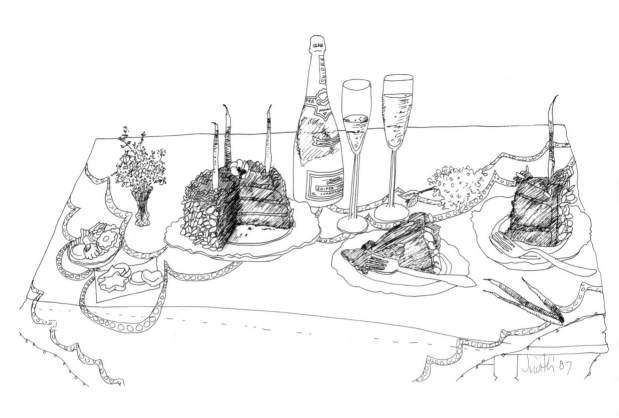

8 · FOOD ALLERGIES

"Environmental medicine experts say that one reason people are developing sensitivities to certain foods is their widespread occurrence in our diets in both the natural and processed forms. Just because you only rarely treat yourself to corn on the cob, for example, doesn't mean you're not eating corn every day. On a typical day you might eat corn flakes, a corn muffin, and processed food products containing both corn starch and corn syrup. Also, many of the daily vitamin C supplements are derived from corn."

IT IS A CLASSIC case of overreaction. Your body incorrectly senses that the food that has just been eaten is a foreign substance to be repelled. Cells begin to exhibit diseaselike symptoms as they react and overreact to the food.

Allergists conservatively estimate that up to 15 percent of the population suffers from a minimum of one allergy, frequently one that is serious enough to warrant medical attention.

Symptoms can range from a mild tension headache or irritablility to criminal actions and full-blown psychotic behavior. Most common are fatigue, headache, insomnia, rapid mood swings, confusion, depression, anxiety, hyperactivity, heart palpitations, muscle aches and joint pains, bed wetting, rhinitis (nasal inflammation), urticaria (hives), shortness of breath, diarrhea, and constipation. Reactions can be immediate following exposure to the allergen or delayed for many hours after contact.

Allergic symptoms are so diverse that the reactions can occur in virtually any organ in the body. Reactions in the brain or central nervous system may lead to behavioral changes and to paranoia or depression. A response in the gastrointestinal tract may translate into bloating, diarrhea, or constipation. Different food combinations can cause multiple reactions in the same person. If a person has an allergy to wheat that manifests itself in the brain, while their gastrointestinal tract is sensitive to milk, they may experience both fatigue and irritable bowel syndrome from a breakfast of whole wheat toast and milk.

Medical literature is filled with case studies in which children experience irritability, hyperactivity, insomnia, lack of concentration, poor memory, fatigue, and lethargy. After isolating and omitting all of the allergens from their diets, these sensitive children often improve. Not only do their physical symptoms clear up, but their behavioral imbalances also return to normal. With the control of the allergy, a normal personality is gradually established and maintained.

Read ingredient labels when buying food. All forms of a potentially offensive food can cause an allergic reaction, not just the whole form. Corn sugars and syrup, including dextrose and glucose, for example, will cause symptoms in many corn-sensitive patients. In many instances, researchers find, corn sugars will cause a more immediate reaction than will corn starch or corn as a vegetable.

Environmental medicine experts say that one reason people are developing sensitivities to certain foods is their widespread occurrence in our diets in both the natural and processed forms. Just because you only rarely treat yourself to corn on the cob, for example, doesn't mean you're not eating corn every day. On a typical day you might eat corn flakes, a corn muffin, and processed food products containing both corn starch and corn syrup. Also, many of the daily vitamin C supplements are derived from corn.

ALLERGIES AND HEREDITY, STRESS, AND PHYSICAL IMBALANCE

You can inherit allergic sensitivities. If both parents suffer from allergies, their children have at least a 75 percent chance of inheriting a predisposition to this hypersensitivity. When one parent is allergic, the chances of an inherited allergy remain as high as 50 percent. The child does not have to inherit the same allergic response. What is inherited is a genetic makeup that is more likely to have allegic reactions in general. For example, the mother may have chronic indigestion while the child's allergy manifests itself as acne. A mother may be sensitive to corn while her child is sensitive to yeast. Infants can develop allergies to the same foods as their mothers while still in the womb, through the placenta, or through breast milk after birth.

COMMON FOOD ALLERGENS AND TYPES OF FOOD ALLERGIES

The foods we eat most frequently are also the most common causes of allergies. These include milk, wheat, corn, eggs, beef, citrus fruits, potatoes, tomatoes, and coffee.

Food allergies fall into several categories.

- **The fixed food allergy**

    Each time you consume a specific food, you react. For example, whenever you eat beef, a reaction occurs.

- **The cyclic allergy**

    This is the most prevalent type of allergy. It occurs when you've had an abundance of a particular food. If exposure to the food can be reduced to no more than once every four days, little or no reaction occurs. The food, in other words, can be infrequently tolerated in small amounts. So, in a cyclic allergy, a person can remain symptom-free as long as he or she eats the offending food infrequently.

    Of course, other factors can influence the degree of this sensitivity. Infection, emotional stress, fatigue and overeating can increase susceptibility. The condition of the food (raw or cooked, fresh or packaged) may also be an important factor. Pollution, the presence of other environmental allergens, or marked environmental temperature change can also help trigger or subdue a reaction.

    A food eaten by itself may be tolerated. But if it is combined with other foods at the same meal, an allergic response may develop. The length and severity of the symptoms will depend in part on how long the allergens remain in your body after ingestion.

- **The addictive allergic reaction**

Here the person craves the foods they're allergic to. In essence, he or she becomes addicted to it. When the individual is made to go without the food, depression and other withdrawallike effects may appear. Moreover, eating the food may momentarily alleviate the symptoms, only to aggravate them later. Over time, the symptoms of the addictive allergy may grow increasingly complex.

This type of allergy often remains hidden or masked—even to the individual who is suffering from the problem. Because of its insidious nature, the person never suspects that the foods that seem to alleviate their symptoms might contain substances to which they're allergic, since they usually feel better right after eating them.

But allergies do not always fit neatly into one of the three categories. A fixed allergy in infancy can develop into an addictive allergic reaction later in life. Milk is a good example of such a food. When first introduced to a baby, it may cause an acute reaction in the form of hives or spitting up. However, if the parents don't recognize this as an allergic reaction and continue to keep milk in the diet, the symptoms may take on a more generalized and less obvious form.

What is first experienced by the body as an acute reaction will finally— in the body's attempt to adapt by assimilating the new foreign substance— lead to more chronic symptoms such as arthritis, fatigue, depression, or headaches.

For example, if you eat milk or milk products every day, symptoms of allergic reactions may blur with your natural personality traits and may become an accepted, even unnoticed part of your everyday life.

Eventually, you may develop a chronic condition, like arthritis, migraines, or depression. Your daily dose of milk would never be suspect at this stage. Your body has upped its tolerance levels in trying to adapt. At the same time, milk's harmful effects have been subtly registered. You keep on with a daily dose of milk, your own substance for abuse, to keep withdrawal symptoms at bay. Acute reactions are gone—except when the milk is withdrawn completely. Chronic reactions have replaced them.

Hidden or masked food allergies, no different from allergies generally, tend to be to the very foods we eat most frequently. In the United States, dairy products, including milk and eggs, are high on the list. Corn, wheat and potatoes are also common allergens, as is beef. Yeast, which occurs in many foods, is often at cause. Finally, many people have a hidden allergy to coffee. Considering that coffee is also an addictive substance and that Americans often drink it all day long (over 100 billion cups consumed annually), it is astounding to contemplate the overall adverse health effects of this one substance alone.

REDUCING THE ALLERGIC THRESHOLD

Most food allergies can be traced to an impaired digestive system. Proper digestion requires that the body secretes sufficient hydrochloric acid and pancreatic enzymes into the stomach to process foods. These substances break down large protein molecules into small molecules so they can be absorbed and utilized. When too few digestive juices or enzymes are secreted, the large protein molecules go directly into the bloodstream. The immune system reacts to these large molecules as if they were foreign invaders—the allergic response. To alleviate these allergies, we must set our nutritional house in order. Nutritional deficiencies and digestive imbalances must be corrected.

In addition, all the other stresses that can affect a person's "allergic threshold" should be reduced or eliminated as much as possible. These include environmental stresses such as air, water, and food pollution; inhalants such as perfume, aerosol hair spray, or room freshener; and emotional stress. The more healthful the physical and mental environment, the greater are our chances for achieving and maintaining a state of well-being.

In most cases, the more severe a person's food sensitivity becomes, the more numerous the allergens that induce it. One clinical study reported that the average person suffering from hay hever was allergic to five foods as well. A total picture of your allergen exposure, environment, habits, and history are vital for effective treatment.

The end result of repeated or prolonged sensitization of the body by recurrent allergic reactions is termed *breakdown*—the point at which diseaselike symptoms appear. They may be erroneously diagnosed as the onset of an illness. But the biochemical breakdown, although it manifests itself suddenly, was actually initiated years before by prolonged exposure to allergens.

ALLERGIES AND ENVIRONMENTAL POLLUTION

Environmental pollution may play a role in food allergies by pushing already hypersensitive individuals over their allergic thresholds. Over the past two centuries the barrage of chemicals introduced into our environment has disrupted the balance of our ecosystem. Residues of many toxic chemicals such as pesticides, herbicides, and insecticides are ingested into our bodies along with food additives and preservatives that are added during commercial food processing.

In many cases, the contamination of food is an irreversible result. Foods such as oranges, sweet potatoes, and butter can be dyed. Other processed and packaged goods like Jell-O, ice cream, sherbet, cookies, candy, and soda can contain large amounts of food additives.

Most of our commercially raised meats and poultry are riddled with residues of antibiotics, tranquilizers, and hormones. It is even common practice to dip certain fish in an antibiotic solution to retard their spoilage. A person allergic to these antibiotics and drugs may be unknowingly ingesting them continuously, provoking either long-term or short-term reactions or illnesses, the source of which might remain unidentified. It is estimated that more than 10 percent of all Americans are sensitive to food additives. But remember, even when a person eats only organically grown foods, they may still be food allergic.

THE MECHANISMS OF ALLERGY

Conventional allergists believe that the mechanism of food allergy is triggered by direct contact of the food antigens—the substances the body produces to fight the "foreign food invader"—with immune system antibodies in the gastrointestinal tract. The usually swift reaction that results is called an immune system-mediated response. This is the only kind of allergic reaction that conventional allergists recognize.

But there is a second mechanism recognized by clinical ecologists, through the absorption of the allergen from the gastrointestinal tract into the bloodstream. Circulating in the blood, allergens can react with elements other than antibodies. The resulting reaction can occur in the blood, in the nervous system, or the musculoskeletal system. Sometimes referred to as a sensitivity or intolerance, to distinguish it from a classic allergic reaction, this second mechanism can be extremely complex. However, tests to uncover these more subtle intolerances are available and are discussed in the next chapter, "Food Allergy Testing and Treatment."

Hypersensitivity to foods can come at any time of life and continue to any age, although the onset occurs most commonly in infancy and early childhood. This is largely because the gastrointestinal systems of the very young are less efficient than in the adult. One researcher refers to the progression of allergies from childhood to adulthood as the "allergic march." Symptoms can move from one organ system to another. A child may suffer from asthma as a result of drinking milk. During teen years the allergy may take the form of pimples. Unfortunately, many people erroneously believe that they have outgrown their allergy because they no longer suffer from the original symptom. They don't consider that their current problems may have the same underlying cause. Their allergic symptoms may continue to vary throughout their lives because of an underlying imbalance that remains constant. Hyperactivity as a child may be the result of ingested food additives. In later years, these same ingredients may cause migraines and fatigue.

FOOD ALLERGIES AND MENTAL HEALTH

If food and chemical sensitivities were routinely considered in each case of chronic disease, there would be a tremendous increase in well-being in this country.

An overly analytical medical system insists instead on classifying patients into narrowly defined disease states. Environmental aspects, including a patient's diet, are considered to be nonmedical. The person's whole experience—including diet, environment, life-style, emotional life, and work life—may also be considered to be outside the physician's domain, although few physicians would deny that the cause of almost any patient's illness will involve one or more of these factors to some degree.

It may be that up to 70 percent of symptoms diagnosed as psychosomatic are probably due to some undiagnosed reaction to foods, chemicals, or inhalants. Different allergic reactions occur. There are localized physical effects like gastrointestinal disorders, eczema, asthma and rhinitis (nasal inflammation). There are acute systemic effects like fatigue, migraine headaches, neuralgia, muscle aches, joint pains, and other generalized symptoms. And there are acute mental effects such as depression, rapid mood swings, hallucinations, delusions, and other behavioral abnormalities.

It has been estimated that over 90 percent of schizophrenics have food and chemical intolerances. More specifically, 64 percent are sensitive to wheat; 51 percent to corn; 51 percent to cow's milk; 75 percent to tobacco; and 30 percent to petrochemical hydrocarbons.

Researchers now believe that food allergies may directly affect the body's nervous system by causing a noninflammatory swelling of the brain, which can trigger aggression. Despite studies at various correctional centers showing clearly the connection between diet and behavior, little is being done to change the dietary standards of correctional facilities throughout the nation. Routine screening programs for food allergies and nutritional deficiencies in chronic offenders do not exist.

While many other factors—not food alone—mitigate criminal, antisocial behavior, or mental illness, a case can be made for testing for and evaluating food sensitivities in any overall treatment, prevention, or rehabilitation program.

FOOD ALLERGIES AND
MIGRAINE HEADACHES

Migraines are an example of a condition in which recognition and elimination of food allergens can make a tremendous difference. The trick is to recognize the possibilities.

Right now, about 25 million people who consult their physicians each year complain about bad headaches. Although there are various types of headaches, about 50 percent of these people suffer from migraines.

Migraine sufferers usually experience pain on only one side of the head, lasting from several hours up to several days. (The word migraine means "half head.") Migraine sufferers average two headaches per month interspersed with symptom-free periods between attacks. While conventional medicine has very little to offer the migraine sufferer, clinical ecologists see migraine as a disorder frequently resulting from food allergies. The nontraditional medicine offered by the clinical ecologist may offer a unique opportunity to relieve the suffering.

Headaches due to food or chemical sensitivities often can be treated simply by eliminating the allergy, once it has been identified, with an elimination or rotary diet. (See Chapter 9, "Food Allergy Testing and Treatment.") Yet, as a rule, food sensitivities are not investigated in the diagnosis and treatment of headaches.

Today, the theory favored by environmental medicine specialists to explain how allergy-related migraines may occur describes an antigen-antibody reaction, initiated by an allergen, and starting as an immune reaction in the tissues where antibodies are localized. The allergic reaction induces the release of chemical mediators like histamine and noradrenalin. The excruciating pain associated with migraines occurs as a direct result of the allergic response: The antigen-antibody reaction affects the temporal arteries in the skull, causing the vessels to expand, with resultant thinning of the vessel walls and subsequent fluid leakage. As a result of the edema (fluid retention), the brain begins to swell, pressing against the inflexible skull structure. The intense pain is mainly due to the stretching of surrounding sensitive tissues in the area of the swelling.

While the pain may sometimes appear immediately after eating a particular food, it may also be delayed until hours afterwards. For this reason it is not unusual for a person to fail to identify the correlation between what they're eating and the onset of their headache. A food may even seem to relieve migraine symptoms temporarily—a classic example of an addictive allergic reaction.

Of course, allergic headaches typically occur as the result of combinations of factors, rather than from food allergies alone. Emotional stress, for example, may play a large role in triggering an episode. Thus, even when a food allergy is at cause, the specific food source may not produce the same symptoms on every occasion, depending on the array of associated circumstantial factors. In some individuals stress may be compounded when the allergic reaction triggers further emotional symptoms. A vicious cycle is created. Sudden changes in temperature or light may also affect one's susceptibility, as well as the presence of any other health problems.

Environmental medicine specialists have found that some of the foods that occur most frequently in the typical American diet are also the foods most commonly implicated in food allergy-related headaches. The list includes wheat, eggs, milk, chocolate, corn, pork, cinnamon, legumes (beans, peas, peanuts, and soybeans), and fish. Moreover, individuals with food allergies should avoid or limit their intake of fermented products like red wine, champagne, and aged cheese because of the presence in these foods of a substance called tyramine. Tyramine has been associated with migraine occurence in some cases.

Childhood Migraines

Children suffering from migraine tend to be sensitive, nervous, and temperamental, with various behavior disturbances as common predisposing factors. Preceding the actual attack, the child may be noticeably lethargic and may refuse to eat, possibly complaining of abdominal discomfort as well. Often, the child's temperature is elevated and may gradually rise to as high as 104°F. during an attack. This fever may draw attention away from the diagnosis of migraine in favor of a diagnosis of acute infection, especially when other symptoms are present, such as abdominal pain, nausea, and vomiting. Acute appendicitis may be erroneously suspected. The array of symptoms typical of migraines in children are often misdiagnosed, particularly as these differ substantially (especially with respect to the prodrome) from adult symptoms.

Migraine headaches, unfortuantely, are not uncommon in childhood or even in infancy. And while migraine sufferers most can most often trace the onset of the headaches to the period of early adulthood, early symptoms occur during childhood in nearly one-third of cases.

Children five years of age and under often suffer from what are called "allergic syndromes," sometimes involving bronchial asthma with migraine symptoms as a secondary condition.

In the vast majority of childhood cases of migraine, hereditary factors seem to be present—with a close relative also having migraines.

In addition to food allergies, a variety of other factors may precipitate a migraine attack during childhood, including: sleeplessness, irregular meals, fatigue, extended exposure to bright sunlight and visual stimulation (e.g., movies or television).

In many cases a particular food or group of foods will be at cause. If so, the best way to identify that food will be by means of an elimination diet—and not by the standard skin tests. Among children, the most common sources of food allergies include chocolate, milk, wheat, eggs, and pork. In one recent study, over 90 percent of the children tested with severe frequent migraines recovered after following strict elimination diets. Moreover, the secondary symptoms from which the children also suffered, including asthma, eczema, abdominal discomfort, and behavioral disorders also improved.

Too often, conventional medical practitioners tend not to look toward nutritional solutions in cases involving allergies, including allergy-related migraines. In part, this is because the medical training they have received does not extend deeply into nutrition. And yet, a preponderance of evidence continues to point to the importance of nutritional solutions for an increasingly wide range of health problems.

FOOD ALLERGIES AND FATIGUE

Probably no allergic disorder is more puzzling and pervasive than "tension fatigue syndrome." Indeed, for many of us, varying daily levels of tension and fatigue are the norm; tranquility and energy, the rare exceptions. To compensate, we choose artificial solutions for moderating energy, from the first caffeinated gulps of coffee in the morning to the quick sugar, caffeine, or drug fix during the day, and the alcoholic "equalizer" in the evening. The result is that energy levels are either depressed or falsely elevated most of the time. In many cases, these quick pick-me-ups are responses to allergic disorders with their roots in food and nutrition.

Next to headaches, tension fatigue syndrome is the most common manifestation of cerebral and nervous system allergy. Yet, too often, this far-reaching malady is not even recognized by physicians or allergists.

Its symptoms are usually assigned a psychiatric origin and treated with drug therapy or some other conventional modality, when in fact, a simple elimination and rotation diet is the best medicine.

There are several reasons for this all too common oversight. First, there are similarities between tension fatigue syndrome and psychiatric disorders. And second, there is the failure of standard scratch tests to identify many food and chemical reactions. The scratch tests simply have not been shown to be effective in the diagnosis of food and chemical sensitivities. And yet they continue to be used by allergists.

Of course, tension, extreme nervousness, irritability, depression, and emotional instability may be symptoms of psychological disorders in some cases. But too often this is the only possibility that is considered by conventional practitioners. In too many cases, the end result is that a psychological origin is erroneously attributed while the actual physical cause remains unrecognized and the chronic allergic reactions persist.

The allergy may be due to any number of foods, and it is only through careful testing that a definitive diagnosis can be made. In all cases where such symptoms appear, food allergies should be ruled out first—before further traditional medical sleuthing occurs. This can save an awful lot of trouble and mistaken diagnoses.

Early research has suggested that an allergic syndrome may be responsible for certain nervous symptoms in adults and children by actually irritating the central nervous system. Thus, if certain allergies act directly on the nervous system, they can cause characteristic behaviorial and physical abnormalities.

Tension fatigue syndrome in a child is sometimes caused by an inhalant sensitivity; however, it is more often due to an unrecognized food intolerance. Reactions to food commonly occur along with other allergic disorders like migraine and asthma, or they can also occur alone.

The symptoms experienced in tension fatigue syndrome can include fatigue, weakness, lack of energy and ambition, drowsiness, mental sluggishness, inability to concentrate, bodily aches, poor memory, irritability, fever, chills and night sweats, nightmares, restlessness, insomnia, and emotional instability. Mental depression is another common symptom, ranging from mild to severe episodes of despondency and melancholia. Generalized muscle aches and pains, especially in the back of the neck or in the back and thigh muscles may also be present, as well as edema (fluid retention), particularly around the eye, and tachycardia (rapid heart beat). Gastrointestinal symptoms often associated with this syndrome are bloating, abdominal cramps or pain, constipation, diarrhea, and a coated tongue. Chills and perspiration are also frequently experienced in association with fatigue during food testing of symptomatic patients.

The disorder can begin at any age. It can last from several months to several decades. In some adults the extreme fatigue, bodily aches, depression, and mental aberrations that come from this continuing allergic state can be so severe that they interfere with work and domestic life.

As headache attacks or gastrointestinal upset caused by allergy increase in frequency, the fatigue is more likely to remain even between episodes. Fatigue soon becomes the allergic individual's major complaint. The allergic origin of the fatigue and weakness associated with migraines or gastrointestinal and respiratory disorders commonly remains a mystery.

It's not unusual for allergic individuals to sleep up to 15 or more hours for several successive nights to try to overcome their fatigue. Unfortunately, in most cases, these efforts prove futile. The fatigue experienced in allergic fatigue is quite different from the fatigue that naturally follows physical exertion. It cannot be relieved by normal or even excessive amounts of rest. It can only be relieved by eliminating its cause—the allergen.

Instead, the majority of these allergic individuals, many of whom have often sought a variety of medical avenues for relief, are eventually labeled neurotics.

What causes the syndrome? Before the diagnosis of allergic fatigue can be definite, a complete medical workup should be done to exclude both organic and functional origins. This should include a comprehensive case history, complete physical examination and diagnostic laboratory blood testing. Other causes for nervous fatigue include chronic infections and metabolic disorders, including diabetes, hypoglycemia, hypothyroidism, neurological disorders, heart disease, anemia, malignancy, and various nutrient deficiencies. Even if another disease is found, allergic fatigue can be still be a causal factor. In some cases, fatigue is caused both by an allergic reaction and an underlying chronic disease state.

The Monday Morning Blahs

It is common for people to binge over the weekend on foods to which they are sensitive. This destructive habit is all too often responsible for the Monday morning blahs. If you are feeling blue by coffee break on Monday, sit down and examine what you've eaten during the previous days. Clinical ecologists suggest that rotary diets may help pinpoint food allergies in patients complaining of fatigue when no other cause is obvious. Very often, patterns of stomach upset will disappear following a careful dietary change, and once the new diet has been maintained over a period of several weeks, fatigue and muscle weakness will be replaced by increased amounts of high energy.

FOOD ALLERGIES AND OBESITY

Many obese men and women believe that they are overweight due to heredity, or because they have a thyroid or metabolic problem, or because they simply eat too much. They may blame their lack of self-control or become convinced that they have psychological problems. And yet, some experts believe that roughly two out of every three obese individuals suffer from some form of allergy.

Of course, allergy may be only one of several factors affecting an obese person's weight. The presence of a thyroid condition or psychological problems can cause or aggravate a weight problem. Obesity is also related to many diseases including high blood pressure, heart disease, kidney problems, and diabetes. For obese individuals with allergies, the problems of each condition may adversely affect the other. Typically, someone who is obese will have allergic responses more often than his or her nonobese counterpart. The extra weight is a burden on the immune system, and the weaker the immune system, the more one may be affected by one's allergies. Obese individuals also may have increased difficulty breathing, with particularly severe implications for allergic persons with asthma. In many cases, problems will occur due to allergies in combination with other factors.

We store chemicals in the body in fat. Very often, allergies are triggered by a response to chemicals stored in this way. Because the obese person may naturally hold more chemicals in the body, he or she may tend to experience more frequent allergic responses. This also may explain why he or she feels worse, or has strong food cravings, at the beginning of a diet. Chemicals are stored in fat, and as the fat is burned, a large quantity of chemicals is passed into the blood stream, often causing such cravings.

The mechanism by which an allergy can trigger obesity may be that of the hidden addictive allergy, whereby a person is addicted to the very foods to which they are allergic. Often, these are high calorie foods, such as chocolate, cheese, or sugar. So, they may gain weight because they eat these high calorie foods too frequently.

Hunger itself can be an allergic response and compulsive eating and intense cravings for particular foods may also result from hidden allergies. In some cases, compulsive eating of the food one is allergic to may really be an attempt to stave off withdrawallike symptoms induced by going without the food for too long. Such withdrawal symptoms might include headaches, drowsiness, irritability, or depression.

Dr. Marshall Mandell, a physician who has written extensively on dietary problems, also notes that some individuals may experience specific food cravings because they know that particuar foods have a short-term positive effect on their mood, or provide them with a quick boost of energy. Such positive changes are only short-lived and are usually followed by a drop of energy, a feeling of fatigue, or some other negative mood change such as depression.

Allergies can cause weight problems if they interfere with the body's natural ability to regulate itself. As noted by Dr. Arthur Kaslow, physician and author, both humans and animals naturally attempt to maintain their bodies in a state of biochemical equilibrium known as homeostasis. Unless there is a flaw in their regulatory system, human beings will maintain their proper weight by eating the amounts and types of foods their bodies need to function properly. When the body needs food, it will send out a hunger signal. When it needs water, it sends out a thirst signal. If this mechanism breaks down, an individual may feel hungry when he or she does not really need food. It is possible that allergies can temporarily impair the cells responsible for sending out these signals.

As noted by several experts, including Drs. Marshall Mandell and Thomas Stone, another way that allergies can affect an individual's weight is by causing edema (fluid retention). The edema may be localized to specific parts of the body, such as the ankles, hands, abdomen, or face, or it can spread throughout the body. When it is evenly distributed through-out the body, the individual often doesn't realize it, and therefore, doesn't think that fluid retention has anything to do with the weight problem. Eating food to which one is allergic can cause water retention equal to 4 percent of total body weight.

Edema occurs when an allergen in a food to which the individual is allergic causes some of the body's capillary (small blood vessel) pores to enlarge. The fluid from the blood plasma may then seep into neighboring tissues. These tissues swell with this excess fluid. When the allergen leaves the body, the capillaries return to their proper size. But if the individual continually ingests the allergen, he or she will always have this excess fluid in the tissues, significantly affecting the weight problem.

A way to determine the possible role of edema in a person's weight problem is to try to have that person recall whether he or she ever lost more that 3½ pounds on a reducing diet for a week. That is the largest amount you can burn up even if you were only drinking water. If a larger weight loss ever occured, edema may have been the cause.

Any initial weight loss on typical reducing diets occurs largely because the diet may eliminate food to which the individual is allergic. For example, if the individual is sensitive to sugar, and the diet restricts the intake of dessert foods, the individual will lose weight beyond that lost from calorie reductions. He or she would lose the extra water retained due to the sugar allergy as part of the edema. Allergic edema would also explain how some individuals can diet and still not lose much weight. This may happen because some food allergen is still in the diet—causing excessive fluid retention and leading to edema.

The orthodox treatment for weight loss is to go on a calorie restricted diet. But be forewarned! This diet may not work if allergic edema is playing a part in contributing to the weight problem. Even the depression many people experience on a standard reducing diet may be allergy re-lated.

An alternative dieting approach is to suggest that the individual initially follow a diet that is well balanced. Then a clinical ecologist can determine which foods or chemicals, if any, are causing any continued weight problems, and have them avoid those substances. A rotation diet may then be introduced to ensure that new sensitivities do not develop.

To help handle food craving in the short term, exercise is highly recommended. It can increase blood flow, bringing needed nutrients to the cells. It can also calm one's mood. Vitamin C as well as vitamin B_6 can also be useful in blocking allergic reactions.

FOOD ALLERGIES AND ARTHRITIS

Arthritis, or joint inflammation, affects over 50 million Americans and the disease is on the rise. While physicians have identified over 100 types of arthritis, two of the most common are rheumatoid arthritis and osteoarthritis.

Osteoarthritis alone affects over 16 million individuals. It is a condition that usually affects only a few joints in the body. The cartilage in the affected joints becomes rough-edged, and may begin to wear away. Grating sounds in the joint may even be heard.

Rheumatoid arthritis is usually considered a chronic condition. It mainly affects women between the ages of 20 and 40. While it may begin with only mild symptoms, it can become severe and even disabling. The most common joints affected are those in the hands, feet, arms, hips, and legs. Rheumatoid arthritis can also affect connective tissue throughout the body. Other conditions may occur in association with rheumatoid arthritis, including chronic fever, tiredness, poor appetite, weight loss, anemia, and enlarged glands and spleen.

The orthodox medical treatment of arthritis relies heavily on the use of drugs. Americans currently spend $2 billion per year on arthritis drugs. While these drugs may be useful, many also have serious accompanying side effects.

The Clinical Ecologist's Approach to Arthritis

Clinical ecologists take a different approach from that of conventional medicine. Some clinical ecologists estimate that from 80 to 90 percent of all cases of arthritis are either allergy induced or are allergylike reactions to some food the patient has eaten. The arthritis may also be related to an environmental factor to which the patient is sensitive, such as gas inhaled from constant proximity to a gas stove. Examining arthritics for both food and environmental allergies may help reduce current symptoms, prevent recurrences of symptoms and minimize the permanent damage that eventually results from joint inflammations.

Studies have shown that, in some cases, arthritic symptoms will lessen if a patient fasts. (Most food allergy symptoms will clear up during a four-day fast.) Studies also report that after arthritis patients fast, the symptoms may reappear if certain foods are eaten. The most frequent foods that caused the reactions were corn, wheat, and meat.

As is true with other food allergy problems, no one specific food causes arthritic symptoms in all patients. Some patients may be allergic to tomatoes while others are allergic to strawberries, wine, or grapefruits. Elimination of the food source from the diet can become an integral part of any treatment program.

For osteoarthritis, there are other factors to be considered. Usually, osteoarthritis is related to a calcium imbalance. Therefore, the imbalance must also be examined and taken into account. Because calcium is deposited in the joints in osteoarthritis, many people assume that the body has too much calcium, while actually the reverse is usually true. While the lack of calcium may be due to a dietary deficiency, it is also often due to a digestive problem. In such cases, the body is not properly handling the calcium it takes in. Therefore, the calcium is deposited in places where it does not belong. Such patients may need supplemental calcium. Vitamin D and vitamin C may also be suggested, since they can aid in calcium absorption by the body.

Dr. Marshall Mandell, a clinical ecologist in Bridgeport, Connecticut, has successfully treated hundreds of arthritis patients by putting them on a five-day distilled water fast and then allowing their usual foods, one at a time, back into their diet. If a food causes the arthritis symptoms, the symptoms will return when it is reintroduced into the diet and should be permanently eliminated.

This 5-day elimination diet can be adapted to allow individuals a way of self-testing specific foods: Keep a food out of your diet for five days, then reintroduce it. If it causes your problems to recur, eliminate it.

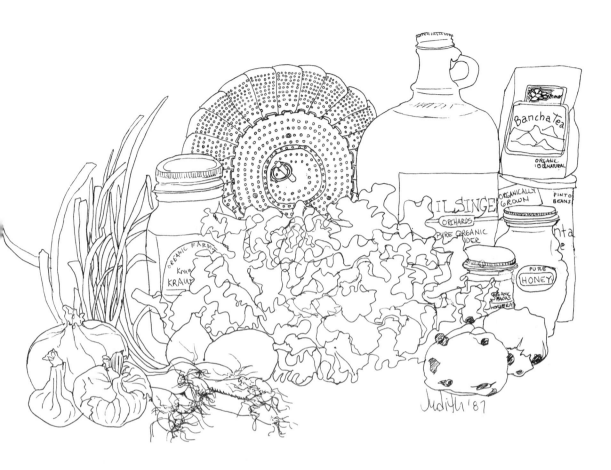

9 · FOOD ALLERGY TESTING AND TREATMENT

"Plan a diet in which you eat no individual food more often than once in four days. After five days, start a food and symptom diary. After reviewing correlations that may crop up through your record keeping, eat any suspected food the next time it comes up in the four-day rotation alone as one full meal. Note symptoms. Eliminate foods that stimulate adverse symptoms from your diet—permanently."

EVERY PERSON IS BIOCHEMICALLY and structurally complex and unique. Obviously, not all disorders have their roots in allergies. Therefore, a change in diet isn't always effective.

However, our environment—including the foods we eat—are responsible for more physical and emotional ill health than most health professionals and the general public realize. Approximately 30 million Americans are estimated to have food and chemical sensitivities.

So proper testing and treatment of these individuals could have an enormous impact on our individual well-being and on society overall. Some techniques for such testing have been around for some time. Other tests are just evolving. The same is true of treatments for those with food allergies.

Patient experience is most important in diagnosing allergies. Environmental medicine specialists now are highlighting the role the allergic individual can and must play in diagnosing and treating his or her own ailment. Articles written in the 1930s reporting the lack of attention paid to the patient regarding their condition could very well be republished in the 1980s. Unfortunately, very few physicians acknowledged this advice in the past, and few acknowledge it today.

TRADITIONAL TESTING

The most common test performed by the traditional allergist is one that really has very little use when seeking food allergies. Still, it is often used. Working well for dust, pollen, mold, animal hair, and insect stings, this is the classic scratch test. The doctor makes 10 to 20 scratches on a patient's arm, using a needle imbedded with the problematical substance being tested. If there is a reaction on the skin, it indicates a sensitivity. But this test picks up reactions only to allergens that stimulate a specific immune response in the body and detects only certain types of antibodies produced by the body with that defensive response.

Another test, developed in the1960s, relies on screening blood samples. Called the radio-allergo sorbant test, RAST for short, this test is much more expensive to perform than the scratch test and can have more false positives and false negatives.

NONTRADITIONAL TESTING

A comprehensive medical history might provide significant clues about your allergic profile. A trained clinical ecologist or environmental medicine specialist may find the needed information from such a medical history alone.

Clinical ecologists also use a skin test, evaluating different-sized doses of a questionable substance. The diluted substance is injected into the skin. After 20 minutes, the physician checks for redness and swelling, measuring the size of the skin raised by the suspected allergen. Progressively larger doses of the same suspected substance are administered in this way until the size of the skin reaction no longer increases. All the while, the patient writes down any other symptoms he or she may be experiencing, like headache, stuffy nose, or nausea.

Physicians can use this approach to determine the size of a particular dose of an allergen that might trigger a reaction, or counteract it. It is therefore useful in testing and in treatment.

While this approach has its advantages, it is time-consuming, expensive, somewhat painful, and can test only the part of the food that can be diluted in water. Other parts of the food (that are fat soluble, for instance) may be at cause that will not respond to the test.

A similar test takes another approach, putting extracts of food mixed with glycerin under the tongue, instead of into the skin by injection. While this test is not painful, it also can be time-consuming and expensive.

Another test, employing a technique called applied kinesiology, is based on the principle that there is a reflex response between a suspected allergen and the patient's body, in the patient's muscles. In this test, a doctor offers food to the patient and then measures or evaluates the energy or muscle function after the food is ingested. Here many foods can be tested in each session. However, the results may not be highly accurate, depending on the nature and experience of both the person administering the test and the person being tested.

Newer tests are being developed all the time. Some, like the cytotoxic test, mix blood samples with food extracts and measure how many white blood cells (cells involved in the body's natural defensive system) burst. In allergy smears, samples of different body fluids or secretions are evaluated in the laboratory to look for a specific type of white blood cell. The various immune system cells may also be evaluated. And in the Arest program, radioactive atoms are used to determine how antibodies respond to particular antigens.

There are also less technical tests, some of which can even be done at home. A fasting test, which should be done under medical supervision, begins by cleansing your system. Symptoms may still be present or, if your allergy is an addiction of some sort, may have worsened by the second or third day of the fast. Then foods are reintroduced one at a time to check for symptoms. This test should not be done for certain already ill patients, the elderly, the hypoglycemic, or young children.

Another test that can be performed at home is the Coca Pulse test. First find your normal pulse range, by taking it every two hours. Then take it again at specific, regular intervals after eating the suspected allergen. If your pulse rises more than 10 points, the food eaten last becomes suspect. The pulse is rising as a reaction to increased adrenalin in your system. The adrenalin, it is believed, usually is being released in reaction to an allergy.

Another home test involves keeping a food diary, and recording everything you eat for a week. Record symptoms and when they occur as well. After the week, look for a relationship between symptoms and food eaten.

Elimination testing is yet another approach. Eliminate the suspected allergen until symptoms clear up over a 12-day period. Reintroduce the food on an empty stomach. Usually symptoms, if they are to develop, will do so within an hour of testing.

A variation on that is the elimination of all common allergens—wheat, corn, dairy foods, citrus fruits, food colorings, sugar, and foods you may crave, over the course of a week. Then reintroduce the foods, one per day. If symptoms develop, the food may be an allergen. Don't eat it for five more days and then reintroduce it to double-check the result.

A final home test—perhaps among the most effective and sensible of all tests—also doubles as a treatment for food allergies. It is called the rotary diversified diet.

Plan a diet in which you eat no individual food more often than once in four days. After five days, start a food and symptom diary. After reviewing correlations that may crop up through your record keeping, eat any suspected food the next time it comes up in the four-day rotation alone as one full meal. Note symptoms. Eliminate foods that stimulate adverse symptoms from your diet—permanently.

The theory here is that food sensitivities become even more pronounced when a food is eliminated and then reintroduced into the diet. With this diet, your symptoms—and with them the responsible food—are clearly highlighted.

This approach is also useful as a maintenance diet, enabling food-allergy prone people to prevent the emergence of new allergies, since they never eat any food too frequently. And even then, if a new food allergy does develop, it is spotted and quickly eliminated.

TREATMENTS

Clinical ecologists offer an alternative to orthodox methods of treating disease. They test the whole person as they exist and react to their total environments.

Our understanding of allergies has been greatly expanded by the clinical ecologist. Because the traditional allergist only recognizes those allergies that are mediated by the immune system, he therefore can only treat a small portion of illnesses the clinical ecologist would classify as allergies. In addition, the traditional allergist has a limited number of alternatives to offer his patients. Other than avoidance of an allergic substance, the traditional allergist has only immunotherapy—"the allergy shot"—to rely on. With this, the physician administers guadually increasing increments of the substance to which the patient is allergic. It will usually take six months until the optimal dose, that is the dosage at which symptoms are blocked, is achieved. The theory is that the patient uses up his antigens on the allergy shot, and therefore has a higher threshold of response before he will respond badly to an allergen again.

The effectiveness of traditional immunotherapy may be limited only to those allergies directly related to the immune system response. Some experts believe this represents only 5 percent of all allergies. And even within this small group, there are some immune system-related allergies that do not respond to the treatment.

Traditional immunotherapy is not useful, for example, with food allergies or animal dander allergies. Nor is it always effective for dust allergies, for while the physician can desensitize the individual to specific particles that are components of dust, the patient may be allergic to other particles that were not in the allergy shot. And the treatment is a time-consuming process, with no results noticeable until the optimal dose is finally discovered.

THE ELIMINATION DIET

A technique that is used by many allergists that does seem to work on food allergies is the elimination diet. Employed for over 60 years, this plan removes the most commonly occurring food allergens from the diet along with any other foods suspected on the basis of case history or positive test results. In the process of eliminating foods, symptoms usually improve. After avoiding all suspected foods for five to seven days, one food at a time is reintroduced back into the diet. At this point, the patient and doctor observe any recurrence or worsening of symptoms. Some doctors introduce a new food at each meal, while others add only one food frequently for seven days before adding another. If an item causes a symptom, it is then avoided and once again introduced at a later date.

THE ROTARY DIVERSIFIED DIET

Clinical ecologists have improved upon the elimination diet by devising a combined diagnostic and preventive regimen called a rotary diversified diet. In it, certain foods may have to be totally avoided (if one has a fixed allergy), while some may be eaten every four to seven days without ill effects (if one suffers from a cyclic allergy). Rotation diets can be designed to deal with individual food sensitivities. But no food is eaten more frequently than every four days. Rotation diets also help to minimize the stress that preexisting allergens cause, at the same time preventing future sensitivities from developing. They are also valuable in diagnosing masked food allergies, since our bodies react acutely to allergens reintroduced after four to seven days of abstinence. Part Three of this book offers a unique rotary diet based on all these factors in combination with optimum nutrition and a gourmet palate.

Since most food allergies are cyclical rather than fixed allergies, that is they come and go in varying degrees of severity, a rotation diet is part of the treatment for many allergic patients. Foods to which the patient is sensitive are eliminated and the remaining foods are eaten no more frequently than once every four days. Foods you ate on Monday might be repeated on Friday or over the weekend, but not before. For some individuals who are highly sensitive, a 5-, 7- or even 12-day cycle may be necessary.

The rotation diet ensures against the development of new food sensitivities in a way that simply substituting one food for another does not. For example, if an individual was allergic to wheat, and eliminated it from his diet, but began to eat rice every day, he might develop a sensitivity to rice. Periodic retesting may be recommended several months after you've made the change to a rotation diet. By retesting your sensitivity to some of the eliminated foods, it may sometimes be possible to reintroduce them on a rotational basis.

A rotary diversified diet often also is recommended to check for obesity and edema (fluid retention) related allergies. Salt, sugar, and tap water is avoided. Then, for each week over a five-week period, the individual tests a common allergen such as dairy foods, wheat, corn, eggs, yeast, pork, soy products, chocolate, or apples. One would avoid each of these foods for four days. If, after five days, the individual has lost five or more pounds, which is then regained when the food is eaten, the test food should be considered an allergen and avoided for at least two months. Then, the food can be reintroduced on a rotational basis, checking to see that it is no longer causing problems. One can continue to test different foods throughout the five-week process.

When following a rotational diet, one should continue to weigh oneself daily, in order to check for edema. Once one has passed the withdrawal period, the avoidance of allergens and a rotation diet can help break food cravings and compulsive eating patterns.

NEUTRALIZING DOSE THERAPY

Another technique to treat allergies used by clinical ecologists is the neutralizing dose therapy. This method is especially useful in cases where avoidance of chemicals and medicinal inhalants is difficult, as during the pollen season, or when multiple food allergies are present. A neutralizing dose is determined for each allergen, and when it is injected or administered under the tongue, this dilution can bring about relief from the allergic symptoms.

These treatments are administered in a series during which the dose of the allergen is progressively increased, causing a desensitization to this substance. (They work on the same theory as allergy shots or vaccines. The only differences are in the dilution of the substance and the wide variety of the substances that can be tested in this way.) Eventually, the person can tolerate contact or ingestion of the allergen with only a mild reaction or no reaction at all.

With the neutralizing dose treatment, the allergist is first determining the amount of a particular allergen that causes a allergic reaction. The physician can work with many substances that the traditional allergist would be unable to treat, including foods, chemicals, perfumes, and cigarette smoke. The neutralizing dose approach seems to be effective in eight out of ten patients.

Like the traditional allergy shot, the neutralizing dose can be administered by injection. However, it can also be given as drops under the tongue. Instead of taking approximately six months to find the optimal dose, the physician can usually determine the correct dosage in one or two sessions using this technique. Another advantage of the neutralizing dose is that the patient can be given the drops to take at home. It not only works as a preventive measure, but also can block a reaction that has already started.

If a parent discovers that a child who is sensitive to wheat is acting hyperactively, and the parent finds out the child was given cookies at school, the parent can terminate the allergic response—the hyperactivity—by administering the drops. On the other hand, if a parent knows the child will be going to a birthday party and knows the child will most likely encounter an allergic food, the parent can administer the drops in advance to forestall an allergic reaction.

TOTAL ENVIRONMENTAL CONTROL

Elimination, rotation diets, and neutralizating dose therapy help in the diagnosis and treatment of many allergic disorders. However, for more serious problems that still resist such treatment, total environmental control in a hospital setting may be required.

This may be the case where the allergy is masked or the patient history reveals too little. A person's system can be cleared of all allergens in four to seven days. This is accomplished in the controlled hospital setting, by having patients fast on distilled water only for at least three days, then traditional tests are administered. The controlled environment also assures that they are not exposed to any environmental contaminants.

BOOSTING THE IMMUNE RESPONSE

Since allergies most often represent an immune system that has gone awry, another important aspect of treatment is finding ways to boost the patient's immune system.

Allergies occur when the immune system has been weakened. Therefore, any strengthening of the immune system should improve resistance to current allergies and reduce susceptibility to new ones. There are several ways in which the immune system may be strengthened. Making sure you are getting sufficient amounts of rest is essential, as is regular exercise. Keeping stress levels to a minimum will also help. You must also be receiving the right nutrients in the right amounts.

Many nutrients have been found to enhance the effectiveness of the immune system. These include vitamin C, beta carotene, vitamin E, selenium and glutathion. These are all antioxidants, which help to eliminate free radicals from the body.

Free radicals are highly reactive molecules created as a by-product during the process by which the body converts food into energy. They can easily latch on to cell membranes and DNA, causing cell damage. Free radicals also can develop from many sources, including X rays, heated vegetable oils and through exposure to ultraviolet light.

Garlic has been found to be an immune stimulant, having both antifungal and antibacterial qualities. Garlic is most effective when eaten raw. It may be either added to one's food or taken as a supplement in tablet or capsule form.

The essential fatty acids are also important to a proper immune response. Dr. Donald Rudin, along with other researchers, recognizes the importance of omega 3 fatty acids, which are found in such oils as linseed and walnut, and in many fatty fishes, like salmon, in warding off both diseases and allergies.

In addition to acting as immune stimulants, there may be other reasons why nutritional supplements may be useful for those with allergies. Dr.

Stuart Freyer has noted that 200 to 500 mg. of pantothenic acid plus 50 mg. of B complex vitamins can be useful for allergic individuals. Vitamin C, in addition to its importance as an antioxidant, also has an antihistamine effect, which may benefit those with allergies by reducing the swelling of tissue and cell membranes. One study found that asthmatics taking 1,000 mg. of Vitamin C daily had 25 percent fewer asthmatic attacks than those receiving a placebo. Another study found that asthmatic children benefited from magnesium supplementation.

STRESS MANAGEMENT

Since stress lowers the immune response, reducing stress should help in food allergy elimination. Stress management techniques are available, including progressive relaxation and biofeedback, to recondition the body to learn a new, more healthful way to respond to and deal with stress.

Many other techniques—from self-hypnosis and affirmations ("I have a healthy strong immune system") to visualizations (imagining immune system cells gobbling up invader allergens), meditation, yoga, and t'ai chi, may prove useful to promote physical and mental relaxation and reduce the stress in our lives.

Stress management techniques can serve to improve the digestion of allergy sufferers. Exercise, in particular, can be an excellent stress reducer. It can lower the levels of anxiety and boost the immune system by helping to eliminate water and toxins from the body and to speed the transfer of nutrients to the cells. It also normalizes blood sugar levels.

Aside from its many other negative affects on the body, sugar is an immune system weakener. One study found that it interferes with the white blood cells' ability to break down many harmful substances. A lack of dietary protein also can damage the immune system. Adequate protein is needed to provide the body with amino acids so that it can produce white blood cells.

PROPER DIGESTION

In addition to a weak immune system, some types of digestive imbalances usually have a role in the development of allergies. Since proper digestion requires the secretion of sufficient hydrochloric acid and pancreatic enzymes for easy absorption and utilization of the nurtrients in the food we eat, when there is too little of this secretion this process can be altered. One result may be that some portion of the nutrition in the food we eat is not made available to us. The large molecules of protein that should have been broken down by the digestive juices or enzymes go directly into the bloodstream. The immune system reacts to these large molecules as if they were foreign invaders, causing an allergic response to the particular food. To alleviate such allergies, it is vital to restore the digestive system to optimum functioning. Balancing the digestive enzymes may be a way to do this.

Thoroughly chewing one's food is essential to proper digestion since there are digestive enzymes in the saliva that break down starches. If food is bolted down, these enzymes do not have enough of a chance to work, and more will have to be done by the intestinal enzymes. The enzymes may then go out of balance.

A lack of stomach acid also may contribute to digestive disorders. Often, this is the case in allergic children. Also, with age, many adults suffer from a decrease in stomach acid. This can be corrected by taking hydrochloric acid tablets with meals. However, individuals should not attempt to self-medicate in this area. The problem may be either too much or too little stomach acid. Hence, if the individual takes antacid tablets when he or she has low stomach acid or takes hydrochloric acid when he or she is overly acidic, the result may be a worsening of the problem.

CREATING AN ALLERGY-FREE ENVIRONMENT

While we are primarily interested in food allergies in this section of *The Complete Guide to Sensible Eating*, allergies and sensitivities to a host of other environmental stimuli are rampant. They range from reactions to the mercury fillings in your teeth to others: pollen, goose feathers and down, animal hair, dust, wool, car exhausts, or household chemicals.

All of these can increase your allergic threshold (the point at which your body starts overreacting) and make you prone to food or other allergies as well. They do this by increasing stress, encouraging free radical formation, weakening your immune system, or playing havoc with proper nutrition, digestion, and absorption.

A careful review of these potential sources of problems can uncover a number of areas of concern along with possible solutions. Your physician, allergist, or clinical ecologist can help inventory these allergy sources and suggest alternative approaches for dealing with or eliminating them.

Often, an allergy-sensitive individual may manifest sensitivities to a variety of environmental areas. The physician may use an adaptation of the rotary or elimination diet to pinpoint and correct environmental sensitivities.

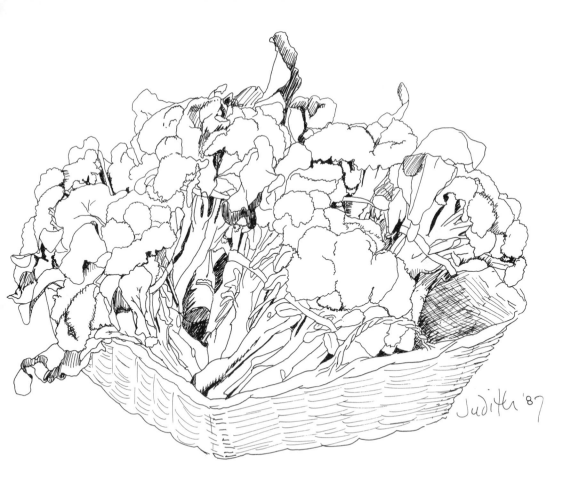

10 · VEGETARIANISM

"When we sit down to a freshly mixed salad filled with dark green leafy vegetables, a variety of sprouts and carrots, millet with tahini-oat gravy and sautéed tempeh with garlic, we are receiving complex carbohydrates, essential fatty acids, complete protein, various B complex vitamins, calcium, iron, and a host of other nutrients....A nonflesh diet will, in the long run, lower your risk of developing many diseases and raise your chances of maintaining good health."

IS IT POSSIBLE TO eat without partaking of the poisoned fruits of technology? A natural food diet, which relies on unrefined grains, legumes, seeds, nuts, and fresh produce, and steers clear of unnatural additives (including sugar and salt), is a step in the right direction. A diet that cuts down or eliminates meat is even closer to an unadulterated, healthful ideal.

There is abundant scientific evidence that proves the adequacy and, in fact, the superiority of a vegetarian diet. The medical literature is filled with studies indicating the protective qualities plant foods possess against many common degenerative diseases currently sweeping the Western world. More importantly, modern medicine is discovering that many of these diseases are directly linked to animal products consumption.

Being a vegetarian offers a wide variety of benefits, but to fully understand this dietary option it is useful to understand that there are a number of diets included under the broad term "vegetarianism."

TYPES OF VEGETARIANS

Vegans, the strictest of the vegetarians, thrive solely on plant foods, specifically vegetables, fruits, nuts, seeds, grains, and legumes. This regimen omits all animal foods, including meat, poultry, fish, eggs, dairy products, and honey.

Lacto-vegetarians eat milk and milk products in addition to vegetable foods.

Lacto-ovo-vegetarians consume eggs along with milk products and vegetables. This basically is a nonflesh diet.

Pescovegetarians eat fish in addition to the plant sources. In Asia, hundreds of millions of people follow this type of diet, living on staples of rice and fish.

Pollovegetarians omit red meat from their diets, but eat poultry in conjunction with plant sources.

All these diets include an abundance of complex carbohydrates, naturally occurring vitamins and minerals, polyunsaturated fats, fiber, and easily digestible quantities of protein. A statistical analysis shows they closely resemble the diet recommended in the "Dietary Goals for the U.S." set by the Senate Select Committee on Nutrition and Human Needs.

MAN, THE HERBIVORE

Underlying any scientific evaluation of vegetarianism is evidence that humans are not biochemically suited to eat meat. Indeed, we possess all of the features of a strictly herbivorous animal. Our flat teeth are not sharp enough to tear through hide or bone. Our lengthy digestive tract resembles that of the classic herbivore. Most carnivores are anatomically constructed to quickly get rid of the meat they eat before it putrefies, and to eliminate the majority of their dietary cholesterol. We aren't. Our digestion begins in the mouth as the salivary glands secrete an enzyme designed to break down the complex plant cells. Carnivores don't have this enzyme. They secrete an enzyme called uricase that breaks down the uric acid in meat.

THE DANGERS OF MEAT

Although designed to subsist on vegetarian foods, man has perverted his dietary habits to accept the food of the carnivore, and thus has increased the risks of developing a number of disorders and diseases.

For instance, saturated fat and cholesterol, which are found in high amounts in many meats and other animal fats, increase the risk of hardening of the arteries and heart disease.

The leading cause of death in America, heart disease, is three times more likely to occur in meat eaters than vegetarians. Consuming meat doubles your chances for colon and rectal cancer, while tripling them for breast cancer. The high-protein intake of beef eaters places undue stress on the liver and kidneys, two important organs of detoxification. It may deplete your calcium supply, leading to osteoporosis, and the uric acid it contains can settle in the joints inducing painful gouty arthritis.

In addition, there are hidden poisons in meat and poultry that, when eaten, place undue stress on our digestive systems. These toxins burden our immune systems, our defense against disease. They include hormones, antibiotics, tranquilizers, additives, preservatives, and pesticides that are added to the meat in breeding and processing the animals. Such long-term bodily pollution creates a vast overall negative effect on our health, making us susceptible to a host of pathological abnormalities. Health benefits commonly noticed by vegetarians include improved digestion and decreased gastrointestinal disturbances, including less gas and constipation.

If meat is so bad for our health, how has it become the principle staple of the American diet? Alex Hershaft, president and founder of the Vegetarian Information Service, was asked that question at a Senate Subcommittee on Health and Scientific Research. He replied: "The answer goes to the very heart of what's wrong with the decision-making machinery of the federal government, where issues are decided less on the basis of their scientific merit than of their economic and political consequences. Few politicians are willing to face up to the $35 billion meat industry and to the several million farmers who make their living from raising animals for food."

Time after time, the public is warned against the nutritional deficiencies of "ill-planned vegetarian diets," or we read that "most nutritionists agree that vegetarian diets can be adequate, if sufficient care is taken in planning them."

The fact is that *any* ill-planned diet should be avoided, no matter what foods are eaten. Sufficient care should be taken in the planning and preparation of all meals—vegetarian and nonvegetarian alike.

The misguided meat eater reading the warnings that surround vegetarianism by rivals of that diet, such as the American Dairy Association, will incorrectly assume that as long as they are healthy, they don't have to give up anything in their diets—even pork, fat, or sugar. We have blindly assumed for too long that so-called "healthy" foods cannot hurt us and that meat is magical. These, quite simply, are myths that have been fabricated and propagated by the meat and dairy industries.

No one food is indispensible or magical. Animal flesh, for instance, is nearly void of carbohydrates, has little or no fiber, and is a poor source of calcium and vitamin C. It is naturally high in saturated fats and cholesterol. Meat eaters derive their complex carbohydrates, dietary fiber, and other nutrients from the same source as vegetarians—vegetables. When meat is omitted, you sacrifice all the harmful ingredients it has while still being able to acquire needed protein from plant sources. Lacto-vegetarians, for example, eat dairy products as sources of calcium and B_{12}. While one cup of whole milk contains 288 mg. of calcium, thiamin, iron, and trace minerals, nuts and other seeds contribute fat, protein, B vitamins and iron. Dark green leafy vegetables are sources of calcium, riboflavin, and carotene and should be eaten in generous amounts.

Depending not on variety but on meat instead for one's nutritional requirements can lead to a variety of health problems. We maintain a false sense of security because meat provides an adequate amount of high-quality protein. But amino acids, the component parts of protein, are only one of the things that make us thrive.

Vegetarians can dispense with animal products because a varied diet of whole grains, nuts, seeds, vegetables, and fruits will automatically provide all nine essential amino acids (the eight essential amino acids plus one, histamine, which is essential for children) in a quality and quantity equal to or sometimes surpassing the "incredible edible egg," nature's most complete protein food.

THE VEGETARIAN SPECTRUM

When we sit down to a freshly mixed salad filled with dark green leafy vegetables, a variety of sprouts and carrots, millet with tahini-oat gravy, and sautéed tempeh with garlic, we are receiving complex carbohydrates, essential fatty acids, complete protein, various B complex vitamins, calcium, iron, and a host of other nutrients. A variety of colorful, wholesome, unprocessed foods encompassing a flavorful spectrum provides the greatest nutritional package.

Americans have a number of misguided ideas about vegetarianism and how it might affect their health. Some, for instance, fear that a vegetarian diet is fattening. This would, of course, be true if one exceeded one's proper caloric needs, no matter what foods are eaten. People think of certain vegetarian foods as especially fattening, and they're often wrong. The biggest victim of this misconception is the potato. A medium-sized plain potato has only about 70 calories, and is packed with essential amino acids and Vitamin C. Excess calories come only from the garnishes that usually accompany the potato, from globs of butter, sour cream or oil, to chili, cheddar cheese, and bacon.

A nonflesh diet will, in the long run, lower your risk of developing many diseases and raise your chances of maintaining good health. Vegetarian diets are especially health promoting during periods of physiological or physical stress in which more nutrients are needed than at other times. These include pregnancy, lactation, periods of rapid growth as during childhood and adolescence, and times of illness and convalescence. Everyone from the very young to the very old can probably benefit from such a diet.

REASONS FOR CHOOSING VEGETARIANISM

Although health improvement is the primary reason why an increasing number of people are giving up meat, there are a number of other reasons for adopting a vegetarian diet.

Economics. The rising cost of living in general and of meat in particular has forced many people to adopt a vegetarian meal plan. Ounce for ounce, plant foods are more economical than other foods. They supply more fiber and a wider variety of vitamins and minerals. The same amount of protein costs one-fifth as much when obtained from plant sources as from animal sources.

In addition, agribusiness—huge agricultural companies—has dominated the animal food industry; its high technology and centralization have created unemployment and forced many small farmers out of business. Many people choose not to support these companies by not buying meat. The switch to a no- or low-meat vegetarian diet can benefit the individual without disrupting the overall economic structure by tending to support small farmers rather than giant agribusiness conglomerates.

Natural resources. The production and processing of animal products demands an enormous amount of land, water, energy, and raw materials. The rapid depletion of these precious, finite resources is of great concern. The grim reality of the fragility of our ecosystem encourages responsible vegetarian life-styles, which do not involve wasting more resources than they use, as does the meat industry.

Food resources. The idea of eating simply so that everyone may eat is supported by the animal-free diet. Our land is capable of supplying food for nearly 14 times as many people when it is used for human food crops as when it is being used to feed livestock, as animals are a grossly inefficient source of nutrition. They need to consume approximately 16 pounds of grain in order to yield one pound of flesh. It has been estimated that our current supply of plant foods could nourish more than double the world population if we managed it better. This substantial waste of protein, calories, and other essential nutrients contributes to global imbalances and starvation. Ultimately, our demand for meat must be drastically curtailed if we are to positively affect the worldwide hunger problem.

Reverence for life. Many people are now refusing a dietary style that supports the cruel treatment and wanton slaughter of million of animals. Since every person who consumes animal products perpetuates the unnecessary and agonizing existence and brutal death of these innocent creatures, these vegetarians actively defy the harsh reality of this inhumane treatment by adhering to plant food diets.

Religious belief. There are various contemporary and ancient faiths that advocate abstinence from meat. Some favor spiritual awareness and reincarnation, others emphasize ethical considerations and health benefits. In the East, these faiths include the Hindus and Buddhists; in the West, they include the Seventh Day Adventists.

Personal Taste. Meat consumption is an acquired habit, not an organic necessity. It starts in childhood for most people, backed by the encouragement of generations of misinformed parents. Our natural taste is actually for the full-flavored, wholesome taste of vegetarian cuisine. This is shown by the fact that most people lose their taste for flesh once it is omitted from their diet. Innumerable culinary delights can be concocted from a wide variety of plant foods, including herbs and spices, and these delicious dishes prove that the only limitations that exist are man-made.

There are numerous reasons why more people than ever before are adopting the vegetarian diet. Such a simple change in our individual style of eating not only enhances our health and well-being, but also strongly influences our economic, political and environmental systems. The dietary regimen we follow is an important aspect of our existence, making a statement for each of us that either supports or attacks the earthly sphere and natural order in which we dwell. The choice is ours.

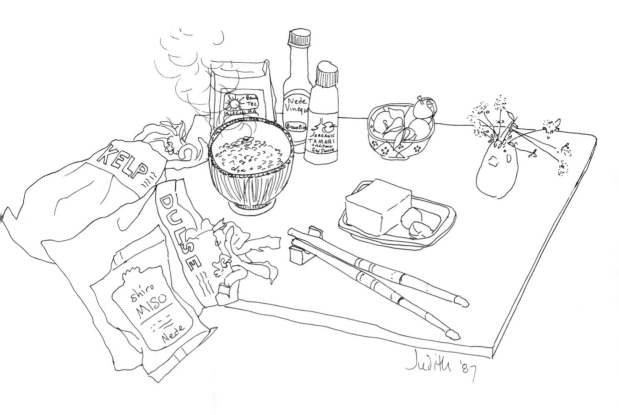

11 · A GUIDE TO VEGETARIAN FOODS

"Rice, from a nutritional point of view, means brown rice—whole grain rice which, unlike white rice, has not had its bran, and with it much of its nutrition, removed. But be careful about your source of brown rice. Commercially produced rice is among the most heavily chemically treated food crops."

BEING A VEGETARIAN MEANS more than subsisting on lettuce. A variety of wholesome food combinations are possible within this dietary option. Creative preparation can yield an infinite array of culinary delights.

WHOLE GRAINS

To the vegetarian, grains are a particularly important food staple. Use a variety of them; each has a rich flavor to impart. But to enjoy these grains' true taste, choose those grown free of chemical fertilizers and sprays. Also, the less whole grains are processed, the greater their nutritional value.

Whole grains contain everything needed to nurture themselves, from germ stage to sprout to mature plant. Plant a whole kernel of any grain and, given the right combination of earth, water, and air, it will naturally sprout and grow to maturity. Not so with *refined* grains. Bury a milled kernel and cultivate it as much as you like; nothing will grow because the kernel is already dead.

Milling the root of whole grains only refines away a wide range of trace minerals and vitamins in the outer layers, resulting in grains that are bulkier and less healthy. Refined grains, robbed of the minerals and vitamins found in the discarded outer layers, strain the body's delicate mechanism of digestion. Nearly all of the B vitamins, vitamin E, unsaturated fatty acids, and quality proteins are found in whole grains, but refining removes most of these nutrients. Even in so-called enriched foods, only a few B vitamins and iron are replaced; the remaining B vitamins, as well as a rich variety of minerals and proteins, are "refined" out.

There are three ways to prepare whole grains for eating: sprouting, soaking, and cooking until tender. All grains can be sprouted in two to three days, or until the sprout reaches the same length as the original seeds. You can reconstitute some semi-processed grains such as bulgar wheat by soaking them overnight or pouring boiling water over them and allowing them to fluff up.

When you cook grains, first rinse them in a colander or strainer, then pour the grain into a pot of water, and swirl it with your hands, removing the hulls and bits of dirt that may float to the surface. Drain the grain through a strainer, dry pan-fry it in a heavy skillet, and add two parts boiling water. Cover the skillet, reduce the heat, and let the grain simmer for about a half hour (time varies with the grain).

Preparing grains in a pressure cooker, the proportion of water to grain is roughly $2^{1}/_{2}$ parts water for each part of grain. Add grain and water to the cooker and bring them rapidly up to full pressure. When the regulator on the lid makes a jiggling sound, the cooker has reached full pressure; reduce the heat to simmer and maintain the same pressure throughout the cooking. Allow the pressure to return to normal before loosening the lid, then open the pot and gently stir the grains, mixing the kernels toward the bottom with those at the top. Let them sit for a few minutes, then mix again.

Most grains at least double in size from their dry to cooked states. This means that 1 cup of cooked grain can feed two or three enthusiastic grain eaters or three to four people eating grain along with other foods. To achieve a sweeter flavor and crunchier texture, try dry-toasting the grain or sautéing it before cooking. To dry-toast, start with a cold skillet, preferably cast iron. To sauté, you must first heat the skillet and then quickly, evenly, coat it with oil. (If the oil smokes, it's too hot.) Whether dry-toasting or sautéing, stir the grain until a few kernels pop and a delicious aroma begins to rise.

Barley has much to offer as a solo grain dish. Some of the best barley in the world—consistently high in protein and minerals—comes from the rich soil of the Red River Valley of North Dakota and Minnesota.

Since unhulled barley is almost impossible to cook, practically all barley available in food stores has been "pearled" so as to remove its tenacious hull. The factor to consider here is just how much pearling has taken place; too much results in a whiter product robbed of the nutrients in its outer layer. Look for the darker barley available in most natural food stores.

Allow 30 to 35 minutes to cook simmered barley using $2^{1}/_3$ parts liquid (water, stock, etc.) to 1 part grain. The barley can also be browned before adding it to the boiling liquid. Pressure cooking (2 parts water to 1 part grain) takes approximately 20 minutes. If the resulting grain seems too chewy, simply add $^{1}/_4$ cup more water, cover, and simmer until soft. You might also try cooking barley with other grains, such as brown rice and wheat berries.

Barley can be sprouted, but first it has to be dehulled (try seed houses and grain suppliers). Harvest the sprout when it's about the same size as the grain. Barley flour can be obtained already milled or ground fresh from the pearled grain. It is often pan-roasted before being used in breads, muffins, and cakes. Recently, researchers have found that barley, eaten daily, was successful in lowering cholesterol levels by 25 percent.

Buckwheat is actually not a true grain but a grass seed related to rhubarb. When raised commercially as a grain crop, buckwheat is unlikely to have been fertilized or sprayed. Fertilization encourages too much leaf growth; spraying stops the bees from pollinating. The best buy is whole, hulled, unroasted (white) buckwheat grains, known as groats. Roasted (brown) and cut groats are less nutritious, and the roasting can easily be done just before cooking without disturbing the flavor or the B vitamins.

Buckwheat cooks quickly, so it is rarely pressure cooked. Simmer for 15 to 20 minutes in the same saucepan or skillet you first roasted it in, using 2 parts water to 1 part buckwheat. If you prefer a porridgelike consistency, use 3 parts water. Cooked buckwheat can serve as a stuffing for everything from cabbage leaves and collard greens to knishes. Buckwheat flour combined variously with whole wheat, unbleached white, and soy flours is a delight to pancake lovers. Whole grain buckwheat flour is always dark; light-colored buckwheat flour is made from sifted flour rather than from unroasted groats. A Japanese pasta called soba (containing anywhere from 30 to 100 percent buckwheat flour) is now readily available in natural food stores and in Oriental markets. Its subtle flavor and light effect on the stomach should encourage pasta enthusiasts to give it a try. It needs no heavy sauces; try a simple garlic or onion and oil topping.

You can prepare a buckwheat cream for morning cereal from buckwheat flour sauteed in oil in a heavy skillet. Allow it to cool and then return it to the heat, gradually adding water and bringing it to a boil. This mixture is then stirred and simmered about 10 minutes or until it reaches the desired consistency.

Sprout buckwheat from the unhulled groats in half an inch of soil or on wet paper toweling and allow it to reach a height of three to four inches. The sprouts or young grass, called buckwheat lettuce, can then be juiced or chewed. The bioflavinoid rutin, which is reported to speed the coagulation of blood, helping stop bleeding, is very high in sprouted buckwheat.

Corn, a staple food for thousands of years, has changed from a small shrub with only a few kernels to today's hybrid varieties with six-foot stalks bearing several ears that contain over a hundred kernels apiece. Both white and yellow varieties of dried corn are readily available, but in the American Southwest the blue and varicolored older types of corn are still grown. "Sweet" corn is normally boiled or steamed in water; field corn is likely to be ground into meals and flours. Field corn is allowed to dry out completely, which changes the simple sugars of the grain into starches.

Yellow cornmeal contains about 10 percent protein and is higher in vitamin A than the white variety. The only difference between a meal and a flour from yellow corn is its degree of coarseness. The germ of cornmeal starts deteriorating in a matter of hours, so you should grind your own meal or flour as you use it for cornbreads, muffins, Southern spoon bread, johnnycakes or whatever. You can fry it in a pan and then cook it with a 5 to 6 parts water as a hearty "mush." Adding cornmeal to whole wheat flour in a tempura batter gives it a delicious crunchiness.

Another favorite form of this versatile grain is creamed corn. You can make creamed corn by cutting off the kernals just far enough down to allow the milky, sugary liquid to flow. Pour in enough water or milk to cover, a dash of salt, and cook the mixture gently for a few minutes. Corn flour can also be used in small amounts in whole grain pastas. A variety of Texas Deaf Smith County sweet corn can be sprouted successfully until the sprout is about a half-inch long.

The many virtues of *millet* are often overlooked because of its reputation as "the poor person's rice." Being the only grain that forms alkaline, millet is the most easily digestible. It is also an intestinal lubricant. Its amino acid structure is well balanced, providing a low-gluten protein, and it is high in calcium, riboflavin, and lecithin.

Millet is cooked the same way as most grains, with 2 parts water or stock to 1 part grain. Pre-roasting releases a lovely aroma and adds texture to the cooked grain. Leftover cooked millet is a highly versatile stuffing for anything from hollowed-out zucchini tubes to mushroom caps.

Millet meal and millet flour are quality protein additions to any bread recipe. Millet meal also makes a good hot cereal. Sprouted millet makes an excellent base for morning cereal; just harvest the sprout when the shoot is the same size as the grain.

Oats must be hulled before they can be eaten; after hulling they are cracked or rolled into the familiar cereal forms. Rolled oats are shot with steam for a number of seconds and then passed through rollers; thus some nutrients are lost. Rolled oats will cook faster than whole oat groats, but whole oat groats are the most beneficial. Known variously as Irish oatmeal, Scotch oats, or steel-cut oats, whole oat groats are soaked overnight before being cooked as porridge. (None of these or any other cereals or porridges should ever be prepared in a pressure cooker; they tend to clog the vent on the lid of the cooker.) Whole oats are wonderful in soups. You can add both rolled and whole groats to all sorts of breads and patties.

Oat flour, available at most natural food stores, can be used in equal proportions with whole wheat flour to bake up a tasty batch of muffins. Oat sprouts can be used in soups, salads, and baked goods; just harvest the sprout when it is as long as the groat.

Rice, from a nutritional point of view, means brown rice—whole grain rice which, unlike white rice, has not had its bran, and with it much of its nutrition, removed. Brown rice is available in short, medium, and long grain varieties, the difference being largely esthetic. The shorter the grain, the more gluten, which means that short grain rice cooks up stickier and long grain comes out fluffier. There's even a sweet rice grain, the most glutinous of all. Excellent quality long and medium grain brown rice comes from southeast Texas and Louisiana; this rice is hulled by a special process that protects the bran layers.

Rice is traditionally simmered, the proportions of water to grain being as follows: short grain—$2^{1}/_{2}$ to 1; medium grain—2 to 1; and long grain—$1^{1}/_{2}$ to 1. All three varieties take from 25 to 35 minutes to cook fully. Stir regularly to prevent the grains that are on the bottom from scorching.

For pressure cooking, the proportion of water to grain is different: short grain—2 to 1; medium grain—1¹/₂ to 1; long grain—1¹/₄ to 1. When the rice is cooked, allow the pressure to return slowly to normal. Some of the cooling steam will add moisture to the grain.

Brown rice is a versatile grain aside from its variety of lengths. Rice cream is made commercially by a dry-roasting method, after which the grain is stone ground to a consistency somewhat coarser than rice flour. You can prepare it as a porridge from the whole grain itself, or from prepacked rice-cream powder. Combine the rice with 4 cups of lightly salted boiling water and stir constantly over a low heat to prevent lumping. Rice flour is used extensively in baking, especially by those on gluten-restricted diets. Rice flakes make quick additions to soups or casserole bases when no other leftovers are available.

The flaking process for grains and beans was originally developed to improve animal nutrition. The grains are cooked for 15 to 20 seconds under dry radiant heat and then are dropped onto rollers and flattened into whole grain flakes. Since no wet methods of processing are used, there is only very minimal leaching and modifying of nutrients. And flaked grains and beans cook in half the usual time. You can add them to breads and casseroles for protein, texture, or taste. In chili, wheat flakes serve to complete the protein of the bean.

A rice-based grain milk called *kokoh* is available prepacked at natural food outlets. This mixture of roasted and ground rice, sweet rice, soybeans, sesame seeds and oatmeal is good as a morning cereal or tea.

But be careful about your source of brown rice. Commercially produced rice is among the most heavily chemically treated food crops.

Rye is mostly known in its flour form, used in bread loaves often flavored with caraway seeds. Especially in its sprouted form, rye is rich in vitamin E, phosphorus, magnesium, and silicon. Like wheat sprouts, rye sprouts sweeten as they lengthen because the natural starches turn to sugar. For salad purposes, use the rye sprout when it's the same size as the grain; allow it to lengthen up to one inch for a sweeter intestinal cleansing sprout and for cooking. Rye can also be harvested as a grass and chewed for its juice.

The whole rye berry is a good grain, adding chewiness and nutritious value, to combine with rice (use about 1 part rye to 2 parts rice). Rye flakes can be added to soups and stews, or used as a cereal if soaked overnight. Rye flakes, like wheat and oat flakes, make good homemade granolas. For cream of rye, somewhat coarser in texture than rye flour, add 4 parts water to 1 part grain and simmer it over a low heat for about 15 minutes.

Triticale, a highly nutritious grain with a relatively high protein content (approximately 17 percent) and a good balance of amino acids, can be cooked whole in combination with other grains, especially rice (2 parts water to 1 part triticale). Sprouted, it can be used in salads or breads; flaked, in granolas and casseroles. Triticale flour has become a favorite of vegetarians because of its unusually nutty sweetness and high protein content. As a flour it must be mixed with other flours containing higher gluten contents, since its own protein has a low gluten content.

Today, *whole wheat* holds a preeminent position among grains because of its versatility and high nutritive qualities. Containing anywhere from 6 to 20 percent protein, wheat is also a source of vitamin E and large amounts of nitrates. These nutrients are distributed throughout the three main parts of the wheat kernel or berry. The outer layers of the kernel are known collectively as the bran; there is relatively little protein here, but it is of high quality and rich in the amino acid lysine. The dietary fiber of wheat bran is also the site of about half of the 11 B vitamins found in wheat, as well as the greater portion of the trace minerals zinc, copper, and iodine. Next comes the endosperm, the white starchy central mass of wheat kernel, which contains some 70 percent of the kernel's total protein, as well as its calorie-providing starch. Finally, there is the small germ found at the base of the kernel, which, in addition to containing the same B vitamins and trace minerals as the bran, is the home of vitamin E and the unsaturated fatty acids.

If you use the wheat berry in conjunction with other grains such as rice, you get the entire nutritive value of the grain. Try pan-roasting 1/3 cup of wheat berries with 2/3 cup rice and then simmering them with 2 cups water for 25 to 30 minutes until both grains are tender. You can also eat whole wheat as wheat flakes, cracked wheat, bulgur, couscous, sprouts and flours (both hard and pastry). The flaking process preserves most of the nutrients of the original form.

Wheat flakes lend themselves especially well to chili dishes, where their addition to the beans provides a completed protein. If added dry to the vegetarian chili about 20 minutes before serving, they will break down into tiny pieces to satisfy the appetites of even the most ardent chili con carne aficionados. Cracked wheat (simple coarse-ground wheat) is most often used as a morning cereal cooked with about 3 cups salted water to 1 cup wheat; it is often added cooked or uncooked to breads and muffins.

Bulgur is a variety of whole grain wheat that is parboiled, dried (often in the sun), and then coarsely cracked. This Near and Middle Eastern staple has found its way to America in a distinctive salad called taboulie. Bulgur does not require cooking but is simply reconstituted by spreading the grain an inch deep in a shallow pan and pouring enough boiling water over it to leave about half an inch of standing water; once the water is absorbed, stir the grain several times with a fork until it's cool. It can then be chilled, combined with greens such as parsley, fresh mint, and watercress, and marinated in a dressing of sesame oil, lemon juice, and tamari.

Couscous is a form of soft, refined durum wheat flour ("semolina") that has been steamed, cracked and dried. It can be prepared for eating by adding 1 cup of couscous to 2 cups of boiling salted water with a teaspoon of butter or margarine if desired, reducing the heat and stirring constantly until most of the moisture is gone. Remove the couscous from the heat and let it stand covered about 15 minutes, fluffing it up several times with a fork.

Wheat also makes an excellent sprout, containing substantially larger amounts of all the vitamins and minerals found in the dormant kernel. The sprout, which sweetens as it lengthens, can be used in desserts.

Whole wheat flour can be made from hard (high protein, high gluten) or soft (lower protein and gluten, high starch) wheat or from spring or winter wheats. Hard wheats are excellent for making bread. The spring wheat contains a higher gluten content than the winter wheat. Soft wheat, either spring or winter, is known as pastry wheat because it yields a fine, starchy flour. Wheat flours are available at natural food stores in many pasta forms—from alphabets to ziti—often combined with other flours such as buckwheat, corn, rice, soy, and Jerusalem artichoke.

Standard white flour is purely endosperm, with most of the bran and germ removed, which means a loss of up to 70 percent of the essential nutrients of wheat. In addition, white flour may be bleached by chlorine dioxide, which completely destroys the vitamin E. "Enriched" flours are actually attempts at making up for these losses; but only four nutrients—compounds of thiamine, niacin, riboflavin (vitamin B_2), and iron—are replaced. Most unbleached white flour has had much of its bran removed, but at least it has not been bleached. Soft wheat pastry flour, which can be substituted for unbleached white flour in any recipe, is a nutritionally superior, whole, refined flour.

Whole grain flours can become rancid. Rancidity occurs when the unsaturated fats in the flour are exposed to the oxygen in the air. The vitamin E in the whole wheat flour acts as a natural preservative, but within three months it is exhausted. This problem can best be handled by storing the flour in a cool dry place immediately after milling. There are a number of small natural food companies that mill and distribute their fresh-ground flour. Home grinding machines are now available at many natural food stores.

Wheat gluten (*kofu*, in Japanese cookery) has long been a popular vegetarian source of protein in many places around the world. It is prepared by mixing whole wheat flour and water in a 2½ to 1 ratio and kneading it into a stiff dough. This dough is then covered with cold water and kneaded underwater; as the water clouds up with starch sediment, it is replaced and the procedure is repeated about five or six times until the water remains clear. Then the remaining gluten dough is steamed or cooked in a double boiler for 30 minutes. Kofu may be eaten as is, flavored with soy sauce, or baked in casserole loaves combined with other grains, such as rice and beans.

Amaranth and Quinoa are two grains new to the American diet that have recently come on the market.

Amaranth is a native grain. It has been cultivated in the American southwest for hundreds of years. The plant yeilds a tiny seed that should be prepared similarly to rice. When cooked, it has a very soft, nutlike consistency.

Quinoa, a staple of the Inca Indians, is a delicate, light-textured, high-protein grain that resembles tiny granules of tabouli or couscous. Known as "the mother grain," it is high in complete protein, cooks in 10 to 15 minutes, and approximately triples its volume when cooked, somewhat mitigating its current high price (up to $4 a pound) in health food stores.

BEANS (LEGUMES)

The members of the bean family are important, inexpensive sources of protein, minerals and vitamins. Legumes can be cooked whole, flaked like grains, sprouted, ground into flours, even transformed into a variety of "dairy" products.

As a general rule, 1 cup of dry beans will make about 2½ cups of cooked beans, enough for 4 servings. Some beans should be soaked, preferably overnight; these include adzuki beans, black beans, chick peas (garbanzos) and soybeans. As an alternative to overnight soaking, you can bring the beans (1 cup) and water (3 to 4 cups) to a boil, remove the pot from the stove and cover, let the beans sit for an hour, then cook the beans by simmering after first bringing them to a boil, or by putting them in a pressure cooker.

When using beans for a soup dish, allow five times as much water as beans at the beginning of the cooking process. Don't salt the water until the beans are soft (or after the pressure in the cooker has come down), because the salt will draw the moisture out of the beans.

Adzuki are small red beans that have a special place in Japanese cuisine as well as in traditional Japanese medicine, where they are used as a remedy for kidney ailments (when combined with a small pumpkin called *hokkaido*). Very high in B vitamins and trace minerals, adzukis should never be pressure-cooked because it turns them bitter.

After overnight soaking, simmer adzukis with a strip of kombu (a kind of kelp) for about 1 to 1½ hours until tender, with 4 to 5 cups water to each cup of beans. One favorite preparation: add 1 cup each of sautéed onions and celery to the tender beans and then puree them together in a blender. The resulting thick, creamy soup can be thinned with water or bean juice and flavored with a dash of lime juice, tamari, and mild curry.

Black beans and their close relative, *turtle beans,* have served as major food sources in the Carribbean, Mexico, and the American Southwest for many years. These beans should not be prepared in a pressure cooker since their skins fall off easily and may clog the valve. A smooth, rich black bean soup, a specialty of Cuba, is made by cooking the soaked beans until tender, adding sauteed garlic, onions, and celery, and then pressing the mixture through a colander (or, more easily, quickly blending it in an electric blender). A small amount of lime juice may be added to lighten the taste.

Black-eyed peas, a Southern favorite, provides a delicious complete protein-balanced meal. Among the quickest-cooking beans, they become tender in 45 minutes to an hour. Eating this bean on New Year's Day is said to bring good luck throughout the year.

Chick-peas, or *garbanzos*, are so versatile that they have been the subject of entire cookbooks. High in protein, they are also good souces of calcium, iron, potassium, and B vitamins. They can be roasted, like peanuts, or boiled. After a very thorough roasting, chick-peas can even be ground and used as a coffee substitute. *Hummus* is a thick paste that combines mashed chick-peas, hulled sesame-seed tahini, garlic, and lemon juice. Bean patés using chick-peas as a base offer many creative opportunities for creating complete proteins, by combining different beans. Cooked grains, ground seeds and nuts, raw vegetables, herbs, and miso may all be combined with the cooked beans to produce a sophisticated and appealing paté or paste.

Great northern beans and their small counterpart, *navy beans*, cook in less than an hour and require no presoaking. They are often used for hearty soups. Cook the beans with 5 to 6 parts water or stock to 1 part dry beans. Firmer vegetables, such as carrots, rutabagas or turnips should be added ½ hour before the soup is finished; other vegetables, such as onions, celery and peppers, should be added 15 minutes later, either sauted or raw.

Kidney beans, standard in all sorts of chilis, will cook in about an hour, after having been soaked overnight. The fragrant brown bean juice produced in cooking the beans makes the addition of tomato virtually unnecessary. Once the beans are tender, try dicing onions, garlic, and red and green peppers; saut them lightly in sesame oil until the onions are translucent, then add them to the beans. Season them to taste. Rich Mexican chili powder seems to lend more flavor to the beans than does a scorching Indian one. Tamari, a dash of blackstrap molasses or fresh-grated ginger root can further enhance the beans. For a perfect final texture, add dry wheat flakes to the chili about 20 minutes before serving; this allows time for the flakes to cook and disintegrate, thickening the dish while complementing the protein of the beans.

Lentils come in a rainbow of colors, but generally only the green, brown, and red varieties are available in the United States. All are inexpensive and nutritious sources of iron, cellulose, and B vitamins. Lentils require no presoaking and disintegrate when cooked, leaving a smooth base to which you can add fresh or sautéed vegetables (including carrots, turnips, onions, and peppers). They sprout well in combination with other seeds and produce large quantities. The flavor of the uncooked sprout is similar to that of fresh ground pepper on salad; when cooked it has a more nutlike taste. The sprouts should be harvested when the shoot is as long as the seed.

Mung beans are probably best known in their sprout form, eaten raw or lightly sautéed with other vegetables. They can be cooked as a dry bean, using three times as much water as beans, and then pureed in an electric blender into a smooth soup. The result is rather bland and benefits from the addition of tamari and fresh or dried basil. But as sprouts, mung beans really come into their own. Mung sprouts are rich in vitamins A and C and contain high amounts of calcium, phosphorus, and iron. Th hulls are easily digestible and rich in minerals. Mung sprouts can be harvested any time from the second day, when the shoot has just appeared, to the third or fourth day when the shoot is about four inches long. Mung beans make a good first choice for beginning sprouters.

Peanuts, though commonly grouped with seeds and nuts, are actually members of the legume family. Their high protein content is well known. In the United States eating peanut butter is virtually a national pastime. Peanut butter can—and should—contain 100 percent peanuts; sugars, colorings, stabilizers, and preservatives are neither necessary nor desirable. A single grinding under pressure extracts enough oil from the nut meal to give the peanuts a creamy texture.

Pinto beans are popular in American Southwest dishes and lend themselves especially well to baking. Naturally sweet in flavor, they adapt to many types of seasonings, and once cooked tender, they can be used in casseroles. Pinto flakes cook quickly and reconstitute themselves into tender round beans in about 40 minutes (2 parts water to 1 part dry flakes). Cumin blends nicely with these beans, if used sparingly.

Soybeans, unquestionably the most nutritious of all the beans, have been the major source of protein in Oriental diets for centuries. They are increasingly being viewed as the most realistic source of high-quality, low-cost protein available today on a large enough scale to meet worldwide needs. In addition to high-quality protein, soybeans contain large amounts of B vitamins, minerals, and unsaturated fatty acids in the form of lecithin that help the body emulsify cholesterol.

Thanks to their bland flavor after cooking and their high concentration of nutrients, soybeans can be made into an amazingly diverse array of foods. Western technology in recent years has focused on creating a wide range of synthetic soybean foods. There are protein concentrates in the form of soy powder containing from 70 to 90 percent moisture-free protein, isolates (defatted flakes and flours used to make simulated dairy products and frozen deserts), spun protein fibers (isolates dissolved in alkali solutions for use in simulated meat products), and textured vegetable proteins (made from soy flour and used in simulated meat products and infant foods). Most Western cooks also have come across soybeans in the form of full-fat soy flour, soy granules, and defatted soy flour and grits—all of which are available in natural food stores. Full-fat soy flour, which contains about 40 percent protein and 20 percent naturally occurring oils, makes a fine addition to many forms of baked goods. Soy granules contain about 50 percent protein, as do defatted soy flour and soy grits, which are basically by-products of the extraction of soy oil. Both are used in breakfast cereals, simulated meats, and desserts. Soybeans are also processed into flakes which, unlike raw soybeans, require no presoaking and only about 1 1/2 hours of cooking.

In striking contrast to these highly refined products of the West are the traditional East Asian soy products, tamari soy sauce, miso (fermented soy paste), and tofu. The first two fermented products will be discussed later in this chapter. *Tofu* (soy curd or soy cheese) is a remarkable food. It is very inexpensive when purchased at Oriental markets or natural food shops and even more so if made at home.

You can make your own tofu by grinding soaked soybeans, cooking them with water, pouring the resulting mixture into a pressing sack, and collecting the soy "milk" underneath by squeezing as much liquid as possible from the sack, leaving the bean fiber behind. The soy milk is then simmered and curdled in a solution containing sea-water brine (called *nigari*), lemon juice, or vinegar. Any of these three solidifiers will work well, although commercial nigari is most often used for this coagulation process.

After the white soy curds curdle and float in a yellowish whey liquid, they are ladeled into a settling box, covered and weighted, and allowed to press into a solid cake, which is then ready for immediate use as is—or for further transformation into a virtually unlimited variety of tofu products. Tofu is high in quality protein and is excellent for creating complete protein, especially when combined with grains. Tofu contains an abundance of lysine, an essential amino acid in which many grains are deficient; on the other hand, grains such as rice are high in the sulfur that contains methionine and cystine, amino acids which are absent in soybeans. These soy and grain proteins complement each other naturally.

Tofu is easy to digest, low in calories, saturated fats, and cholesterol. When solidified with calcium chloride or calcium sulfate—as in most commercial American tofu—tofu contains more calcium by weight than dairy milk; it's also a good source of other minerals such as iron, phosphorus, and potassium.

Since it's made from soybeans, tofu is free of chemical toxins. Soybeans are an important feed crop for the beef and dairy industries and the spraying is therefore carefully monitored by the Food and Drug Administration.

In addition to tofu, the soybean can be enjoyed in many other ways. It can be served as a fresh green summer vegetable, simmered or steamed in the pod. Roasted soybeans are now available in many varieties: dry-roasted, oil-roasted, salted, unsalted, and with garlic or barbecue flavors. They contain up to 47 percent protein and can either be eaten as a snack or added to casseroles for texture.

When cooking whole dry soybeans, a pressure cooker can save a great deal of time. Use $2^1/2$ to 3 cups of water over a low flame for each cup of dry soybeans. Once the right pressure has been reached, cook until tender—about 90 minutes. Before cooking soybeans by the ordinary simmering method, soak them overnight in 4 cups of water. Bring them to a boil in 4 more cups of liquid and simmer about 3 hours, adding more water whenever necessary.

An interesting soybean preparation called *tempeh* is made from cooked dehulled soybean halves, to which a *Rhizopus mold* is introduced. The inoculated bean cakes are then fermented overnight, during which time the white mycellium mold partially digests the beans and effectively deactivates the trypsin enzyme, which could inhibit digestion. The soybeans have, by this time, become fragrant cakes bound together by the mold; you can then either deep-fry or bake them into a dish that tastes remarkably like veal or chicken. Tempeh is rich in protein (from 18 to 48 percent) and highly digestible. In addition, like the other fermented soy products and sea vegetables, it is one of the few nonmeat sources of vitamin B_{12}. Tempeh can be made easily in any kitchen. The tempeh starter (*Rhizopus oligosporus*, mold spores) is available from the Department of Agriculture, complete with an enthusiastic brochure on its use.

A further use of this "queen of the beans" is as a sprout. Significant amounts of vitamin C, not found in the dried bean, are released in the sprouts, which are also rich in vitamins A, E, and the B complex, as well as minerals. The yellow soybean does well for sprouting, and the black variety can also sprout prolifically. Rinse the sprouts two to three times a day and harvest them when the shoot is from $1/4$ to $1^1/2$ inches long. As a matter of taste, you may or may not prefer to remove the outer husk before using the sprout. Steaming or boiling the soybean sprouts lightly before eating will destroy the urease and antitrypsin enzymes that interfere with digestion. The sprouts can be ground and used in sandwiches and salad dressings, and they make a fine addition to any sauté of crisp Chinese-style vegetables.

Split peas, both green and yellow, make a simple soup filled with protein and minerals. They do not require soaking. Start with 1 part dry peas and 5 to 6 cups water and cook quickly in about 45 minutes. Once the peas are cooked, the soup will continue to thicken; this leftover paste can be diluted several times in the following days for a quick hot soup. Sautéed onions, tamari, and $1/2$ stick of soy margarine complete the soup.

NUTS AND SEEDS

Nuts and seeds are fine sources of protein, minerals (especially magnesium), some B vitamins, and unsaturated fatty acids. They can be eaten as snack foods or used with other foods to add interesting flavors, textures, and nutritional values.

A general sprouting procedure for seeds and nuts: soak the dried seeds for about 8 hours (approximately 4 parts water to 1 part seed). Don't throw away the soaking water; use it as a cooking liquid, or water your houseplants with it. Rinse the seeds with cool water and place them in a sprouter.

Keys to successful sprouting include keeping the sprouts moist but never soaked, keeping them moderately warm, rinsing them as often as possible, and giving them enough room so that air can freely circulate around them. Actually, only about five minutes a day is needed for growing a successful sprout garden. Use the sprouts as soon as possible. They have a refrigerator life of seven to ten days. Sprouts can also be dried easily for use in beverages, nut butter, and spreads. Place the sprouts on cookie sheets for a few hours in a warm room, or keep them in a warm oven until they're dry.

Then grind them in a blender and store this nutritious food concentrate in a jar and refrigerate.

Many people think of *alfalfa* as a barnyard grass, which it is. Because its roots penetrate deep underground to seek out the elements it craves, alfalfa is one of the best possible fodders. But the fresh, mineral-laden leaves of this plant are especially nutritious for humans when juiced. Alfalfa seeds purchased at a natural food store may seem expensive, but a few of them go a long way—$1/2$ teaspoon of dry seeds yields an entire trayful of sprouts. The sprouts have a light sweet taste and are particularly rich in vitamin C, as well as in chlorophyll (when allowed to develop in light). They also have high mineral values, containing phosphorus, chlorine, silicon, aluminum, calcium, magnesium, sulfur, sodium, and potassium. Alfalfa seeds sprout well in combination with other seeds and have a high germination rate. They can also be used when dried.

Almonds will sprout only from the fresh unhulled nut after soaking overnight; they must be kept very moist until their sprouts reach a length of about one inch (four days). They can then be used to make almond milk: a combination of 1 cup of almond sprouts (or merely almonds soaked overnight) blended with 4 times as much water or apple juice. Almonds, which have an exceptionally high mineral content, are delicious raw or roasted with tamari. The raw nut can be sliced, slivered, or chopped, and even can be ground into almond butter.

Brazil nuts, like other seeds and nuts, have a high fat content. But because they are also high in protein, they are actually not much higher in calories per gram of usable protein than are whole grains. They also offer unusually high amounts of the sulfur-containing amino acids. For this reason, you can serve them to good advantage as a chopped garnish for fresh vegetables, such as brussel sprouts, cauliflower, green peas, and lima beans. These vegetables are all deficient in the sulfur-containing amino acids but high in the amino acid isoleucine lacking in Brazil nuts.

Cashews are also popular nuts that can be added to many dishes. Use them as a layer in a casserole, or simply roast them lightly and toss them in a bowl of steamed snow peas. Cashew butter, from both raw and roasted nuts, is fast growing in popularity and is well suited for use in sauces, where it can be diluted with water and miso paste. You can mix it yourself in a nutritious soy "milkshake." Blend 2 cups of plain or sweetened soy milk with $1/2$ cup of cashew butter; add 2 tablespoons of carob powder, a pinch of salt, and a dash of vanilla extract and nutmeg.

Chia seeds, now available in natural food stores, have long been a staple in Mexican and American Indian diets, where they were traditionally used to increase endurance on long hunts and migrations. Although a member of the mint family, chia seeds have a mild flaxlike taste. They can be chewed raw or sprinkled into hot or cold cereals. Since they are in a class of seeds called mucilaginous, which become sticky when soaked in water, their sprouting procedure is slightly different. Sprinkle the seeds over a saucer filled with water and allow to stand overnight. By morning, the seeds, having absorbed all the water, will stick to the saucer. Gently rinse and drain them, using a sieve if possible. Then, as with other seeds, rinse twice daily. Also try sprouting the seeds in a flat covered container lined with damp paper towels. Harvest the chia seeds when the shoot is one inch long.

The red variety of *clover*, makes a delicious sprout similar in taste to alfalfa. In its sprout form, this forage plant can be an excellent source of chlorophyll; when the primary leaves are about one inch in length, spread them out in a nonmetallic tray and dampen them. They should be covered with clear plastic to hold in moisture and placed in a sunny spot for one to two hours.

Cress seeds are tiny members of the mustard family. They add a zesty taste to salads when used in their sprout form. They are also mucilaginous seeds and so are sprouted in the same way as chia seeds. Harvest the sprouts at about one inch long and use them in sandwiches instead of lettuce.

Fenugreek seeds were first used to brew tea by the ancient Greeks. This strong tea is an excellent mouthwash, as well as a tasty and nutritious addition to soy or nut milk. The ground dry seed is one of the components of curry powder. When sprouted, fenugreek can be added to soups, salads, and grain dishes. The sprout should be harvested once it is one-fourth inch long, for it will become very bitter soon afterward.

Filberts or *hazelnuts* are tasty nuts that, once chopped, make a delicious garnish for both greens and creamy tofu pudding. These nuts, however, contain an excess amount of calories for the amount of protein they provide.

Flax, also known as *linseed*, is a versatile plant. The fiber of the mature plant is used to make linen and pressed to extract its oil. As a sprout, flax has been used for centuries; it is recorded that at Greek and Roman banquets, flax sprouts were served between courses for their mild laxative effect. Though flax is sprouted as a mucilaginous seed, its sprouts work well in conjunction with wheat and rye kernels. Harvest when the shoots are about an inch long and serve as a breakfast salad. Taken on an empty stomach, this sprout mixture cleanses and lubricates the colon.

The small seeds of the common black *mustard* plant will sprout quite readily and are usually available at herb and spice stores. Small amounts of these sprouts add a spicy flavor to salads and sandwiches. Harvest when shoots are about an inch long.

Pecans are nuts that are cultivated organically in Texas and New Mexico. Though high in potassium and B vitamins, pecans are not good sources of protein; like filberts, they contain too many calories for the amount of protein they offer. Pecans are delicious as tamari-roasted nuts: dry-roast in a heavy skillet and, when they begin to emit a pleasing fragrance, remove to a plate and sprinkle lightly with tamari.

Pignolias, or pine nuts, have an unusual flavor, but are a poor source of protein. Pignolias, found in the cones of the small piñon pine, which grows in the American Southwest, have been used by many Indian tribes as a food staple. Most of the pignolias consumed in the United States, however, come from Portugal. Pan-roasted pine nuts are delicious with green vegetables like peas and beans, and are also tasty in bread stuffings.

Pistachio nuts are familiar to many as an Italian ice cream flavor. For snacking purposes, use the naturally grown pistachio rather than the dyed varieties. Like other nuts, pistachios should be consumed only in small quantities, since they are high in calories.

Pumpkin seeds, *pepitas* and *squash seeds* are delicious seeds rich in minerals that can be eaten as snacks or ground into a meal for use in baking and cooking. Eastern Europeans, who eat many more pumpkin seeds than do Americans, use them to help prevent prostate disorders. Save the seeds from a pumpkin or squash and sprout them. Harvest when the shoot is just beginning to show (after three or four days); if allowed to lengthen any further, the sprouts will taste bitter.

Radish seeds, both black and red, make wonderfully tangy sprouts. They sprout easily and work well when combined with alfalfa and clover seeds. They're relatively expensive compared to most sprouting seeds, but you don't need many of these peppery-tasting sprouts to perk up a salad. Harvest these shoots when they're about an inch long.

Sesame seeds, or *benne*, are popular around the world because of their taste and high nutritive content. Most sesame seeds available in the United States are grown in southern Mexico, where few sprays are used, and they are available hulled or unhulled. The unhulled variety is nutritionally superior since most of the mineral value is found in the hull.

The seeds are an excellent source of protein, unsaturated fatty acids, calcium, magnesium, niacin, and vitamins A and E. The protein in sesame seeds effectively complements the protein of legumes, because both contain high amounts of each other's deficient amino acids. Therefore, an especially good addition to a soy-milk shake is *tahini*, or sesame butter.

Used extensively as the whole seed in breads and other baked foods, in grain dishes, and on vegetables, the unhulled seeds can also be toasted and ground into sesame butter, which has a stronger taste and higher mineral content than sesame tahini. Tahini, made from toasted and hulled seeds, is a mild sweet butter. Tahini is used extensively in the Middle East, where the oil that separates from the butter is used as a cooking oil. Tahini is an excellent base for salad dressing and acts as a perfect thickener for all sorts of sauces.

The unhulled seed must be used when sprouting. The sprouts can be used, like the whole seed, in cooked foods or blended into beverages. Harvest when the shoot reaches one-sixteenth inch in length (usually within two days). At this stage the sprouts are sweet, but become bitter with further growth.

Sunflower seeds are sun-energized, nutritional powerhouses rich in protein (about 30 percent), unsaturated fatty acids, phosphorus, calcium, iron, fluorine, iodine, potassium, magnesium, zinc, several B vitamins, vitamin E, and vitamin D (one of the few vegetable sources of this vitamin). Its high mineral content is the result of the sunflower's extensive root system, which penetrates deep into the subsoil seeking nutrients; its vitamin D content is partially due to the flower's tendency to follow and face the sun as it moves across the sky.

Sunflowers were cultivated extensively by American Indians as a food crop. In their raw state, sunflower seeds can be enjoyed as snacks or included in everything from breads to salads. The seeds are also available in a toasted, salted nut butter.

Sprouted sunflower seeds should be eaten when barely budded or they will taste very bitter. However, it usually takes four to five days for the shoot to appear. Unhulled seeds, or special hulled sprouting seeds, are used when sprouting, but the husk should be removed before eating.

Walnuts are a good source of protein and iron. Black walnuts contain about 40 percent more protein than English walnuts (also known as California walnuts in the United States). Walnuts will keep fresh much longer when purchased in the shell. This is true of all nuts. It also brings down the price considerably.

SEAWEEDS

Seaweeds rank high as sources for the basic essential minerals, as do green vegetables such as dandelions and watercress. They all contain calcium, magnesium, phosphorus, potassium, iron, iodine, and sodium. Most Westerners dislike the idea of eating seaweed. If they were to sample what they're missing, though, they'd find a new world of taste and high-quality nutrients—especially trace minerals—in the six varieties of sea vegetables available in most natural food stores and food co-ops.

Agar, or *agar-agar* (called *kantan* in Japanese, and also know as *Ceylonese moss*) is a translucent, almost weightless seaweed product found in stick, flake, or powdered form. You can use it like gelatin to thicken fruit juices or purees. Agar also can be used to make aspics and clear molds of fruit juices, fruits, or vegetables. If you tear 1 to 1¹/₂ sticks into small pieces and dissolve them in 1 quart of liquid, you will produce a pudding-like consistency. More agar can be used to achieve a jellied texture. When used in stick form, agar should be simmered in liquid for 10 to 15 minutes, to ensure that all the pieces have dissolved. This simmering isn't necessary when using the flaked or powdered varieties.

Dulse is the only commercial sea vegetable that comes from the Atlantic Ocean (specifically, the Canadian Maritime Provinces). This ready-to-eat seaweed can be chewed in its tough dry state, but a short soaking to rinse it and to remove any small, clinging shells is worthwhile. Dulse can be added to miso soup.

Another Japanese seaweed is the jet-black *hijiki*, or *hiziki*. This stringy, hairlike seaweed contains 57 percent more calcium by weight than dry milk and has high levels of iron as well. Dried hiziki should be soaked in several cups of water for about 20 minutes, then strained in a colander and lightly pressed to squeeze out excess moisture. Once reconstituted, hiziki is best when sautéed together with other vegetables—especially onion and leeks—or cooked with beans and grains.

Kombu is the Japanese term for several species of brown algae. In English, these are usually referred to collectively as *kelp*. Kombu is especially rich in iodine, vitamin B_2 and calcium. When using the dried form of kombu, rinse it once and soak for 10 to 15 minutes.

Note that all dried seaweeds increase greatly in size when reconstituted. For example, ¹/₄ cup of dried hiziki would yield 1 cup when soaked. Save the water in which the seaweeds are soaked and use it as soup stock. Reconstituted kombu strips can be used whole in the cooking water for beans and grains, or can be cut into thin strips or diced for use in soups and salads.

Nori is the most popular Japanese seaweed, also known as dried purple *laver*. It is sold in the form of paper-thin purplish sheets, with eight to ten sheets per package. Laver has been used as a food by many peoples— including the American Pacific Coast Indians. The Japanese and Koreans are, however, the only people to cultivate these plants and dry and press the mature leaves into sheets.

The nori sheets are toasted over a flame until crisp, during which their color changes from black or purple to green. They are then crumbled or slivered and used as a condiment for noodles, grains, beans and soups. Remarkably rich in protein, nori is also high in vitamins A, B$_2$, B$_{12}$, D, and niacin.

Wakame is a long seaweed with symmetrical and fluted fronds growing from both sides of an edible midrib. Although generally used fresh in Japan, it is only available dried in the West. It is reconstituted in the same manner as kombu: rinsed once, soaked, and pressed of excess moisture. If the midrib is particularly tough, it can be removed. When used in soups, wakame should be cooked for no more than several minutes and should therefore be one of the last ingredients added to miso soup. This delicious vegetable is rich in protein and niacin, and contains, in its dried state, almost 50 percent more calcium than dry milk.

FERMENTED FOODS: MISO AND TAMARI

Miso and tamari, derived from soybeans and grain, deserve special consideration in any sensible vegetarian diet.

The fermentation process in the healthy human intestine isn't that different from what occurs in the production of fermented soy foods. For example, in our digestive tract, maltose and glucose are broken down to form lactic acid, ethyl alcohol, and organic acids. The microorganic cultures responsible for these syntheses enter our own bodies when we digest them in fermented foods and help us to assimilate the nutrients we need.

Miso, a fermented soybean paste, has long been a staple seasoning in the Oriental kitchen. It is produced by combining cooked soybeans, salt and various grains. Barley miso is made with barley and soybeans. Rice miso is made with both hulled and unhulled rice plus soybeans, and soybeans alone are used to make matcho miso. These cooked and slated combinations are dusted with a fungus mold, *koji*, which produces the enzymes that start to digest the bean-and-grain mixture.

Tamari is naturally fermented soy sauce. Originally considered excess liquid, it was drained off miso that had finished fermenting. Today it is a product in its own right and is made from a natural fermentation process of whole soybeans, natural sea salt, well water, roasted cracked wheat and koji spores, all aged for 12 to 18 months. Tamari, like miso, has a range of colors, textures, and aromas as wide and varied as that of wines and cheeses.

Miso and tamari contain between 9 and 18 percent complete protein; the higher the soybean content, the higher the protein. The protein in these products is "predigested": it is already broken down into 17 amino acids, which makes for easy digestion. Also, the digestion-inhibiting enzyme present in raw or poorly cooked soybeans is destroyed by their fermentations. During the microorganic synthesis of miso and tamari, the amounts of B vitamins, riboflavin, and niacin increase. In addition, miso and tamari are among the few vegetable sources of vitamin B_{12}, which is actually manufactured by fungi and bacteria in the fermenting mixtures just as it is synthesized in the human intestine.

Miso and tamari are useful in all cuisines, but because of their high salt content—11 percent for the saltiest of hatcho miso and 18 percent for tamari—they should be used sparingly. Miso diluted with water can be used as a base for a sauce made with tahini; a dash of tamari brings out new flavors in familiar grains. Miso also makes a wonderful soup base to which tofu, mushrooms, seaweeds, and many fresh or cooked vegetables can be added.

All of the natural miso and tamari available in the United States today comes from Japan. If a package of miso you purchase has started to expand, you can be assured its contents have not been pasturized and that the microorganisms are still alive and producing carbon dioxide gas. Get rid of it.

In the future, the United States may begin producing its own fermented soybean foods. A lively market now exists and many people are acquiring the necessary technical know-how. Organic farmers are already producing soybeans, wheat, barley, and rice; the koji starter and engineering skills are always available from the Orient. As fermented soy foods play a larger role in American diets, we may start to develop and adapt our own distinctive varieties.

SALT: SOME ALTERNATIVE SOURCES

A controversy continues about the virtues and dangers of salt. Some people consume large quantites of salt. Many others attempt to get their salt from the juices of celery, spinach, beets, or carrots; very little sodium, however, is derived from these supposedly sodium-rich foods. Still other people decide upon, or are prescribed, low-sodium or even "salt-free" diets. People on low-sodium diets have often been suffering from hypertension or kidney problems. Overconsumption of salt will lead to hypertension: The salt draws water out of blood cells and vessels, which in turn causes dehydration of the tissues and forces the heart to pump much too strenuously. Overconsumption of salt also clogs the kidneys and creates an excess of water that cannot be properly eliminated from the body.

On the other hand, moderate and intelligent consumption of salt helps the body retain heat by slightly contracting the blood vessels, which is why we tend to consume more salt in cold months. Sodium also helps maintain intestinal muscle tone. You should evaluate your own salt needs according to your physical activity, climate, water intake, and—above all—diet. People in meat-eating cultures seldom need extra salt per se, because they get all they need from the blood and flesh of the animals they eat; vegetarian or agricultural peoples, however, tend to have a high regard for salt and use it to cook, pickle, and preserve foods.

If you want to eat salt, you should use the natural sun- or kiln-dried variety, which still contains important trace minerals. Refined "table" salt is made fine by high heats and flash-cooling, and then combined with such additives as sodium silico aluminate to keep it "free-flowing." Kosher salt is an exception; it has larger crystals due to its milder processing, and nothing is added to the better brands. Natural salt—rock salt or sea salt—is not free-flowing, but some brands add calcium carbonate, a natural compound, to prevent caking. All salt is or once was sea salt, so differences between salt obtained from inland rock deposits or from the sea are minor and unimportant.

No natural salt contains iodine, which is far too volatile a substance to remain stable for long without numerous additives. But there is an excellent source of iodine from the ocean: sea vegetables, the most common being kelp. These contain a natural, sugar-stabilized iodine—as well as about 4 to 8 percent salt. They are harvested, roasted, ground up, and marketed as salt alternatives.

Another healthful way of adding salt to your diet is to use *sesame salt*, sold as *gomasio*. This versatile condiment can be used in place of ordinary salt on cooked greens, grains and raw salads. Gomasio can be purchased in most natural food stores, but the serious cook should grind his or her own.

The ridged ceramic grinding bowl called a suribachi is needed to make sesame salt. A proportion of 15 parts sesame seeds (unhulled) to 1 part salt is recommended by Lima Ohsawa in her cookbook, *The Art of Just Cooking*. She suggests that this formula should be adjusted to fit the individual taste and climate and advises a milder salt content for children. Start with 1 cup of sesame seeds, wash them in a fine strainer, and set aside to drain. Roast 1 level teaspoon of salt in a heavy skillet until the strong odor of chlorine is no longer released. Then transfer the salt to the suribachi and pulverize it with the wooden pestle.

Roast the drained sesame seeds in the skillet over moderate heat, constantly stirring until they are light brown in color and they begin to release their characteristic aroma. Transfer these browned seeds to the suribachi and grind lightly with salt until about 80 percent of the seeds are crushed.

Store the mixture until needed in an airtight container. Making gomasio becomes a beautiful ritual well worth the effort.

Another alternative is *salted umeboshi plums*. These small Japanese plums are known for the high quality and quantity of citric acid they contain. The citric acid in plums allegedly helps neutralize and eliminate some of the excess lactic acid in the body, helping to restore a natural balance. An excess of lactic acid in the body is caused by excessive consumption of sugar; if not converted to body energy, the sugar turns into lactic acid and combines with protein to contribute to ailments like headaches, fatigue, and high blood pressure.

In Japan, these organically grown plums are available in a variety of preservative-free forms—from concentrates to salted plums. In most American natural food stores, only the salted plums are available. These are potent alkaline sources, excellent to aid indigestion, colds, and fatigue. Umeboshi also have many culinary uses. Use them to salt the water in which grains will be cooked or use several in tofu salad dressings instead of tamari or sea salt.

SWEETENERS

Carbohydrate sugar is unquestionably essential to life, but try to get it in as unadulterated a form as possible. Common table sugar has been processed to 99.9 percent sucrose, devoid of the vitamins and minerals found in sugar cane or sugar beets. This refined sucrose taxes the body's digestive system and depletes its core of minerals and enzymes as the sugar is metabolized. For this reason and others, white sugar has earned a bad reputation and the label, "empty food."

Carbohydrates include many sugars. The best known is *sucrose*, or white table sugar, which breaks down in the body into simpler sugars— glucose and fructose. There are also starches in whole cereals (together with their own component enzymes, vitamins, minerals, and proteins) that break down uniformly in the body into simple glucose molecules once they have been cooked, chewed, and digested. Compared with these refined starches, refined sugars tend to overstrain the body's digestive system. So, it would seem wiser to get the sugars you need from abundant natural stores in cereals, vegetables, and fruits. Eaten in moderate amounts, starches are not fattening, contrary to public opinion. In fact, according to Dr. Alfred Meiss, "the body's adaptation to starch is nearly perfect" since starch is the "biochemically most efficient" carbohydrate, while "sucrose makes it harder for the body to produce energy over the long run."

When cooking with natural foods, you should simply replace refined sugars with the richer flavors of naturally occurring sugars. *Maple syrup*, for example, or honey or fruit juice can substitute for sugar in almost any home recipe. Maple sugar is expensive and very sweet, so use it in moderation. Use 1/2 cup of maple syrup instead of 1 cup of sugar and either reduce the other liquids in the recipe or increase the dry ingredients accordingly. Maple syrup is believed by some to be a source of the trace mineral zinc. But be sure that the maple syrup you buy has not been extracted with formaldehyde.

All *honeys* are basically the fruit sugar fructose, which consists of varying amounts of dextrose, levulose, maltose, and other simple sugars. The flavor of honey depends on the source of the bees' nectar. All honey you use should be unheated and unfiltered so that its natural enzymes and vitamins are still intact. When cooking with honey in a recipe originally calling for refined sugar, divide the amount of sugar called for in half and adjust the recipe with less liquid or more dry ingredients.

In fact, not too much sugar of *any* kind should be used in cooking or baking, because heat can be destructive to protein in the presence of sugar. This is especially true when using honey or a refined glucose such as corn syrup. Try using fruit juices or purees made from soaked dried fruits to sweeten dishes; a little of these natural sugars will go a long way.

Granulated date sugar, available in many natural food stores, is indispensable when your recipe specifically calls for a granulated dry sugar. This sugar has the distinctive flavor of whole dry dates. Another dry sweetner is *carob*, or *St.-John's bread*. This powder comes from the dried pods of the carob tree and can be purchased roasted or unroasted. Use the unroasted variety and toast it yourself for a fresher taste. In addition to its natural sugars, carob is rich in trace minerals and low in fats. Not much of this strong sweetner is necessary; either mix with the dry ingredients or dissolve in a little water or soy milk before adding to the other liquids. Carob is also available as a syrup. If you are using carob as a substitute for cocoa or chocolate, the equivalent of 1 square of chocolate is 3 tablespoons of carob plus 2 tablespoons of water or soy milk.

From the starches, two grain sweeteners are available: *barley malt* (also made from other grains and containing the sugar maltose) and a rice syrup called *ame* in Japanese. These grain syrups are produced by combining the cooked grains—rice in this instance with fresh sprouts from whole oats, barley, or wheat. This combination is allowed to stand for several hours until it has reached the sweet stage, when the liquid is squeezed off through cheesecloth, lightly salted, and cooked to the desired consistency. This thick, pale-amber syrup works well in pastries and sauces. Its semisolid state can be softened by beating to the consistency of thick honey. It is also sold in health food stores in the West as a chewy taffy.

For those who use dairy products, *noninstant dry milk powder* is a versatile natural sweetener containing the milk sugar lactose.

So-called *raw sugar*, or *turbinado*, is available in many stores, but is only slightly more nutritious than white sugar. It is 96 percent sucrose, compared with the 99.9 percent sucrose in white sugar. The only refining step to which it has not been subjected is a final acid bath that whitens the sugar and removes the final calcium and magnesium salts. This "pure" sugar was, as a juice from either sugar beets or sugar cane, only 15 percent sucrose; in its final form, all natural goodness has been lost.

Several sweeteners produced in the intermediate stages of sugar refining can be used somewhat more nutritionally than white table sugar. Once the cane or beet juice has been extracted, clarified to a syrup form, and crystallized, it is then spun in a centrifuge where more crystals are separated from the liquid. This remaining liquid is *molasses*, which is then repeatedly treated and centrifuged to extract more and more crystal until the final "blackstrap" form contains about 35 percent sucrose. Blackstrap molasses also contains iron, calcium, and B vitamins. Another variety of molasses is known as *barbados*. This milder, dark-brown syrup is extracted from the processes described earlier, resulting in a lighter-tasting product with a higher sucrose content. *Sorghum molasses* is produced by a similar process, but uses as raw material the cane from the sorghum plant. It has a distinctive, rather cloying, taste and is best used in baking, especially cookies.

UNREFINED OILS

For a healthful diet, you should obtain necessary unsaturated fatty acids primarily from unrefined vegetable oils. Like other unrefined foods, these oils still contain all the nutrients present in the grains, beans, or seeds from which they were derived.

Nearly all cooking oils are made by first heating the grains, beans, or seeds; then, to produce "unrefined" oils, they are pressed with a centrifuge and expelled without the use of chemicals or solvents. No further processing occurs, but some firms do filter their "unrefined" oils to remove the remaining particles of the germ. It is better, of course, to purchase unfiltered, unrefined oils with some sediment left in the bottle; too much filtering removes nutrients. Commercial processing also results in the loss of vitamin E, which is found naturally in the oil and is essential for the proper utilization of important unsaturated fatty acids. You therefore benefit very little from refined oils, since they are a poor source of unsaturated fatty acids.

Refined oils also lack the natural odors and flavors that are noticeable in all unrefined oils. The mildest of the unrefined oils are *safflower* and *sunflower*. Unrefined *sesame oil* imparts a unique nutty taste to sautéed foods, while unrefined *corn-germ* oil gives a buttery taste to baked goods. Everyone has appreciated the full-bodied flavor of unrefined *olive oil* in salad dressings. *Peanut* and *soybean oil* are stronger in flavor and can be better utilized in sautéing, which reduces the intensity of their taste. Unrefined *coconut* and *palm oil* are also available in natural food stores; these partially saturated oils are used extensively by Southern cultures for all types of cooking (and in many processed foods).

Another reason for using unrefined oils is that at high temperatures the chemical makeup of an oil is altered and possibly becomes detrimental to health. Many advertisements praise refined oils for their ability to be used at extremely high temperatures, but these high heats are neither necessary nor desirable. Unrefined safflower oil can be used for deep-frying at about 400 degrees, and can withstand higher temperatures than most other oils. Cooking temperatures above this simply aren't necessary. Overheating of unrefined, unfiltered oil causes the germ to scorch and most nutrients to be lost. When substituting unrefined oils for solid fats in recipes, reduce the amounts of other liquids slightly or increase the dry ingredients.

OTHER USEFUL FOODS

Bancha tea is high in calcium. It is a coarse green undyed tea. The leaves, which must have remained on the bush for three years, should be roasted in the oven until browned. *Bancha twig tea*, known as *kukicha*, consists of the twigs of the tea bush and is generally available. One spare teaspoon of kukicha should be used for each cup of tea, which is prepared by simmering the twigs for about 15 to 20 minutes.

Baking powders are used to make "quick breads" that can usually be put together and baked in less than half an hour and that rise by virtue of the baking powder included. It's best not to use too many quick breads, but they occasionally do lend themselves well to the use of concentrated nutrients such as seeds and nuts, and they can contain a mixture of flours such as whole wheat with fresh ground corn, millet, triticale, and soy flour. Never use sodium bicarbonate in making quick breads; its action is not only unnecessary but potentially unhealthy, destroying vitamin C and some B vitamins. Instead, the baking powder you choose should be low-sodium and aluminum-free; aluminum is known to be toxic. Potassium bicarbonate does not destroy vitamin D in the body. Most natural food stores carry this type of low-sodium baking powder, but you can make your own by using 1 part potassium bicarbonate, 2 parts cream of tartar (potassium bitartrate) and 2 parts arrowroot powder. It may be necessary to obtain potassium bicarbonate through a chemical company because it is not generally available at pharmacies.

Nutritional yeast is a natural treasurehouse of proteins, vitamins, and minerals that can be used as a dietary supplement when added to juices or included in cooked dishes. Often called *brewer's yeast* because at one time it was a by-product of the brewing industry, nutritional yeast is the tiniest of cultivated plants. The miniscule plants are grown on herbaceous grains and hops under carefully controlled temperature conditions. The yeast plant grows at an astoundingly fast rate. Once it has multiplied many times and matured, it is harvested and dried in a way that preserves all its nutrients. These yeast "flakes" are one of the most economical sources of the B vitamin complexes—B_1, B_2, B_6, niacin, B_{12}, folic acid, pantothenic acid, and biotin. In addition to these vitamins, yeast flakes contain minerals such as calcium, phosphorus, iron, sodium, potassium, and 16 of the amino acids, all working in conjunction with the B vitamins. Many people take several tablespoons of yeast daily. If yeast is to be used in a beverage such as a vegetable juice, the flakes should first be mixed with a small amount of the liquid and stirred into a paste, then added to the rest of the liquid and thoroughly mixed again. A blender will simplify this method of preparation. Yeast flakes also may be added to baked foods such as breads and casseroles or mixed in small amounts with nut butter or bean paste sandwich spreads.

Thickeners for smooth soups and sauces are usually based on a finely ground starch or flour, the most widely used being whole wheat, rice, and whole wheat pastry. The thickness of a flour sauce is determined by the ratio of flour to liquid. One tablespoon of flour to 1 cup liquid yields a thin sauce; up to 3 tablespoons flour to 1 cup liquid, a thick sauce. *Cornstarch*, corn flour in its finest version, is used in the same way to thicken sauces. *Arrowroot powder*, or flour made from the arrowroot plant, produces a finer sauce than cornstarch. The arrowroot starch should be dissolved in cold water before being added to hot foods to prevent lumping. Once the arrowroot has been added, simmer the thickened sauce to allow all the flavors to merge. *Kudzu* is another high-quality but rather expensive thickening agent. The kudzu plant grows wild in the United States as well as in Japan, where it has long been used in folk medicine, often prescribed for diarrhea and head colds. The crumbly white chunks should first be dissolved in cold water before being added to hot sauces to prevent lumping.

If *vinegar* is called for in a recipe, never use the white distilled or wine varieties; use an apple cider vinegar made from whole, unsprayed apples, undiluted and naturally aged. Refined, distilled vinegar has few of the naturally occurring nutrients (such as potassium) and virtually none of the indefinable subtle flavors of slowly aged cider vinegar. Because of the predominance of acetic acid in white distilled and wine vinegars, use them sparingly. Apple cider vinegar, on the other hand, contains a predominance of malic acid, which when wisely used is a constructive acid, naturally involved in the digestive system. Besides its culinary uses for preparing salad dressings and preserving foods, vinegar has long been useful as an antiseptic and blood coagulant. Rice vinegar is also available at natural food stores and in Oriental markets. It has a distinctive aroma and taste; so use it with utmost discretion in pickling and salad dressings. Thanks to its natural fermentation, it contains none of the problematical properties of commercial distilled vinegars.

Part Three

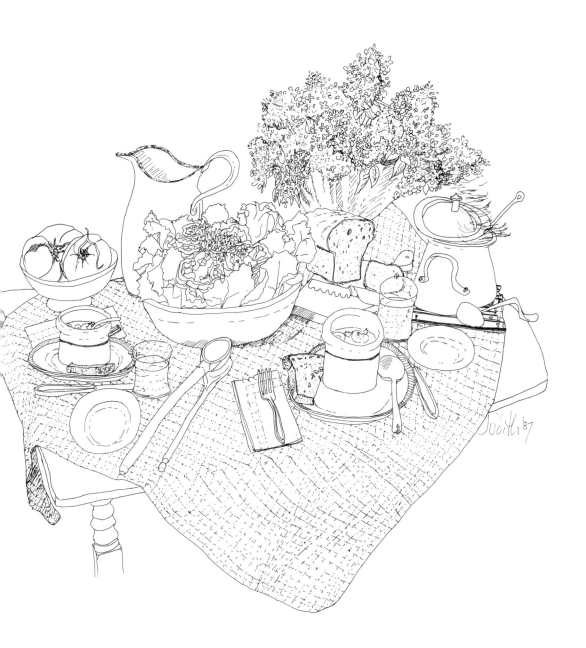

The Egg Project

MORE THAN A DOZEN years ago, I reviewed the available literature on protein requirements for human beings and found that there was an inconsistency between the prevalent beliefs of the scientific community as stated in the medical literature and the personal experience of many individuals. The people who should have been feeling healthy because they were getting more than adequate amounts of protein in their diet were frequently not receiving the healthful benefits from the protein in their diet. There was an escalating incidence of kidney disease in America that had no apparent cause. The prevaling myth stated that all of the protein from animal sources was complete, meaning that it contains all the essential amino acids, and furthermore, that all other amino acids, from plant foods, is incomplete—capable of sustaining life, but not of promoting optimum growth and maturation. Plant food diets were considered to be both faddist and dangerous. Clearly, this view had to be challenged.

I, along with Dr. Hillard Fitsky, who has a background in computer sciences, did a computer-assisted analysis of the 110 or so most commonly consumed vegetarian foods. We matched each one of the amino acids in the given food against the food source that is considered to contain the most complete protein, the chicken egg.

As the research progressed, it became clear that many of the assumptions concerning protein and our selection of foods were grossly in error. First, we found that not all animal protein is high quality and complete. Generally, only 40 percent is high quality. Second, we confirmed that not all vegetarian foods are incomplete. To the contrary, the vast majority of vegetarian foods are complete, containing all the essential amino acids. The bean or legume family in particular tended to have protein in large quantities and of a high quality. This made it easier to understand how the oriental and Indian cultures have been able to sustain themselves and demonstrate remarkable longevity on a limited vegetarian diet.

Taking this logic one step further, I reasoned that if single foods in the grain, legume, and sea vegetable families tended to have remarkably high-quality protein, what would be the result of combining two or three of these together? What I found was that the overall quality of the protein tended to increase tremendously. Not only did I find specific combinations that approximated the completeness of the egg, but some that actually exceeded the egg in terms of the amounts of complete, usable protein they provided.

Of the 5,000 combinations that I was able to compute over a five-year period, all offered protein of a quality nearer to the egg than the closest animal protein food source, milk. Other animal protein foods, including fish, hamburger, veal, chicken, and cheese all proved to offer far less complete and less usable protein than that available in the right combinations of vegetarian foods. Of course, the plant foods had far less calories, none of the cholesterol, the high saturated fat, the toxic growth-stimulating hormones, or the antibiotic residues such as penicillin that you would find in the animal products. They offered instead quality protein, abundant fiber, plentiful B vitamins, vitamin A, vitamin C, minerals, and the full spectrum of other nutrients. In other words, the concept of protein complementation allowed the acknowledged benefits of the vegetarian foods to be viewed alongside an appreciation of their demonstrable protein value even when compared to meat. In effect, it was time to virtually rewrite in a revolutionary way the whole notion of how we perceive protein. Even vegetarians, we found, are generally receiving between two and three times more protein than they require.

In the two chapters which follow, the principles of food combining and food rotation are observed. In both, a four-day rotational program is recommended.

Chapter 12 is specifically designed for individuals interested in managing their weight. It does not take for granted that you are already a vegetarian, and several types of fish are suggested as main courses.

Chapter 13 includes only vegetarian foods and features 50 of my favorite recipes. In preparing these recipes and adjusting your diet in favor of plant foods as protein sources, you will be applying many of the principles discussed in earlier chapters.

In both diets, you will be eating only 3 to 4 ounces of any given food at one time. Whether your goal be to lose weight, to increase the variety of your diet, or to discover the nutritiousness of vegetarian foods, you will find something here that will assist your search.

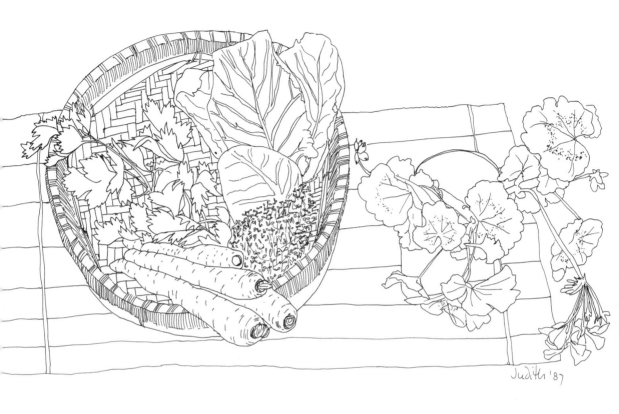

12 · A BEGINNER'S WEIGHT MANAGEMENT DIET

"Another benefit of eating starchy, high-fiber foods is that, because they digest rather slowly, you benefit from the natural sugars they contain over a period of several hours. Unlike that quick jolt of energy that you get from sugar when you have a soft drink, or a dessert, that makes you very high and then very low very quickly, potatoes and other complex carbohydrates provide sustained energy."

HAVE YOU EVER WANTED to start a diet plan but kept finding reasons to put it off? Or perhaps you've tried quick weight-loss programs, only to gain back what you've lost and then some. You can lose that weight and keep it off.

This chapter will explore how you can break the cycle of overeating and crash dieting with a program that's appetizing, nutritionally sound, and designed to last a lifetime.

In this program, you'll learn how to detoxify your body—how to get rid of the poisons accumulated from years of poor eating habits. You will gain tips on how to determine your individual nutritional needs, and how to satisfy them. And you'll learn about food rotation: why it's important, what kinds of foods to eat, and when. This chapter will outline a 14-day plan for you, so you can rebuild your health, lose that weight, and never have to worry about gaining it back.

This chapter is organized around the experiences of a group of average, overweight Americans whom I gathered together so that their real diet experiences might serve to help others beginning on the road to improved health.

Joyce is 55 years old and wants to lose 20 pounds. She describes herself as having been "on every ridiculous diet that one can think of. At my age, or any other age," she says, "it's not healthy to be doing that. It worries me that I weigh so much. I am really serious about learning to diet right, and I am determined to lose the weight. But where do I start?"

BEGIN WITH DETOXIFICATION

There is no need to upset your whole system and your life in the process of losing weight.

In our society, most people don't really eat right for total health. Are you like most Americans? Do you tend to eat too much of foods that undermine your health: animal proteins, saturated fats, fried foods, overly spicy foods, and foods made of refined carbohydrates, such as pizzas, french fries, and different types of confections? Do you indulge, all too often, in bagels, donuts, white bread products, and preserved, pickled or processed foods? These foods have been denatured. That is, much of their vitamins and minerals have been destroyed.

Once you have done all that to yourself, your body, in effect, has become a toxic waste dumpsite. Thousands of man-made chemicals end up in your lean muscle and fat tissues. They don't belong there. They can't be utilized for energy, for repair or growth of your body. On the contrary, they disrupt your normal biochemical processes.

One by-product of this disrupted biochemistry is a malfunctioning metabolism. Your metabolism—the way in which your body burns foods—is the process that allows you to have energy when operating normally, or lack energy when it is out of balance; to gain weight properly, or to gain it excessively. You may be overweight because your body's biochemistry is out of balance.

Yet you don't have to be a biochemist or an endocrinologist to understand the basic rules of proper eating. If you drink a lot of alcohol, you can't compensate by taking a vitamin B_1 tablet. Your body doesn't work that way.

The first step toward proper eating is to detoxify, and rebalance your body so you can start afresh. A Taj Mahal built on quicksand would soon sink. You don't have a strong foundation until you get rid of the debris that litters that foundation. You can't just repaint an old house whose wood is rotted and deteriorated. You first have to repair it; otherwise the decay continues hidden under that fresh coat of paint.

The single most important thing anyone who wants to change his or her diet can do is to detoxify by getting rid of the pollution in the body.

The rewards will be substantial. You will feel better, have more energy, feel lighter, and have an easier time maintaining a normal weight. You will find you have more endurance. Your body will no longer feel sluggish, and you will probably find you need less sleep.

Detoxifying need not be harsh upon either the mind or body. To begin, though, you have to know your relative state of health. Each of us is biologically unique; we all have particular needs and wants. Any diet doctor, who says everyone should have 5 mg. of B_2, and 10 mg. of B_6 is wrong, because no other person has the same biochemistry as you. Even two people who are the same age, the same sex, the same height, and the same weight—even identical twins, will have different biochemical needs.

That's why faddish popular diets, in general, don't work. Too often, they try to provide specific information for a general audience, as if everyone were the same. *We're not all the same.* There is no message I could share with you that would be more important, no specific counsel I could give you, no recipe I could offer, that would have the significance of this statement.

You will maximize your health, normalize your weight, lose weight, and feel good when you understand what you own nutritional requirements are. They have nothing to do with anyone else's.

Steve is 40 years old. He describes his weight problem in the following way: "For as long as I can remember I've been about 10 or 15 pounds overweight. Nothing I do seems to get rid of that excess weight. I can lose weight temporarily, but I've tried everything from grapefruit to horseradish, and nothing really seems to help me get my weight down and keep it down. How do I find out what my own nutritional requirements are?"

THE IMPORTANCE OF PROPER TESTING

The answer to Steve's concern begins with a basic blood chemistry test that evaluates the different components of your blood (the SMA-12, or SMA-24; see Chapter 7, "Detoxification"). It measures a variety of vitamin, triglycerid, cholesterol, and mineral levels. Steve should also have a hair analysis done to determine whether there are toxic levels of different minerals in his system—harmful metal like cadmium, mercury, and lead. An excess of lead or cadmium can come from smoking cigarettes. These metals will directly affect the mechanism in the brain that determines the appetite and satiety levels.

When you get your blood chemistry results back, you may find that your individual biochemical profile indicates a need for some nutritional support and detoxification. What other tests can help you determine your nutritional and health needs?

Everybody should also have a musculo-skeletal examination. An osteopath or a chiropractor can make this diagnosis for you, checking to see whether your muscular system is functioning properly. Frequently, the posture is so poor that there are blocked energy pathways. When you use certain muscle groups improperly, other muscle groups overreact in the body. For example, if you lean on one side while watching television, then the muscles on the opposite side of your body pull in the opposite direction. The result may be a sore back, sore arms and legs, hunched shoulders, or a hunched back.

We are a nation of people who sit, stand, and walk with poor posture. Posture can make an enormous difference in your energy levels and how you feel.

To summarize the way to begin: Step one is to cleanse out the old debris. It is necessary to eliminate the toxic metals, pesticides, herbicides, fungicides, and other synthetic substances from your system. Then you want to determine your own biological nature. What do you need—how much vitamin C, how much B_1? You don't want to put excessive amounts in your system, and yet you don't want to be deficient.

Numerous studies show that as a nation we are deficient in vitamin C, selenium, calcium, magnesium, and vitamin A. Those are easily obtainable from food in the diet. If you're eating what would be considered the average American diet, you're still almost certainly eating poorly.

Barbara is 25 years old. She says, "I've always been about 15 to 20 pounds overweight. A couple of times in my life I've gone on crash diets.

I've lost all the weight I wanted to and felt great for two weeks. But I also have these terrible junk food habits with midnight binges. I think I'm ready to change my entire way of looking at the way I eat food, because what I've been doing is obviously not helping me. I've taken the tests and I've gotten back the results. What do I do now?"

COMBINING DETOXIFICATION WITH REBUILDING HEALTH

A detoxification program will show you which foods and nutrients you can take into your system on a daily basis, to help take away some of the negative effects of eating a high sugar, high calorie, high fat, animal protein diet. You should then go on to a special 14-day eating program. First you detoxify, then rebuild health by losing weight, and then continue to eat right.

What are some good foods for building good health? At the top of the list is a group of foods called sprouts. Sprouts are the knockouts of nutrition. The sprout, quite simply, is one of the most nutrient-rich, powerful, health-building foods in nature. You just cannot find anything healthier. They will help cleanse and rebuild your entire system.

What kind of sprouts should you try? Don't stop with just common sprouts like alfalfa or mung beans. Expand your cuisine. Try high-protein buckwheat sprouts; the sweet sunflower sprout; the aromatic fenugreek sprout; clover sprout; and for a little bite and pinch, try a radish sprout. A mustard sprout will turn your tongue twice around your mouth. It tastes as good as mustard, and yet it has that nice salad feel to it.

Over 15 different seeds for sprouting are available commercially. They're inexpensive and versatile. You can make salads out of them, put them into pita bread, use them in casseroles and put them in soups.

Next, add miso to the list of detoxifying and rebuilding foods. For over 3,000 years, this nutritionally superior food has been helping people to better health. Miso is a fermented product. Like yogurt, its bacteria work well in your intestines. After all, the health of the intestine determines the health of your body. Remember that miso is to be used sparingly, however, because it does have a high sodium content.

Vegetable juices are a third health-giving detoxifier. Generally speaking, take no more than one glass of carrot juice per day. Beta carotine is a precursor of vitamin A in the body. If you drink too much carrot juice, you'll be overloading the liver with vitamin A and your skin may turn yellow. One glass a day is fine. You wil get the beneficial effects of vitamin A, which has been shown to be an anti-viral vitamin; it protects against viruses.

Add to carrot juice: celery, cabbage, parsley, sprouts, or cucumber for a variety of delicious juices. For people who've never really enjoyed vegetables, juices are another way to get good-tasting, high quality nutrition into your diet.

Grains are another group of foods that help the body cleanse itself and rebuild its strength. It is unfortunate that most Americans, unbelievably, never taste whole grain. They taste refined carbohydrates in white bread, or white rice, but never eat brown rice or whole grain bread. Yet these are inexpensive and readily available, even in supermarkets.

Whole grains are loaded with far more nutrition than their refined counterparts. The grain family includes rice, corn, buckwheat, rye, oats and millet, as well as less well-known, newly available grains like triticale, amaranth, and quinoa (pronounced keen-wa), a light, fast-cooking grain from South America now available in some health food stores.

The next group of foods to include as part of your health rebuilding program is the sea family of vegetables. These include hijiki, a form of seaweed that tastes salty like fish.

You can buy seaweed dry and store it for months. There are many types, including konbu, wakami, and nori. To cook them, place a small piece in cold water. After five minutes, replace the water with fresh water; after five more minutes, replace the water again. You now have rinsed the seaweed and it's ready for cooking. You can cut it into pieces, flake it, or put it into casseroles or soups. Include seaweed in your miso soup to increase its nutritional value.

You can add cold seaweed to salad, or serve it with vinegar or lemon juice as an appetizer.

You can wrap up seaweed like grape leaves.

Seaweed is so versatile that entire books are devoted to its use in cookery.

Seaweed is loaded with minerals. In fact, there is ten times more available calcium in hijiki, by dry weight, than in cow's milk.

At this point, we can answer a question raised by Joyce, who speaks for many when she says she's "been told for years that starchy vegetables such as potatoes and yams are fattening." She asks, "but are they?"

RETHINKING THE MYTHS

These foods are low in calories and rich in minerals and vitamins. It's what you put on them that makes them high in calories. A potato alone has only about 80 calories. But people often put about 150 calories' worth of butter or margarine on it. In fact, potatoes are an excellent source of vitamin C, in quantities comparable to that found in oranges.

Another benefit of eating starchy, high-fiber foods is that, because they digest rather slowly, you benefit from the natural sugars they contain over a period of several hours. Unlike that quick jolt of energy that you get from sugar when you have a soft drink, or a dessert, that makes you very high and then very low very quickly, potatoes and other complex carbohydrates provide sustained energy.

There's one last group of healthy, detoxifying foods although, too often, Americans deliberately stay away from them. These are the beans, or legumes.

Why do people leave the room when Aunt Gertrude helps herself to beans? We have kept ourselves away from one of nature's most important sources of vitamins, minerals, and fiber, because we have never really understood how to cook them. Most people, and most restaurants, do not soak beans overnight. Because beans are not soaked overnight, when our body finally digests them, gas is formed in the colon, causing indigestion and flatulence. That uncomfortable feeling needn't be. All you have to do is soak beans overnight and then boil them for one to two hours. That usually takes care of most gas-producing properties. Then be sure to combine them with the right foods: Don't eat fruit or sugary foods with a bean meal.

Beans have more protein than grains or seeds. They are an excellent source of protein, as good in protein quality as animal proteins, yet also high in fiber.

Try adding legumes to your diet. Legumes include black-eyed peas, red beans, kidney beans, great northern beans, lentils, garbanzo beans, alfalfa, lima beans, and split peas, among others. There are over 60 different legumes.

Beans are a great way to help your body. They are low in calories, and high in protein, minerals, and complex carbohydrates.

If you eat this way, you're not going to have a problem with weight. You will be able to lose the extra weight that you are carrying, while you cleanse your body. You won't be taking toxic materials into your body and will meet the body's nutritional needs for proteins, vitamins, essential fatty acids, and minerals. And you will spend less on food. A detoxifying diet is exciting eating. And it's the basis of good health. The foundation is where we start.

Now let's look at what we can do to incorporate all this into a 14-day eating program. Keep in mind that the 14 days could be 1,400 days, 14 years, or the rest of your life. But here is a menu for two weeks to help get you started. Let's begin on Monday. We're going to take this on a four-day rotational basis. I'll explain why later in the chapter.

THE FOUR-DAY ROTATION

Day 1

BREAKFAST Monday morning, start your day with hot cereal breakfast. Today the hot cereal can be oatmeal.

SNACK For a midmorning snack you can have a fruit if you are not hypoglycemic or severely diabetic. If you are, you may want to have a food such as cottage cheese or yogurt.

Take only small quantities of each food. On this eating program, you won't be eating until you're full, but only approximately 3 to 4 ounces of a given food. Thus, you may have as many as 12 to 14 ounces of total food in a given meal. The idea is to space your food over the day rather than eat a lot at one time.

By spacing your food, you will provide your body with energy, protein, carbohydrates, vitamins, and minerals throughout the day. After all, your body needs them 24 hours a day. People who skip breakfast, skimp on lunch, and then have the entire kitchen sink for dinner are only—after all is said and done—utilizing about 12 ounces of the food they eat. They're only able to use a small percentage of the protein they're taking in; the rest becomes fat. When you eat small amounts of food, several times throughout the day, very little becomes fat because your body is using it for energy throughout the day. This is a very important lesson if you want to lose weight and stay healthy.

LUNCH For Monday lunch, help yourself to a sardine salad, an egg salad or a tofu salad. Or, you can have a regular salad with a side order of any vegetables you like. You can choose steamed or stir-fried vegetables, and eat them with a grain, such as brown rice. If you are eating a salad, you might want to try serving your rice cold, the way the Japanese sometimes do. But remember—brown rice is preferable to white.

SNACK For your midafternoon break, let's say between two and four o'clock, you can have a juice, a fruit, or perhaps some marinated vegetable sticks. If you marinate them the night before in a vinaigrette sauce, you will find that your vegetables have a nice tangy quality to them.

DINNER For dinner, you can start off with a soup. Try, for example, split pea soup with an appetizer of seaweed. There are many recipes for either cold or warm seaweed.

As a main entree, have a soy food over rice. In this way you combine a grain in rice form with a legume, soy beans in this case, in the form of either tofu or tempeh. By the way, if you like the taste of chicken and want to give it up, tempeh is a great alternative. It contains no cholesterol and is made from soy beans. It tastes like chicken, has as much protein, is low in calories and high in calcium. It is, in fact, one of the best foods, nutritionally.

Finally, you can enjoy a salad at dinner. It should be a sprout salad on Monday. Make yourself a dressing, one without oil. There are many recipes for oilless dressings. There are also already prepared mixes to which you need only add water, vinegar, or lemon juice.

BEFORE BEDTIME   If you feel hungry before bed, drink some carbonated water with a pinch of lime or lemon in it.

Let's take a look at what Monday's foods will do for you. You will have eaten foods that are low on the food chain, meaning they contain lower concentrations of pesticides and other chemicals than animal protein. You've eaten plenty of fiber. Not only are high-fiber foods low in calories, they will also improve your digestion. You have eaten plenty of calcium and moderate amounts of protein. You've consumed no refined sugar or starch. You've eaten modest amounts of foods that are easily digested, therefore ones that don't overtax your digestive systems, taking away the oxygen and blood that you need in your brain. You've eaten foods from which nutrients are readily and easily available for absorption. Also, because so much chewing is necessary with these foods, you've been helping your jaws and lowering your appetite. The more you chew, the more quickly your appetite is satisfied. Chewing each bite well prevents you from gorging. A short list of foods for the day—Oats, rice, tofu, split peas, sprouts, seaweeds, and, if you wish, sardines or eggs—have accomplished so much to help detoxify and rebuild your health!

Day 2

Hopefully, you are starting off your day with exercise. (See Chapter 15, "Nutrition and Exercise.") Fifteen minutes of aerobic exercise will improve your metabolism and stimulate the cells to burn more fatty acids, reducing overall body fat content and improving muscle tone as well as your overall sense of well-being.

BREAKFAST   For breakfast, begin with a glass of fruit juice. Fresh fruit juice is preferable to frozen or canned juices. Try making yourself fresh-squeezed grape juice. If you do, dilute it with some water, because grape juice is sweet.

Then, enjoy a different hot cereal. Today, try an alkalinizing cereal, millet. With the millet, you can puree in a banana, adding a sprinkle of cinnamon or nutmeg. Add just a little soy milk, fruit juice, or regular milk.

SNACK For a midmorning snack, I generally carry a little extra millet with me in a plastic container, and eat 4 or 5 tablespoons when I get hungry. If I tell myself I'm going to have 5 tablespoons and no more, I count them out, and that's all I have, as a way of controlling the urge to overeat.

LUNCH For lunch today, try a three-bean salad of black beans, kidney beans, and lentils. These beans supply protein, fiber, vitamins, and minerals galore. Also, try a salad of vegetables different than those eaten on Monday. For instance, if on Monday, you ate watercress, rugala and spinach, then on Tuesday, take chickory, romaine, or Boston lettuce. You might have a soup as well. This would be a good opportunity for a black bean soup with a slice of whole grain bread. No butter, no margarine. Just moist, chewy whole grain bread.

SNACK For midafternoon, have a piece of fruit, perhaps with another piece of whole grain bread. Whole grain bread only has around 100 calories and plenty of fiber in it. Therefore, it will be easily and quickly digested.

DINNER For dinner on Tuesday, you might have hot millet, stir fried. Again, I like to make extra millet in the morning and have it all day long. Cooking it is just a matter of heating it up. Add a salad, and a different soup: kidney bean soup or a great northern bean soup.

For your main dish, eat fish. Salmon is a good choice. Fish not only gives you quality protein, but also essential fatty acids that your body needs. Omega 3 fatty acids—the kind found in many fish—have been shown to help the heart by lowering cholesterol levels.

SNACK Later on, you can have your dessert. Never eat your dessert right after your meal: That's improper food combining. You do not want to combine a protein food, such as fish, which may take four or five hours to digest, with a simple sugar food that might have honey or fruit in it that might take only a half hour to digest. Combining sugary foods with protein or fat in the same meal leads to acid indigestion.

Wait till later in the evening and then have a banana. Try freezing it and then putting it into a blender or food processor. Whip it up, and it tastes like banana custard. For a special treat, take frozen cherries and frozen bananas and whip them together in a blender. You will be rewarded with a delicious, nutritious, and tasty dessert, low in calories, and high in complex carbohydrates, vitamins, and minerals. It is also very filling.

Thanks to your banana dessert late in the evening, and your fish, salad, soup and millet earlier, you will feel full without having consumed too many calories. That's eating right for total health.

Day 3

BREAKFAST On Wednesday, begin your day with a hot rye cereal. Add to the rye cereal a fruit of your choice. Make it a fruit you have not eaten on either Monday or Tuesday. Take your cereal with some juice, milk, or soy milk.

SNACK Later in the morning, eat a bit more of the morning cereal cold.

LUNCH For lunch, enjoy a salad. Make it with different vegetables or different sprouts than Monday's or Tuesday's. Toss a handful of garbanzo beans into the salad today. Garbanzo beans are loaded with protein and are very nutritious. Mix some black-eyed peas or great northern beans in with the garbanzo beans to enhance the protein value of the beans.

Then, enjoy a soup made from any legume you didn't already eat on Monday or Tuesday. For example, you might want an aduki bean soup for lunch.

SNACK Later in the day, have some fruit or a vegetable if you still feel you need a snack.

DINNER For dinner, start with miso soup. Then, try a guacamole, or avacado salad, made with mashed avacado, tomatoes, and lemon. Avacado is the fattiest fruit, so use only a quarter of an avacado for your quacamole. If you don't want guacamole, try another nutritious appetizer, babaganoush. This is a dish made from eggplant, garlic, and lemon juice. Anyone who's enjoyed Middle Eastern foods knows the joy of babaganoush.

For your main course, turn again to fish, this time filet of sole. You can also have a side dish of vegetables, such as peas and corn. In the salad, try such vegetables as marinated asparagus tips, broccoli, and cauliflower. That gives you a lot to eat, and you'll feel full, but not filled out, having kept your calories low but nutrients high.

Day 4

BREAKFAST Start off your day with a juice as before—a different fruit juice than the other days this week. For example, if one day you drank orange juice, you shouldn't repeat orange juice for another four days. Instead, you should have apple juice, prune juice, or grapefruit juice.

Then, enjoy a steaming bowl of wheatena or cream of wheat. These cereals are available everywhere. They are loaded with nutrition and high in fiber. But, to get more fiber into your system, to help cleanse your system, eat a bran muffin as well and be sure it's unsweetened.

SNACK   For a midmorning snack, have another bran muffin, since it contains only 70 calories. The muffin will help fill you up, but will also pass easily through your system.

LUNCH   For lunch, start off with some navy bean soup. Have salad, this time a marinated salad, like a cold salad or a seaweed salad. For your main entree have eggs, sardines, or tuna, whichever you didn't have on Monday.

SNACK   For later in the day, enjoy any type of fruit or vegetable, one that you haven't eaten yet on other days.

DINNER   For dinner, begin with a vegetable soup. Then, enjoy a tabouli salad, made with wheat and chopped parsley. As your main entree, we try either sea bass or blue fish, served with hot seaweed. For your vegetable, have some red potatoes. This meal supplies complex carbohydrates, complete proteins, and plenty of fiber, along with chlolrophyl, vitamins and minerals.

SNACK   Later at night, you could have a frozen fruit or juice, if you feel the need.

THE REWARDS OF ROTATION

What was just described is an eating program for the first four days of your diet. This will form the pattern for the subsequent ten days and thereafter. The basic concept is a four-day rotational diet.

Why a rotational diet? Because, very often, people's headaches, mood swings (going from a pleasant to an angry disposition), fatigue, musculoskeletal aches and pains, indigestion, post-nasal drip, puffy eyes, and many other symptoms of not-quite-perfect health are exacerbated or caused by food sensitivities. We can become sensitive or allergic to any food we eat too frequently, including wheat, dairy, beef, chicken, corn, citrus fruits, peanuts, chocolate, soy, or any other food.

If you generally eat one or all these foods every day, you are likely to be food sensitive. This list includes the foods that clinical ecologists and allergists have found most likely to cause allergic reactions, as they predominate in the typical American diet.

Most people are familiar with the kind of allergies in which a person gets a skin rash immediately after eating, for example, strawberries. But there are other kinds of allergies that can be at cause when a child can't pay attention in class, or when an adult feels so tired after eating that he or she just wants to lay down and sleep. The allergies that cause these symptoms are very often caused by food sensitivities and can also lead to unnecessary pounds.

Studies have shown that when we are allergic to a food, we frequently have a faulty metabolism and gain weight above normal.

One of the fastest ways, then, to lose weight healthfully is to go on a four-day rotational diet and eliminate those foods to which we are allergic, or rotate them so that we don't have any one of them more frequently than every fourth day.

For example, if on Monday we ate oats, rice, split peas, the seaweed hijiki, and soy foods such as tofu or miso, we wouldn't have them again until Friday.

On Tuesday, if we ate millet, black-eyed peas, lentils, and kidney beans, we wouldn't have those again until Saturday. On Wednesday, if we ate rye, garbanzo beans, adzuki beans, sole, broccoli, asparagus and cauliflower, we wouldn't eat those foods again until Sunday. If on Thursday, we ate cream of wheat, navy beans, blue fish or sea bass, and red potatoes, we wouldn't consume those foods again until Monday.

Thus, we are creating a four-day rotational diet plan. Virtually all of the environmental medicine experts (they are known as clinical ecologists; *see* Resource Guide Listings at the back of the book) believe that our bodies need four days to recuperate after exposure to a food to which we are sensitive.

By now it should be clear how to turn a four-day rotation into a 14-day eating program. You simply continue the same eating plan for 14 days. In other words, every fourth day you would start from the beginning. You can change your recipes, adding any vegetables or fish you haven't eaten for at least four days or longer. Give yourself two weeks to see the effects of combining exercise (see Chapter 15, "Nutrition and Exercise") with a rotational eating plan, 14 days of eating wholesome, nourishing foods. If you've been allergic to foods, weaning yourself of them will frequently assist weight loss. You will also feel much better, and this will help inspire you to eat right from then on. The four-day rotational diet can be used as the basis for a maintenance dietary program. It's easy, it's inexpensive, and the rewards of eating right for a lifetime will pay off a thousandfold.

This program doesn't just address the problem of weight loss. Excess weight is a symptom of a larger problem, one that can't be solved by going on a crash diet, even if you do lose ten pounds in one week. This program is not an instant solution, but it offers you the chance to revitalize yourself in many areas of health. Weight loss is only one benefit. If you follow these guidelines, you'll feel more energetic and less stressed, and you'll probably live longer. In short, the quality of your life will improve.

If this diet seems to work for you after two weeks, try moving on to the vegetarian food diet contained in the next chapter. Begin by extending your original 14-day program into a 21-day program, using only vegetarian foods during the final week. Then try staying on the vegetarian diet alone. Use the recipes and the three different four-day rotations contained in Chapter 13 to get you started.

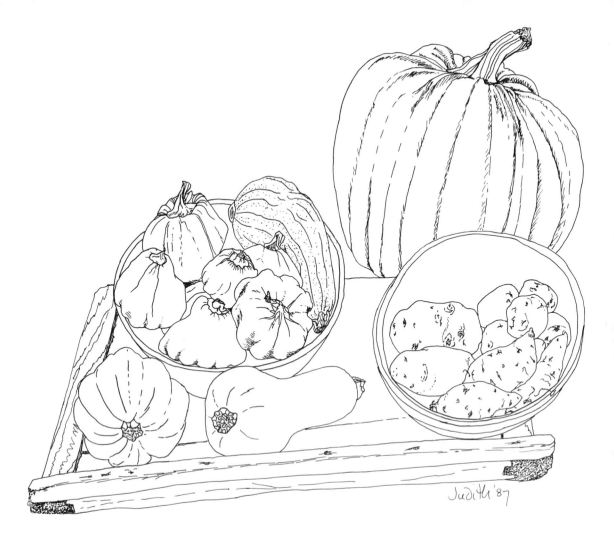

Judith '87

13 · A VEGETARIAN ROTATION DIET AND RECIPES

"Generally, you should eat no more than 3 to 4 ounces of a given food at any one meal. In these quantities, you may eat the same food several times during the day, however. This approach will reduce your overall caloric intake and keep your body functioning with optimal energy."

THE RECIPES IN THIS chapter have benefited from years of research and experimentation. They have been designed to fit easily into a four-day roatational diet plan in which specific foods such as brown rice, soy beans, or wheat are eaten only once every four days. On any one day, a food may be eaten several times in relatively small quantities.

Additionally, the recipes included here have been devised according to the principles of proper food combining in order to allow for optimal digestibility, absorption, assimilation, and elimination. Following a diet using these recipes will provide all the protein and fiber that you need, as well as a full spectrum of vitamins and minerals.

At first, the idea of avoiding animal products in your regular diet may seem foreign. But perhaps you have heard the warnings of the American Heart Association, which link excessive consumption of red meat and dairy products to heart disease, or those of the American Cancer Society linking breast, colon, and prostate cancer to these products. Or you may have heard of the statement issued by the National Academy of Science containing evidence that the ideal human diet is essentially a vegetarian one, high in fresh fruits, vegetables, and grains, while low in animal proteins, fats, and refined foods. You may have grown curious about the benefits of a vegetarian diet as you've become aware of the risks associated with a diet high in animal protein foods, but still you hesitate. Don't worry, you are not alone.

The habit of many years may be fixed in a number of popular beliefs with a strong hold on many of us. First among these is the myth that you have to eat meat to get sufficient amounts of protein. Other fixed ideas include the belief that milk is our best source of calcium, and that only meat and animal products provide vitamin B_{12}. Meat is commonly associated with sexual potency and virility. On the other side of the coin, vegetarian cooking is commonly considered monotonous and unappetizing. Very often, there is an underlying fear of disapproval of friends and family should you become a vegetarian, and the feeling that it is simply too difficult to eat properly without meat as a mainstay.

The recipes offered in this chapter were designed specifically to dispell the myths that a vegetarian diet must be boring, unappetizing, and nutritionally inadequate. While a macrobiotic diet has been of benefit to many people, too often those who are unfamiliar with vegetarianism consider macrobiotic cuisine, as prepared in many restaurants, to by synonomous with vegetarian cuising generally. And yet the major cuisines of the world, including the those of China, India, the Middle East, and Mexico are essentially vegetarian, using meat only sparingly, as a spice rather than an entree. Vegetarian cooking can be both tasty and varied.

Being a vegetarian should not be a burden, nor should it alienate you from your friends and family. Of course, at first you may find it neccessary to make a certain number of life-style changes. You will want to look for a good health food store that is convenient to shop in and provides the products that you need. At first you may have to spend a little more time planning and preparing your meals, but with time it will become second nature.

Two important things to remember are flexibility and gentleness. Rigidly held beliefs and dogmas will lead to an accumulation of stress that can deplete your body of essential vitamins and minerals no matter how well you eat. At the same time as you establish your new diet, see if you can relax too. The important thing to remember is to be gentle with yourself. You are learning something new, and initially you may well make mistakes. If, for example, you go off of the diet at a party or if you go on a "binge," it will not help to beat yourself up for it. Simply chalk one up to experience and plan on doing better the next time. If you are out with friends at a restaurant that does not serve brown rice or vegetarian meals, don't panic. You will learn to see your way through such situations without feeling embarrassed or making those around you uncomfortable. For instance, you can order the baked potato instead of the rice, and a grilled piece of fish instead of the red meat.

The ideal diet involves eating a number of small meals throughout the day. Eating just one large meal can interfere with the proper absorption of nutrients and place a burden on digestion. It can also add surplus calories. Generally, you should eat no more than 3 to 4 ounces of a given food at any one meal. In these quantities, you may eat the same food several times during the day, however. This approach will reduce your overall caloric intake and keep your body functioning with optimal energy. Keep in mind that it is best to meet the body's vitamin, mineral, and protein requirements throughout the day.

Reader! If you wish to prepare additional servings of these recipes, increase the amounts of main ingredients (vegetables, fruits, seeds, grains, legumes, flour, etc.) in proportions equal to the existing recipes. Condiments should only be increased by 1/8 tsp. per additional portion.

First Cycle

DAY 1

BREAKFAST

Warm and Sweet Morning Cereal

6 oz. amaranth
3 oz. fresh pineapple,
   if possible; if not,
   pineapple sweetened
   in its own juice
3 oz. raisins
1 tbsp. honey
pinch cardamon
pinch cinnamon

In a medium saucepan, combine amaranth and water. Lower the heat when the water begins to boil. Allow to simmer for approximately 25 minutes. While the amaranth is cooking, cut the pineapple into $1/2$" pieces. When the amaranth is cooked, add the pineapple and the remaining ingredients. Mix thoroughly. (*Serves 1.*)

LUNCH

Three-Grain Vegetable Bake

3 oz. amaranth
3 oz. basmati rice
3 oz. couscous
3 oz. carrots
$1^1/2$ oz. watercress
3 oz. celery
$1^1/2$ oz. pecans
2 tbsp. safflower oil
2 oz. water
$1/4$ tsp. basil
$1/4$ tsp. rosemary
$1/2$ tsp. fresh mustard
3 oz. golden raisins

Prepare a medium saucepan for each of the grains (amaranth, basmati rice, and couscous). Place 10 oz. of water in the saucepan with the amaranth and cook for 25 minutes. Place 10 oz. of water in the saucepan with the rice and cook for approximately 20 minutes. Place couscous in 10 oz. of water and cook for 10 minutes. Carefully wash carrots and then grate into a small bowl. Rinse watercress and chop. Clean the celery stalks and chop. In a large mixing bowl, combine all the grains and then add remaining ingredients. Mix well. Place mixture in a baking pan. Bake for 20 minutes in a 325-degree oven. (*Serves 2.*)

DINNER

Italian Vegetable Toss

3 oz. carrots
6 oz. zucchini
3 oz. arugula
1 oz. parsley
2 tbsp. safflower oil
1 clove garlic,
   chopped finely
$1/3$ tsp. tarragon
$1/3$ tsp. basil
2 red cabbage leaves
$1^1/2$ oz. pine nuts

Carefully clean the carrots and zucchini. Cut them into bite-sized pieces and steam in either a bamboo steam basket or a stainless steel steamer. Steam for approximately 8 minutes. Rinse arugula and parsley, pat dry with a paper towel and tear into smaller pieces. In a separate small bowl, combine the oil and the herbs. When vegetables are steamed, allow them to cool to room temperature. Transfer them into a large bowl and toss in the arugula and parsley. Pour oil mixture into the bowl as well. Place cabbage leaves on each plate and place mixture on top. Top with pine nuts. (*Serves 2.*)

DINNER (2nd Option)

3 oz. sweet potato
3 oz. amaranth
3 oz. basmati rice
3 oz. zucchini
2 oz. celery
2 tbsp. safflower oil
1/4 tsp basil
2/3 tsp. salt
1/3 tsp. curry
1/2 tsp. tarragon
1/2 tsp. cumin

Aromatic Indian Sweet Potato Bake

Place sweet potatoes in a preheated 400-degree oven for 40 minutes or until done. (You can test it by inserting a fork.) In a medium saucepan, place the amaranth in 10 oz. water. Cook for approximately 25 minutes or until done. In another saucepan, prepare the rice similarly in 10 oz. of water, and then cook for 20 minutes. While the grains are cooking, carefully wash the zucchini and celery. Cut the zucchini into 1/2" cubes. Slice the celery into 1/4" pieces. When the sweet potato is cooked, allow it to cool so you can handle it. Then scoop the sweet potato out of its skin and place it in medium-sized mixing bowl with the cooked rice, amaranth and the remaining ingredients. Turn the mixture into the baking dish. Bake for 15 minutes in a preheated 375-degree oven. (*Serves 2.*)

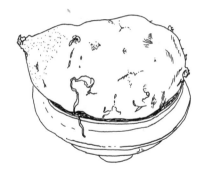

DAY 2

BREAKFAST

6 oz. brown rice
1 1/2 oz. coconut, shredded and unsweetened
1 1/2 oz. cashews
1 1/2 oz. dates
1/2 tsp. cinnamon
2 oz. water
1 oz. chopped apples
1 1/2 oz. sunflower seeds

Crunchy Sweet Rice

In a medium saucepan, cook brown rice in 14 oz. of water. Lower heat when it comes to a boil. Cooking time is about 30 minutes. When rice is cooked, add coconut. Chop cashews and dates finely and add to rice. Add cinnamon. Take half of the mixture and puree along with 2 oz. of water for a few seconds. Then add the pureed mixture back to the rest of the rice. Sprinkle sunflower seeds and apples on top. (*Serves 1.*)

LUNCH

3 oz. kidney beans
3 oz. cauliflower
3 oz. asparagus
3 oz. celery
2 oz. mushrooms
2 oz. zucchini
1 1/2 oz. filberts
2 oz. water
2 tbsp. sunflower oil
1/4 tsp. basil
2/3 tsp. dill
1/3 tsp. chili powder
1/5 tsp. celery seed
1 garlic clove chopped
1/2 tsp. salt

Vegetable Filbertasia

Soak the beans in a large bowl in 16 oz. of water overnight. In the morning, rinse the beans and replace with 16 oz. of fresh water in a medium pot. Cook for 1 3/4 hours to 2 hours until done. Carefully rinse the cauliflower, asparagus, celery, mushrooms and zucchini. Steam cauliflower and asparagus for 10 minutes. Chop celery, slice mushrooms and zucchini. Chop filberts medium fine. Put filberts in a blender with water, oil, spices and salt. Place all the vegetables in a serving pan. Top with filbert/kidney bean sauce. Serve at room temperature. (*Serves 2.*)

DINNER

3 oz. butternut squash
1 1/2 oz. shallots
1 1/2 oz. peanuts
2 oz. water
1 garlic clove, finely
    diced
1 tsp. fresh ginger,
    diced
1/2 tsp. basil
1/2 tsp. salt
2 tbsp. sunflower oil
3 oz. avocado, sliced

Nutty Butternut Squash

Cut squash in half, remove the seeds and discard them. Place squash in a baking pan with 1/3" water, cut side down. Bake for 40 minutes at 400 degrees. When squash is cool enough to handle, remove its skin and cut into 1" pieces. Place in a medium-sized mixing bowl. Chop shallots medium fine and add to the squash. Place peanuts, water, herbs, salt and oil in a blender. Mix well. Add this sauce to the squash and the shallots. Place mixture in a greased, covered baking pan at 350 degrees for 20 minutes. When done, place avocado slices on top as garnish. (*Serves 2.*)

DAY 3

BREAKFAST

6 oz. millet
1 1/2 oz. almonds
pinch cinnamon
1 1/2 oz. brewer's yeast
1 tsp. vanilla
1 tsp. maple syrup

High-Protein Cinnamon Millet

In a medium saucepan, cook millet in 13 oz. of water. When the water comes to a boil, lower heat. Stir occasionally. Cooking time is approximately 30 minutes. In another saucepan, blanche the almonds by placing them in scalding water in order to remove the skins. Then chop them. Add cinnamon, brewer's yeast, vanilla and maple syrup as well as the almonds. (*Serves 1.*)

LUNCH

Thick and Spicy Potato Chowder

9 oz. potato
4 c. water
3 oz. tomato
3 oz. green pepper
3 oz. carrots
3 oz. broccoli
1/5 tsp. cumin
1/5 tsp. basil
3 tbsp. sesame oil
1 1/4 tsp. salt
3 oz. scallions,
  chopped

Scrub or peel potatoes and place in 4 cups of water in a medium saucepan. Boil for approximately 15 minutes. When the potatoes are cooked, place in a blender with the water in which it was cooked, the seasonings and the oil and salt. Wash the tomatoes, pepper, carrots and broccoli. Chop into bite-sized pieces. Transfer the potato mixture back into a saucepan. Add the chopped vegetables. Cook over a low heat for an additional 10 to 15 minutes. Top with scallions. (*Yields 4 to 5 cups approximately.*)

DINNER

Almost Spaghetti Squash Dinner

3 oz. spaghetti squash
3 oz. scallions
6 oz. tomato
3 oz. green pepper
1 1/2 oz. onion
2 oz. mushrooms
2 tbsp. olive oil
1/4 tsp. basil
1/2 tsp. rosemary
1 tsp. fresh garlic,
  minced
1 tsp. salt

Cut squash in half, remove the seeds and discard them. Place the halves in a baking pan with 1/3" of water, cut side down. Bake for 40 minutes at 400 degrees. When the squash is cool enough to handle, remove the pulp or "spaghetti." Carefully wash the scallions, tomato, pepper, onion and mushrooms. Chop them medium fine. In a large skillet, place the oil and sauté the vegetables along with the seasonings and salt for 5 minutes. Combine all the ingredients in a large bowl. Mix carefully and then transfer to a serving dish. (*Serves 2.*)

DAY 4

BREAKFAST

Banana Barley

6 oz. barley
2 tbsp. barley malt
3 oz. mashed banana
2 oz. raisins

In a medium saucepan, cook barley in 14 oz. of water for 20 minutes or until done. Add barley malt, mashed banana and raisins. Mix well. Serve hot. (*Serves 1.*)

3 oz. soy beans
3 oz. kale
3 oz. cauliflower
3 oz. carrots
2 oz. yellow squash
1¹/₂ oz. brazil nuts
1¹/₂ tbsp. soy oil
¹/₃ tsp. garlic, minced
1¹/₂ oz. chives
¹/₄ tsp. coriander
¹/₄ tsp. tarragon
¹/₂ tsp. salt

Rainbow Vegetable Salad

In a large bowl, soak beans overnight in 16 oz. of water. In the morning, rinse the beans and transfer to a medium soup pot with 16 oz. of fresh water. Cook for 2 hours or until done. Carefully rinse kale, cauliflower and yellow squash. Tear the kale and cut the vegetables into bite-sized pieces. Steam in a bamboo steamer basket or stainless steel steamer for 8 minutes. Chop brazil nuts finely. Combine all ingredients in a medium-sized mixing bowl. Mix well. Serve hot or cold. (*Serves 2.*)

3 oz. lima beans
3 oz. broccoli
3 oz. tofu
2 oz. onions
1¹/₂ oz. brazil nuts
2 tbsp. soy oil
1 clove garlic, minced
1 tsp. coriander
1 tsp. parsley
¹/₂ tsp. salt
1 tsp. fresh mustard

Brazilian Broccoli Bake

In a large mixing bowl, soak lima beans overnight in 16 oz. of water. In the morning, rinse the beans and transfer them into a medium soup pot with 16 oz. of fresh water. Cook for 1¹/₂ hours or until done. Rinse broccoli and cut into ¹/₂" flowerettes. Rinse tofu and cut into ¹/₂" cubes. Peel and slice the onion. Place all ingredients in a large mixing bowl. Add ¹/₂ of the brazil nuts, the oil and seasonings. Add the mustard. Mix well. Place in a greased baking dish with lid. Top with remaining brazil nuts. Bake for 20 minutes in a preheated 350-degree oven. (*Serves 2.*)

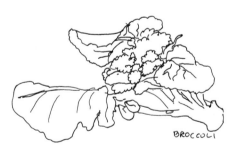

BROCCOLI

Second Cycle

DAY 1

BREAKFAST

Carob Gruel

6 oz. oatmeal
1¹/₂ oz. raisins
1 tbsp. carob powder
pinch nutmeg
¹/₄ tsp. cinnamon

In a medium saucepan, boil 15 oz. of cold water. When water begins to boil, add oatmeal and lower heat. Stir frequently. Cooking time is approximately 10 minutes. Add remaining ingredients one minute before the oatmeal is fully cooked. Serve hot. (*Serves 1.*)

LUNCH

Light 'n' Easy Squash Salad

3 oz. couscous
3 oz. mushrooms
3 oz. carrots
3 oz. summer squash
1¹/₂ oz. parsley
¹/₂ clove garlic,
   chopped
2 tsp. thyme
¹/₂ tsp. basil
¹/₂ tsp. salt
1¹/₂ oz. pine nuts
4 cherry tomatoes for
   garnish

In a medium saucepan, cook couscous in 9 oz. of water for 10 minutes or until done. Wash mushrooms, carrots and squash carefully. Slice the mushrooms, carrots and squash into bite-sized pieces. Steam in a bamboo steamer basket or stainless steel steamer until tender but crunchy. Take into consideration that the carrots will take longer to steam than the squash and the mushrooms. Rinse parsley and chop finely. Chop garlic. Combine all ingredients in a large salad bowl. Garnish with cherry tomatoes. (*Serves 2.*)

DINNER

Vegetable Cornucopia Soup with Black-Eyed Peas

3 oz. black-eyed peas
3 oz. basmati rice
1 oz. hijiki, dry
1¹/₂ oz. watercress
2 oz. parsnip
3 oz. carrot
2 oz. celery
2 oz. onion, chopped
1 tsp. tamari
2 garlic cloves, finely
   diced
3 tbsp. safflower oil
1 tsp. coriander
1 bay leaf
1 tsp. salt

In a large bowl, soak peas overnight in 3 cups of water. In the morning, rinse well and transfer to a medium soup pot with 4 cups of fresh water. Bring beans to a boil, lower to medium heat and cover. In a medium saucepan, cook rice in 10 oz. water for 20 minutes. Meanwhile soak hijiki in 8 oz. of water and rinse twice. Rinse the watercress and tear into smaller pieces. Clean the parsnips and carrots well and cut into bite-sized pieces. Clean celery and slice in ¹/₄" pieces. When peas have cooked for 1¹/₂ hours, add the cooked rice and remaining ingredients. Cook over a low heat for 25 to 30 minutes or until beans are tender. (*Yields 4 to 5 cups.*)

Tossed Garden Salad

3 oz. red leaf lettuce
2 oz. endive
2 oz. red pepper
1 oz. alfalfa sprouts

Wash lettuce, endive and pepper. Cut into bite-sized pieces and put into a salad bowl. Top with sprouts. (Serves 2.)

DAY 2

BREAKFAST

Tropical Rice Breakfast

6 oz. brown rice
1½ oz. raisins
1½ oz. sunflower
    seeds
1½ oz. coconut
½ banana, mashed
2 oz. of your favorite
    fruit juice, optional

In a medium saucepan, cook brown rice in 14 oz. of water. When water comes to a boil, lower heat. Cooking time is approximately 30 minutes. During the last ten minutes of cooking, add the raisins, sunflower seeds and coconut. When it is completely cooked, add the mashed banana. When serving, you may add the fruit juice if you wish. (Serves 1.)

LUNCH

Butternut Arugula Salad

3 oz. butternut squash
3 oz. arugula
3 oz. alfalfa sprouts
1½ oz. currants
2 tbsp. sunflower oil
½ tsp. dill
½ tsp. parsley
½ tsp. salt

Peel the butternut squash. Cut it in half and remove the seeds. Discard the seeds. Place the squash cut side down in a baking pan with ⅓″ of water. Bake for 40 minutes at 400 degrees. When squash is cool enough to handle, cut it into bite-sized pieces. Place in a medium mixing bowl. Rinse arugula carefully to get all the dirt off. Tear off the stems and discard. Then add the arugula to the squash. Add the remaining ingredients. Toss gently so as not to mash the squash. Serve hot or cold. (Serves 2.)

Herby Italian Noodles with Rice

DINNER

3 oz. brown rice
3 oz. buckwheat
  noodles
3 oz. avocado
3 oz. marinated
  artichokes
2 tbsp. sunflower oil
2 tsp. scallions,
  chopped
1 tsp. parsley,
  chopped
1 garlic clove, minced
1/2 tsp. basil
1/2 tsp salt
1 oz. black olives,
  garnish

In a medium saucepan, cook brown rice in 12 oz. of water for 35 minutes or until done. Cook noodles according to directions on package. Chop the avocado and artichokes into bite-sized pieces and place in a medium mixing bowl. Add the remaining ingredients. Toss gently. When the rice and noodles are done, place them on your plates. Top with the avocado mixture. Serve at room temperature. (*Serves 2.*)

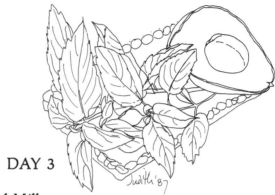

DAY 3

Almond Millet

BREAKFAST

6 oz. millet
1 oz. dried banana
1 1/2 oz. almonds
1 1/2 oz. brewer's yeast
1 tbsp. maple syrup

Cook millet in 13 oz. of water in a medium saucepan for 30 minutes. Add dried banana. Chop almonds. Add them to the millet along with the brewer's yeast and maple syrup. Serve hot. (*Serves 1.*)

Savory Mushroom Dip

LUNCH

3 oz. potato
3 oz. mushrooms
1 1/2 oz. onion
1/2 oz. sesame seeds
3 1/2 oz. water or
  broth
3 tbsp. olive oil
1 tsp. salt
1/4 tsp. cayenne
1/2 tsp. cumin
1/4 tsp. coriander
vegetable sticks
  (celery, carrots,
  daikon, etc.)

Peel potatoes. Wash them. Slice approximately 1/4" thick and place in a medium saucepan with enough water to cover. Cook until the potatoes are tender when you stick a fork in them. Rinse and slice mushrooms and onion. Sauté in a medium skillet until the onions are a golden brown. When the potatoes are cooked, place them in a blender with all the other ingredients. Puree well into a diplike consistency. Serve with a variety of vegetable sticks. (*Yield is 12 oz.*)

DINNER

3 oz. onion
1¹/₂ oz. olive oil
¹/₄ tsp. basil
¹/₄ tsp. oregano
¹/₄ tsp. cumin
6 oz. tomato
3 oz. yellow pepper
2 oz. zucchini
2 oz. tomato paste
3 oz. water
1 garlic clove, minced
¹/₂ tsp. salt
6 oz. spaghetti

Spaghetti Deluxe

Peel and slice onion. Sauté the onion in the oil with the herbs in a 2-quart saucepan for 5 minutes. Chop the tomato, pepper and zucchini finely and then add them to the saucepan along with the tomato paste, water, garlic and salt. Continue to cook, covered, for 15 minutes on low heat. Cook spaghetti in 20 oz. of water in another saucepan for 10 to 12 minutes or until done. Combine with vegetables in a medium mixing bowl. Serve hot. (*Serves 2.*)

TOMATO

DAY 4

BREAKFAST

1¹/₂ oz. brazil nuts
4 oz. soy milk
1¹/₂ oz. apple cider
1 tbsp. carob powder
¹/₂ banana
pinch cinnamon

Chock Full of Protein Drink

Chop brazil nuts finely. Combine all of the ingredients in a blender, including the brazil nuts, and blend well. It tastes really good when the mixture is smooth and creamy. If you like your drinks sweeter, you may use the whole banana. (*Serves 1.*)

LUNCH

3 oz. lentils
2 oz. carrots
3 oz. corn (may be
    fresh and removed
    from the husk or
    frozen)
3 oz. fresh chives
3 tbsp. soy oil
¹/₂ tsp. garlic powder
¹/₂ tsp. coriander
¹/₂ tsp. rosemary
¹/₂ tsp. basil
³/₄ tsp. salt
several parsley sprigs
    for garnish

Hearty Lentil Soup

Cook lentils in a medium soup pot with enough water to cover. Bring to a boil and then set on medium heat with the lid on. Cooking time is approximately 1 hour. Scrub carrots and cut them into bite-sized pieces. After the lentils have cooked for approximately 20 minutes, drop the carrots into the pot along with the corn and remaining ingredients. When the mixture has cooked for an additional 30 minutes, take half of the mixture out of the pot and put it into a blender. Puree it for 15 seconds and then pour it back into the pot. Cook for an additional 10 minutes. Garnish with parsley sprigs. (*Yields 4 to 5 cups.*)

Nutty Bean Salad

3 oz. black beans
1¹/₂ oz. walnuts
2 oz. celery
2 oz. carrots
1¹/₂ tbsp. soy oil
1 garlic clove, minced
1 tsp. tarragon
¹/₂ tsp. sage
¹/₂ tsp. salt

In a large bowl, soak the black beans overnight in 16 oz. of water. In the morning, rinse the beans and transfer them to a medium saucepan with 16 oz. fresh water. Cook for 1¹/₂ hours or until done. Chop walnuts very finely. Rinse celery and scrub carrots. Cut celery and carrots into bite-sized pieces. Place oil in a wok or skillet and heat. Place all ingredients into the wok or skillet and sauté for 5 minutes. Serve at room temperature. (*Serves 1.*)

DINNER

Hot and Crunchy Veggie Mix

3 oz. snap green beans
3 oz. cauliflower
3 oz. brussel sprouts
1¹/₂ oz. walnuts
¹/₅ tsp. sage
¹/₂ tsp. dill
¹/₂ tsp. parsley
juice of ¹/₂ lemon
pinch cayenne
2 tbsp. soy oil
³/₄ tsp. salt
2 oz. water

Wash beans and cut them into bite-sized pieces. Steam in a bamboo steam basket or stainless steel steamer for 10 minutes or until tender. Rinse cauliflower and brussel sprouts and cut into bite-sized pieces. Steam for 8 minutes. In a blender, place the steamed beans, walnuts and the remaining ingredients. Pour sauce over the cauliflower and brussel sprouts. You may serve this dish either hot or cold. (*Serves 2.*)

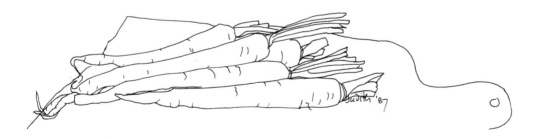

Third Cycle

DAY 1

BREAKFAST

6 oz. couscous
3 oz. apple
2 oz. raisins
½ tbsp. honey
½ tsp. cinnamon
3 oz. favorite fruit
   juice, optional

Sweet Cinnamon Couscous

In a medium saucepan, cook couscous in 14 oz. of water. Bring to a boil, stirring often. Then lower heat. Cook time is approximately 10 to 12 minutes. Wash and slice apples. When couscous has cooked, add apple slices and remaining ingredients. Mix well. Transfer to serving bowls. Add fruit juice if you wish. (Serves 1.)

LUNCH

3 oz. mung beans
6 oz. zucchini
4½ oz. summer
   squash
2 oz. Spanish onion
2 oz. carrots
1 oz. parsley
a garlic clove, finely
   diced
3 tbsp. safflower oil
¾ tsp. salt
½ tsp. basil
¼ tsp. oregano

Milano Bean and Vegetable Soup

Place mung beans in a large bowl with 3 cups of water. Allow the beans to soak overnight. In the morning, rinse the beans well and transfer into a large soup pot, adding 4 cups of fresh water. Bring beans to a boil and lower to medium heat. Keep the lid on. Scrub the zucchini and summer squash, peel the onion and the carrots. Chop the vegetables into bite-sized pieces. Rinse parsley and chop finely. After the beans have been cooking for approximately one hour, add the vegetables and the remaining ingredients. Remove half of the mixture and transfer into a blender. Puree for 15 seconds. Return the puree to the rest of the soup to finish cooking for another 30 minutes. (Yields 4 to 5 cups.)

DINNER

3 oz. amaranth
3 oz. basmati rice
1 oz. watercress
1 oz. dill
1½ oz. parsley
1½ oz. carrot
2 tbsp. safflower oil
juice of ½ lemon
½ tsp. salt
2 oz. water
⅓ tsp. tarragon

Superb Vegetable Rice Salad

In a medium pot, cook amaranth for 25 minutes in 10 oz. of water. In another pot, cook the rice in 10 oz. of water for 20 minutes. Rinse the watercress, dill and parsley and chop medium fine. Scrub the carrots well and chop into bite-sized pieces. Place all the ingredients in a medium mixing bowl and mix well. (Serves 2.)

DINNER (2nd Option)

3 oz. amaranth
3 oz. hijiki seaweed
    (1 oz. dry; 3 oz.
    soaked)
3 oz. carrot
3 oz. zucchini
2 oz. daikon
2 tbsp. safflower oil
2/3 tsp. salt
1/4 tsp. garlic
1/4 tsp. coriander
1/2 tsp. cumin
1 1/2 oz. pecan

Oriental Zucchini Salad

In a medium saucepan, cook amaranth in 10 oz. of water for 25 minutes. Rinse hijiki and soak 3 times. Scrub carrots and zucchini. Peel daikon. Cut carrots, zucchini and daikon into bite-sized pieces and steam in a bamboo steamer basket or stainless steamer for 8 minutes. In a skillet or wok, sauté the hijiki with the safflower oil and the herbs for 5 minutes. Combine all the ingredients together in a medium bowl. Add the pecans. Mix well. (Serves 2.)

DAY 2

BREAKFAST

6 oz. brown rice
1 1/2 oz. coconut
1 1/2 oz. cashews
1 tbsp. your favorite
    fruit conserve (no
    sugar, just fruit)
1 oz. chopped figs

Fruity Rice Breakfast

In a medium saucepan, cook brown rice in 14 oz. of water. When water comes to a boil, lower heat. Cooking time is approximately 30 minutes. When cooked, add the coconut and cashews. Mix well. Remove from the heat. Add the conserves and the figs. Mix again. Transfer to bowl. (Serves 1.)

LUNCH

6 oz. split peas
6 oz. brown rice
3 oz. broccoli
3 oz. carrots
3 oz. zucchini
2 oz. onions
3 tbsp. sunflower oil
1/2 tsp. curry powder
3/4 tsp. salt

Curried Vegetable Rice

In a medium saucepan, cook split peas in enough water to cover. Bring to a boil then lower heat. After peas have cooked for 15 minutes, In another saucepan, cook rice in 14 oz. of water for 30 minutes. Clean vegetables well and cut into bite-sized pieces. After peas have cooked for 15 minutes, add the chopped vegetables, cooked brown rice and remaining ingredients. Cook for an additional 15 minutes. (Yields 4 to 5 cups.)

Sunny Squash

3 oz. butternut squash
3 oz. buckwheat
   noodles
3 oz. asparagus
2 oz. watercress
1 tsp. parsley
1 clove garlic, minced
5 tbsp. sunflower oil
3/4 tsp. salt

Cut squash in half, remove the seeds and discard them. Place the squash in a baking pan with 1/3" water, cut side down. Bake for 40 minutes at 400 degrees. When the squash is cool enough to handle, remove the squash from the skin and set aside in a medium-sized bowl. Drop the noodles into salted boiling water and cook for 5 minutes. Set aside. Rinse the asparagus. Steam in a bamboo steamer basket or stainless steel steamer. Cut into 2" pieces. Rinse watercress and chop. Add noodles to the squash along with the asparagus, watercress, and remaining ingredients. Mix well, tossing gently. (*Yields 4 to 5 cups.*)

Basic Tossed Salad

3 oz. romaine
3 oz. carrots
2 oz. red cabbage
2 oz. tomato

Rinse vegetables and cut into bite-sized pieces. Combine everything together in a salad bowl. (*Serves 2.*)

DAY 3

Heart-Warming Breakfast

6 oz. cream of wheat
2 oz. chopped dates
1 oz. coconut
1 1/2 oz. brewer's yeast
1/2 tsp. cinnamon

In a medium saucepan, cook cream of wheat in 12 oz. of water for 10 minutes or until done. Stir occasionally on medium heat. When cooked, add the remaining ingredients. Transfer to bowl. (*Serves 1.*)

Baked Potato Sesame

3 oz. potato
3 oz. spaghetti
1 1/2 oz. scallions
1 tsp. dill
3 oz. tahini sauce
1 1/2 oz. sesame seeds
1 1/2 tbsp. sesame oil
1/4 tsp. coriander
1/2 tsp. salt
1 garlic clove, minced

Bake potato for 40 minutes at 400 degrees. When cool enough to handle, cut into 3/4" cubes. Cook spaghetti in a medium saucepan in 20 oz. of water for 10 minutes. Rinse scallions and chop them medium fine. Mix potato and spaghetti in a medium mixing bowl. Add the remaining ingredients. Transfer to a baking pan and bake for 15 minutes in a preheated 375-degree oven. (*Serves 2.*)

DINNER

3 oz. adzuki beans
1¹/₂ oz. almonds
3 oz. scallions
3 oz. red pepper
1 tsp. parsley
3 oz. tomato
2 tbsp. sesame oil
¹/₄ tsp. oregano
1 tsp. salt
¹/₂ tsp. thyme
1 clove garlic, minced
several leaves of
    romaine lettuce

Crunchy Vegetable Bean Salad

In a large bowl, soak beans overnight in 16 oz. of water. In the morning, rinse the beans and place them into a medium pot with 16 oz. of fresh water. Cook for 1 hour or until done. Blanch the almonds by bringing 18 oz. of water in a small saucepan to a boil and dropping the almonds into the water. Remove from the heat. Let the almonds remain in the boiling water for 5 minutes and then run cold water into the saucepan. Squeeze the skins off and let the almonds dry. Sliver the almonds. Rinse the scallions, red pepper, parsley and tomato. Cut them into bite-sized pieces. In a medium mixing bowl, put the beans, almonds and vegetables. Toss gently. Add the remaining ingredients and mix well. Serve cool on a bed of romaine lettuce. (*Serves 2.*)

DAY 4

BREAKFAST

6 oz. banana
2 oz. raisins
3 oz. tofu
4 oz. barley malt
¹/₂ oz. carob powder
1 tsp. vanilla
3 heaping tsp. Ener-G-
    Egg Replacer
6 oz. apple juice
pinch cinnamon
pinch nutmeg

Creamy Banana Tofu Pudding

Place all ingredients in a blender. Puree until smooth and creamy. Transfer to a medium saucepan and cook over medium heat for 5 minutes, stirring frequently. Allow to chill for 45 minutes. (*Yields 20 oz.*)

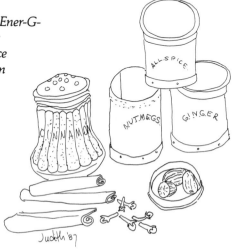

LUNCH

3 oz. chick-peas
1/2 oz. dulse, dry
3 oz. cauliflower
3 oz. tempeh
2 oz. onion
6 oz. tomato sauce
2 tbsp. soy oil
a garlic clove, minced
1/4 tsp. salt
1/2 tsp. basil
2 oz. water

Mid-Eastern Tempeh

In a medium bowl, soak the chick-peas overnight in 16 oz. of water. In the morning, rinse the chick-peas and transfer into a medium soup pot with 20 oz. of fresh water. Cook for 1 3/4 to 2 hours or until done. Rinse dulse 2 or 3 times in cold water. Rinse cauliflower and cut into flowerettes. Cut tempeh into 1/2" cubes and put all the ingredients together in a medium mixing bowl. Peel and slice the onion and add to the mixture. Toss gently. Add the remaining ingredients and mix well. Transfer to a greased baking pan and bake for 20 minutes in a preheated 350-degree oven. (*Serves 2.*)

DINNER

3 oz. lima beans
3 oz. lentils
3 oz. okra
3 oz. cauliflower
1 1/2 oz. brazil nut
    butter
1 1/2 tbsp. corn oil
1 1/2 oz. water
1/4 tsp. tarragon
1/2 tsp. sage
1/2 tsp. salt
1 garlic clove, minced
Note: Brazil nut butter
    is made with
    "Champion" juicer
    or similar grinder.

Double Bean Delight

In a large bowl, soak beans overnight in 16 oz. of water. In the morning, rinse and replace with 16 oz. of fresh water in a medium soup pot. Cook for 1 1/2 hours or until done. In another pot, cook lentils in 12 oz. of water for 25 minutes. Rinse and cut vegetables into bite-sized pieces. Steam in a bamboo steamer basket or stainless steel steamer for 8 minutes or until tender. Transfer all ingredients into a medium mixing bowl and gently toss. Add the remaining ingredients and mix well. Transfer to a baking pan and bake for 15 minutes in a 350-degree oven. (*Serves 2.*)

Additional Desserts

Multi-Fruit Oatmeal Pudding

3 oz. pears
3 oz. oatmeal
6 oz. pear juice
1 banana
2 heaping tsp. Ener-G-
    Egg Replacer
pinch cinnamon
3 oz. apples

Place all ingredients, except for apples, in a blender. Puree. Transfer puree into small saucepan and cook over medium heat for approximately 5 minutes. Wash and cube apples. Add them to puree and stir frequently. Place in a medium mixing bowl or individual dessert dishes and allow to chill in the refrigerator for at least 45 minutes. (*Yields approximately 18 oz.*)

Tropical Pudding

6 oz. pineapple
6 oz. apple juice
3 tbsp. honey
2 tbsp. Ener-G-Egg
    Replacer
2 tbsp. coconut
pinch nutmeg
4^1/$_2$ oz. papaya
1^1/$_2$ oz. pecans

Place all ingredients, except for papaya and pecans, in a blender. Puree. Transfer puree into small saucepan and cook over medium heat for approximately 5 minutes. Peel papaya, remove seeds and cube. Chop pecans. Add both to the puree and stir. Place in medium mixing bowl or individual dessert dishes and allow to chill in refrigerator for at least 45 minutes. (*Yields approximately 16 oz.*)

Mango Strawberry Canton

4 oz. mango
4 oz. strawberries
12 oz. apple juice
2 heaping tbsp. agar-
    agar
1 tsp. vanilla
2 oz. dates, chopped

Peel mango and remove pit. Put in the blender with 2 oz. strawberries. Add apple juice and blend. Transfer to medium saucepan and bring to a boil. Lower heat and add agar-agar. Stir and dissolve agar-agar and simmer for 5 minutes. Add vanilla and chopped dates. Transfer to mixing bowl or individual dessert dishes and place in the refrigerator until juice begins to gel—about 10 minutes. Drop in the remaining strawberries. Chill for 1 hour. (*Serves 2 to 4.*)

Papaya Brown Rice Pudding

3 oz. brown rice
6 oz. papaya
1^1/$_2$ oz. coconut
1^1/$_2$ oz. figs
10 oz. pineapple
    coconut juice
2 heaping tsp. Ener-G-
    Egg Replacer
2 oz. blueberries

In a medium saucepan, cook brown rice in about 10 oz. water for 25 minutes. When cooked, place in blender. Peel papaya and remove seeds. Add to blender along with remaining ingredients, except for blueberries. Puree until creamy and smooth. Transfer to medium saucepan and cook over medium heat for approximately 5 minutes. Stir frequently. Transfer to medium mixing bowl or individual dessert dishes and place in refrigerator to chill for 45 minutes. (*Yields approximately 15 oz.*)

Blueberry Kiwi Pudding

3 oz. millet
5 oz. blueberries
2 oz. kiwi
^{1}/$_2$ banana
6 oz. apple strawberry
    juice
2 heaping tsp. Ener-G-
    Egg Replacer
1 tsp. lemon juice
1^1/$_2$ oz. slivered
    almonds

Place millet in a small saucepan with approximately 10 oz. water and cook for 20 minutes. When cooked, put in blender with the remaining ingredients, except for almonds. Puree until smooth and creamy. Transfer puree to medium saucepan and heat for 5 minutes over medium heat, stirring frequently. Transfer to medium mixing bowl or individual dessert dishes and allow to chill in refrigerator for 45 minutes. (*Yields approximately 23 oz.*)

Strawberry Tofu Pudding

4¹/₂ oz. strawberry
6 oz. tofu
3 tbsp. maple syrup
1 tsp. vanilla

Place all ingredients in the blender. Puree until creamy and smooth. Transfer into one medium mixing bowl or individual dessert dishes. Place in refrigerator and allow to chill for 45 minutes. (*Serves 2.*)

Peach Canton

6 oz. peaches
12 oz. apple blackberry juice
2 heaping tbsp. agar-agar
2 tbsp. Barbados molasses
3 oz. pitted black cherries

Wash and cut peaches into small pieces. Place half of the peaches in a blender with juice. Place mixture in a medium saucepan and bring to a boil. Lower heat and add agar-agar. Stir and dissolve agar and simmer for 5 minutes. Add molasses. Transfer to a medium mixing bowl or individual dessert dishes and place in refrigerator until juice begins to gel—around 10 minutes. Add remaining peaches and cherries. Chill for 1 hour. (*Serves 2.*)

Peachy Tofu Pudding

6 oz. peaches
3 oz. tofu
3 oz. barley malt
1 tsp. vanilla
6 oz. peach juice

Wash and cut peaches. Place all ingredients in blender and puree until smooth. Transfer to medium saucepan and place on medium heat for 5 minutes, stirring frequently. Transfer to medium mixing bowl or individual dessert dishes and allow to chill in refrigerator for 45 minutes. (*Yields 18 oz.*)

Blueberry Banana Pudding

6 oz. blueberries
1 banana
3 oz. tofu
3 oz. apple juice
4 oz. nectarines, sliced
2 oz. almonds

Place blueberries, banana, tofu and apple juice in a blender. Puree until smooth and creamy. Transfer to medium mixing bowl or individual dessert dishes. Top with nectarine slices and almonds. (*Serves 2.*)

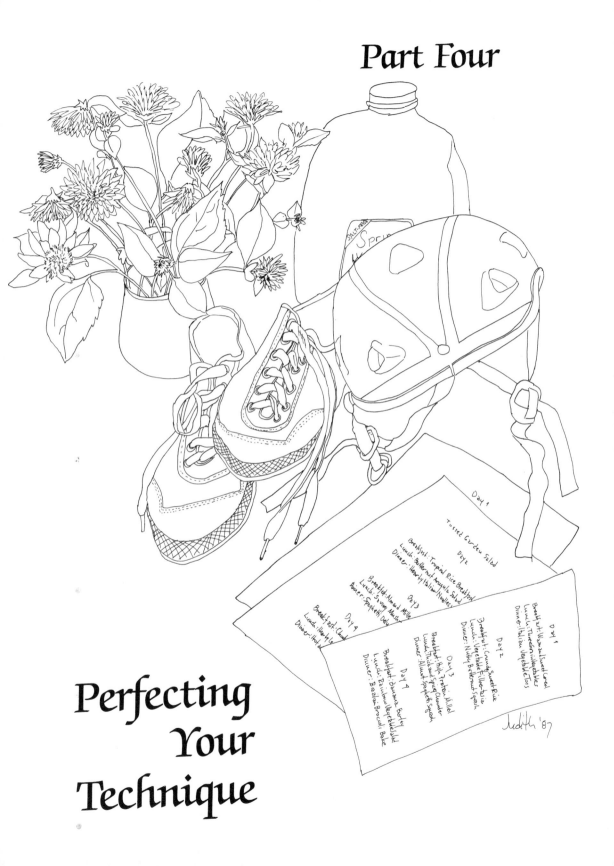

Part Four

Perfecting
Your
Technique

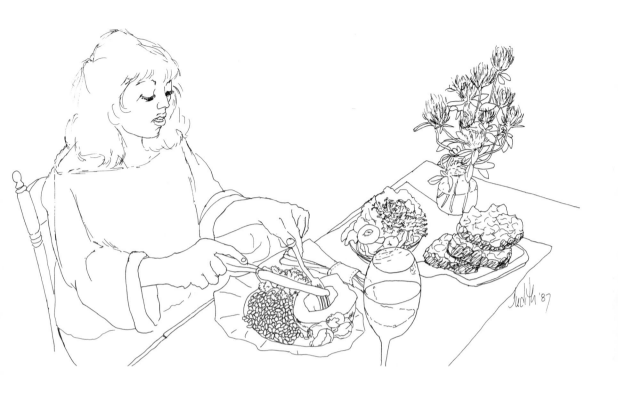

14 · WEIGHT MANAGEMENT

"Counting calories is not as important as thoughtfully choosing the kinds and amounts of food you eat. The typical American diet needs to be adjusted to include more complex carbohydrates, fewer proteins, and less fat. Begin your new eating plan by eliminating the three whites from your diet: white sugar, white flour, and salt. Then eliminate processed food including most canned, frozen, or prepared convenience foods. Read labels and do not eat anything you can't pronounce."

THERE ARE VIRTUALLY HUNDREDS of diet programs available today. Most are based on high-protein, low-calorie regimens, or involve products that are supposed to melt away fat, change the metabolism or stimulate muscle development. Before embarking upon any of these, first examine the notion of what is proper weight, making sure your perception of what constitutes your ideal weight is not mistaken.

THE SCOPE OF THE PROBLEM

You may not realize it, but it requires from two to four years of being over-fat before you become overweight. Excess fat will first infiltrate the muscle tissue before it spills out as subcutaneous tissue, that which you can see underneath the folds of skin. By the time the fat is visible on your arms and face, the problem has already reached the advanced stages and the buttocks, thighs, belly, upper arms, and back have already been saturated. To assume that a crash diet based on fasting, or calorie restriction is going to reverse this process can be a dangerous assumption to make. The end result of easy solutions may only be repeated failures. The key to weight management, and ideal weight control, is not diet alone but exercise in combination with diet.

THE ROLE OF EXERCISE

Exercise is more important in maintaining proper weight than counting calories. You have heard that for every 3,500 calories in excess of your body's metabolic requirements you will gain a pound, while for every 3,500 calories under that requirement you would lose a pound. These were both cumulative figures. So that, for example, if you were eating one extra slice of bread per day, you would have gained over ten pounds by the year's end, at the rate of 70 extra calories per slice, 490 calories per week. But this represents a gross misunderstanding of how our bodies work. Diets based on such a seemingly rational, logical, though mechanistic view of the body sound simple. Yet they don't work—because the body does not work that way—so rationally, logically and, worst of all, so mechanically. Look at all the thin people who eat great quantities of food and never gain an ounce. Look at all the fat people who just have to think about food, or smell food, and gain pounds.

We need to determine what causes weight problems and treat the causes, not the symptoms. The way to do this is to understand how the body works, and then use its own natural mechanisms to produce the desired results. Exercise is the key.

THE SETPOINT

Primitive man gorged when food was available and starved when there was none. His body had built-in survival mechanisms that stored fat when he gorged and then conserved energy when food was scarce. The conservation mechanism slowed down his metabolism, making use only of enough energy to keep him alive and functioning. That mechanism is still with us and still working. Decreasing your caloric intake, skipping a meal or even eating irregularly may trigger the starvation mechanism. Your body's protective response is to go into its conservation mode—to conserve energy and preserve the fat, just in case starvation is really imminent. When the body gets food, it puts it in a "bank," to ensure against any possible further deprivation. Each of our bodies seems to have a certain natural level, or setpoint, that it strives to maintain to keep itself functioning.

Researchers are now looking at how the body gains and retains weight and are redefining their understanding of weight control. What are the causes of weight gain? The answer seems to lie in a weight-regulating mechanism located in a control center in the brain called the hypothalamus. It determines the level of fat that it considers ideal for the body. It proceeds to maintain that level, come what may. That level, selected by the weight-regulating mechanism, then becomes the setpoint. The setpoint is analogous to a thermostat. A thermostat set at 70° kicks off and activates the heating system when the temperature falls below 70°. Similarly, a setpoint of 140 pounds activates the weight-regulating mechanism to store more fat if the body weight falls below that 140-pound level. In its effort to maintain the setpoint, the weight-regulating mechanism works in two ways: It controls the appetite and it regulates our metabolism and the storage of energy.

First, appetite control determines when you feel hungry. It sends you a message to eat. You may have no control over the urge to eat—the hypothalamus makes sure of that—but you do have complete control over your response. You can choose when and how to respond. What you eat and how much you eat are totally up to you. The hypothalamus will continue to stimulate the feeding mechanism and decrease satiety, you will continue to feel hungry and eat, until the desired setpoint level is achieved, and your weight is back to where it was.

Second, a weight-regulating mechanism signals the body when to conserve energy and store it, or use it up. If you eat a large amount of food, it increases the rate at which the body burns calories. If you eat a small amount, the body decreases the rate. In each case, the goal is to preserve the setpoint. This explains why people on diets may lose weight temporarily, but ultimately regain it, and then keep their weight at close to the former, albeit unsatisfactory level. It's called the yo-yo syndrome, and every dieter is familiar with it. Usually that weight has been typical for them for many years. It is their setpoint. The body is accustomed to it, feels safe and secure at that level, and consequently does what it can to maintain it. People who are overweight commonly observe that they don't really eat that much. Indeed, studies have confirmed that underweight people comonly eat more than overweight people. What we distill from this is that overweight people may have a body chemistry geared to making fat even from a low-calorie diet. It seems that they are just better at storing fat than at burning fat. Their bodies are programmed to make fat and protect their setpoints. This also explains why some other people never seem to gain weight. Their setpoints are low, their ability to use energy is efficient, and so they don't store fat. You cannot cheat the setpoint. You can, however, change the setpoint, but only through aerobic exercise.

THE AGING FACTOR

From the age of 30 on, your metabolism decelerates about 5 percent every seven years. In other words, if you were eating the same number of calories at 50 years of age that you ate at 30, you would be gaining several pounds every year. But weight itself is not an indication of optimal body health. A person weighing 200 pounds, who lifts weights and exercises, may have only 3 to 4 percent body fat. Many football players, for example, would fall into this category. But if these individuals stopped all their physical activity and one year later they weighed the same, their entire body structure would be different. They would look and feel obese, because their muscle would have turned to fat. Muscle that is not used, atrophies. Weight itself should not be taken as the primary indicator of health. What is important is the percentage of lean muscle tissue and the percentage of fat to total body mass. Ideally, most men should be approximately 15 percent body fat, most women no more than 18 to 20 percent. However, most studies indicate that most men are between 22 and 24 percent, most women between 26 and 34 percent.

LEAN BODY MASS

Lean body mass increases when intramuscular fat is replaced with muscle. Muscles have special enzymes that burn calories during exercise. The more muscle you have, the more enzymes you have that burn calories. As the amount of muscle increases, the amount of fat decreases, and the capacity for burning more calories is further enhanced. So when muscles move, they burn calories and increase lean body mass. It's a new cycle, but this time it's not vicious!

AEROBIC EXERCISE AND THE FIT CYCLE

Although there are probably genetic tendencies that predetermine that one of us will have a low setpoint and be thin, or a high setpoint and be overweight, it is still possible for most people to "re-set" their fat thermostat. The key to reprogramming your setpoint lies in understanding and acting on the relationship between the kind and amount of exercise you do (your energy output) and the kind and amount of food you eat (your energy input). The trick lies in changing from a fat cycle to a fit cycle.

Running and other aerobic exercises can help you enter the fit cycle. Aerobic exercises uses large muscles in a repetitive rhythmic pattern.

To measure the effect of aerobic exercise on your body you will need to "watch"—or more appropriately—"feel" your heart rate, by measuring your pulse. There are three different heart rates to monitor.

RESTING HEART RATE

The resting heart rate is the rate at which your heart has been pumping after you sit quietly for at least 15 minutes. It is usually 15–20 beats per minute slower than your "normal" heart rate.

Measure by taking your pulse for 10 or 20 seconds and then multiplying the result by 6 or 3, respectively. The average resting heart rate for men is 72–78 beats per minute, for women it's faster: 78–84. The better your aerobic circulation, the lower this rate will be.

Studies seem to indicate that people with resting heart rates above 70 have a greater risk of heart attack. By beating fewer times per minute, an efficient heart has more time to rest between beats. Hence, at each contraction or beat, it may be pumping more oxygen to the body's cells.

TARGET HEART RATE

To produce a beneficial cardiovascular effort during exercise, you should elevate your heart rate sufficiently to strengthen heart muscles while at the same time avoiding any damage to the heart or cardiovascular system.

Take your pulse throughout your aerobic workout to make sure you are neither under- nor over-exerting yourself. Generally, your target rate is determined by taking 220 and subtracting your age and then multiplying the result by 70 percent. So a 31-year-old person would have a rate of 220 minus 31 times 70 percent or 132.

Whatever you do you should not exceed 140 beats per minute when you're just starting an aerobic exercise program.

RECOVERY HEART RATE

This rate records your heart beat five minutes after you've stopped exercising. It gives you some indication about whether you have gone one or more beats too far. If this rate is 120 beats per minute (150 in those over 50 years old), you need to cut back during your next workout.

To achieve a training effect on cardiovascular functioning or to lower your setpoint toward "thinness," you must do the exercise continuously for 20 to 60 minutes at your target heart rate at least three times a week.

During aerobic exercise, the body uses free fatty acids primarily and glycogen secondarily as fuel. While exercising, you do not use many calories. For example, you would have to walk $11^1/_2$ miles to burn up 3,500 calories or one pound. Weight loss is the effect of a *cumulative* process in which calories are being used on a more regular and frequent basis. This cumulative use of calories produces ongoing changes in the body's chemistry, lowering the setpoint, increasing the lean muscle mass with its fat-burning enzymes, and increasing the metabolism so the body burns calories at a higher rate. For hours following the exercise period, the body continues to burn calories at a higher rate. The effects of exercise on the body last long after the exercise period has ended. This will be true as long as you continue to do aerobic exercise at least three days a week. Remember, duration is more important than distance or intensity.

Although many people may intellectually recognize the need for and benefit of aerobic exercise, too often they would rather spend their time doing other things, or hope to take a pill to reduce because it requires no particular effort or ongoing commitment. Making a change in your lifestyle to accomodate exercise *does* require effort and commitment. Your health and well-being are worth the price.

Exercise increases muscle, which has fat-burning enzymes. The more you exercise and develop muscles, the more lean body mass and less fat. All this will happen in addition to the much heralded cardiovascular and psychological advantages of aerobic exercise. Lowering the setpoint is a bonus.

Your individual exercise program will start the same way whether your goal is overall fitness or weight management. The proper sequence for a holistic workout is outlined in Chapter 15, starting with relaxation techniques and measurement of the pulse at rest. In addition, you will want to take your body measurements before starting any exercise program.

If you step on the scale after a few weeks of exercising, you may notice an increase in pounds. Don't be dismayed. That is a good sign. It means you are increasing muscle in relation to intramuscular fat (muscle weighs more than fat). Interpret the increase as getting better and stronger, not heavier. Then throw away the scale. Pounds do not measure fitness. Your tape measure and your clothes are better indicators of changes in your body. You will lose inches, usually in the "right" places.

EATING PLANS

Counting calories is not as important as thoughtfully choosing the kinds and amounts of food you eat. The typical American diet needs to be adjusted to include more complex carbohydrates, fewer proteins, and less fat. Begin your new eating plan by eliminating the three whites from your diet: white sugar, white flour, and salt. Then eliminate processed food including most canned, frozen or prepared convenience foods. Read labels and do not eat anything you can't pronounce.

There is one point that most books on dieting fail to mention. That is the importance of getting in touch with your appetite thermostat. Your body tells you when to eat and when to stop, and you don't always hear it or listen to it.

The best eating plan is to eat more frequently—smaller meals, every four to six hours, so that both hunger and satiety can be experienced. Do eat breakfast, just keep down fat and sugar consumption. More people who skip breakfast are overweight than underweight. Get in touch with your eating drives. Keep lunch light, preferably eating complex carbohydrates, which are low in calories and high in satiety. Soup is a satisfying lunch, especially a water-based soup full of vegetables, grains, and legumes. Salads are good for lunch, but after eating one you could feel hungry again quite soon. Add whole grain bread to complement it. Beware of salad dressings; most are high in fat, sugar, and calories. Eat enough breakfast and lunch to take away the strong hunger drive, but not enough to feel full. If you are hungry before the next meal, have a snack. Eat only in response to hunger, not for entertainment.

Another divergence from traditional diets, but designed to pay attention to your body's natural eating drive, is to eat one meal a day to complete satiety, until you do not want to eat anymore. The evening meal is preferred, so it will hold you throught the evening until bedtime. This is the most difficult time to avoid snacks.

Beware: The weight you eventually reach may not necessarily be the weight you desire. Be realistic and be philosophical. The genetic determinants of setpoint may limit what you can realistically accomplish. If you follow the principles of exercise and diet for a reasonable period of time, and your weight stabilizes at a point higher than your fantasy weight, accept it and enjoy being yourself, as you are.

If you continue to exercise aerobically and eat a healthful diet, your weight-regulating mechanism will stabilize your weight and keep it at the new setpoint. Eating and exercising in this way will soon become a natural way of living for you. You won't need a maintenance diet or some other interim discipline to follow. Once you've set your own course, there will be no other course to follow and no need for fad approaches to dieting.

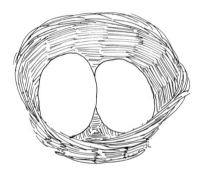

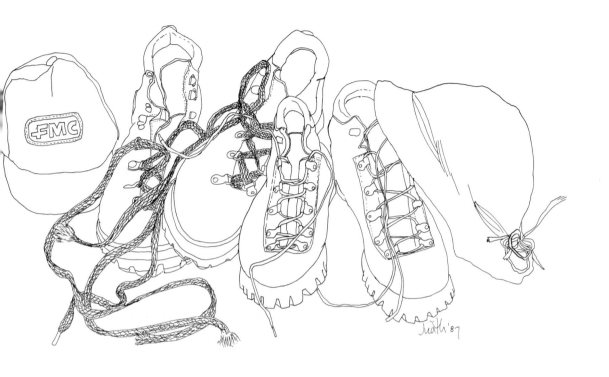

15 · NUTRITION AND EXERCISE

"Walking can be done by almost anyone, almost anywhere. For some, including the elderly, pregnant, arthritic, or those with heart disease, it is the only form of reasonable cardiovascular exercise. All you need is some comfortable old clothes, a good pair of running (walking) shoes, and a hat to protect you if the weather is hot and sunny or cold and windy. About 1½ hours of walking will give you the same aerobic effect as 30 minutes of running."

ANY DIET SHOULD BE tailored to each person's specific requirements, with attention paid to your body's specialized needs as well as to the type and amount of exercise to which you are accustomed. The additional stress of exercise requires adjusting your nutritional intake to replenish the fuel used up during exercise.

FOOD ALLERGIES AFFECTING EXERCISE

Food allergies are discussed at length in the allergy chapters of the book. Few things can adversely affect our energy level during exercise more than allergies. An allergy will weaken your immune system, making you more vulnerable to infection and deterioration. If you overexercise, you will probably incur joint and muscle inflammation, yet a properly functioning immune system will allow your body to quickly repair itself.

FAT AND PROTEIN

When you exercise regularly, your body burns a higher than normal percentage of fats, even while you sleep. To give your body an adequate supply of essential fatty acids, steer clear of animal fats and eat extra oils selected from a variety of available vegetable sources. Rely primarily on unrefined oils found in foods such as raw seeds, raw nuts, avocados, and grains. Refined oils increase your risk of consuming too many free radicals—unstable molecules that can attack your cells, speed up the aging process, and weaken your body.

Protein is an inefficient fuel that is pressed into service only after preferred fuels are depleted. It is digested slowly and tends to dehydrate your body by using lots of water for its digestion and elimination. Under normal circumstances, you can only digest and utilize three ounces of food at a time, so regulate your protein intake to avoid the taxing waste of energy that follows overconsumption. Complex carbohydrates are much more efficient and should serve as your key foods for replenishing glycogen, the energy fuel.

CARBOHYDRATE LOADING

Carbohydrate loading is an eating regimen followed by some athletes in preparation for a long competition, such as a running marathon. A typical schedule for a runner begins seven days before the event with an exhausting bout of exercise, depleting the stores of glycogen in the body. To further aid the glycogen depletion, the runner eats a low-carbohydrate, high-protein and high-fat diet. Three days before the event, he packs in as many carbohydrates as possible to replenish the glycogen, keeping protein and fat at moderate levels. The body is stressed by this deprivation of carbohydrate fuel, and it responds to that stress by overcompensating and storing extra supplies of glycogen in the muscles. Thus, the marathon runner has more energy and can run longer before tiring.

One modification of this classic loading technique is to substitute tapered rest for the exhaustive bout of exercise during the week preceding the event. Also, the last week might feature a high complex carbohydrate diet. A further modification sometimes suggested is for the runner to rest and eat a high complex carbohydrate diet 48 to 72 hours before the event.

What was just described is preparation for an extraordinary event that few of us would even participate in. For regular exercise, or competition in general, guidelines for eating are: 1) Eat enough so as not to feel hungry during the event. Eat modest amounts of complex carbohydrates up to $2^1/2$ hours before exercising. Stay away from fat and protein. Avoid salty or spicy foods, simple sugars, and unfamiliar foods that could irritate or upset you. 2) Allow time for your stomach and small intestines to empty. 3) Drink water or diluted fruit juice until one hour before the event, then continue to drink water only.

You may wonder if, after drinking so much water, a runner, walker, or biker will need to stop and urinate. The fact is the kidneys slow down during exercise, so the body will retain fluids for use by other tissues to reduce heat build-up that comes with exercise and produce sweat. The body, in effect, turns off the water-eliminating system and turns on the water-retention system.

SUPPLEMENTS

In general a person who eats a well-balanced diet will not need vitamin or mineral supplements for their exercise needs. However, not all the vitamins and minerals naturally available in foods will be available to everyone, due to food sensitivities, poor absorption, chemical imbalances and improper food combining. Persons affected by these factors may need supplements, even megadoses, of vitamins and minerals to bring a particular deficiency up to par or to strengthen a weak point.

Exercise stresses the body, with B complex vitamins in particular burned off by stress. It is recommended that B complex vitamins as well as vitamin A, which helps stimulate the immune system, be taken as part of an exercise regimen. The antioxidants, vitamins C and E, and selenium, are also recommended before and after exercise. Calcium and magnesium, in a 1:1 ratio, are commonly used to benefit muscles. Iron deficiency is common among women and athletes, and runners should be tested for iron deficiency before training begins.

SALT INTAKE AFTER EXERCISE

A common misconception is that your body loses salt through perspiration after exercise. In fact, it loses only water, leaving the body's salt in higher concentrations than before. You need more water after exercise, not more salt, to help prevent fatigue, irritability, and exhaustion. Salt pills are not recommended.

A BIG DINNER OR A BEDTIME SNACK?

If you are serious about exercise, dinner should be your smallest meal of the day. In the late afternoon or early evening, your body is in a state of recuperation and repair from exercise. Burdening it with a heavy meal hampers this process.

You shouldn't eat anything substantial for at least two hours before you go to sleep because little will leave your stomach within an hour after eating. Once you're in a prone position, whatever is in your stomach has difficulty moving into the intestine. If you are hungry late in the evening, try a very light food such as fruit, or have a liquid refreshment like an herbal tea.

POST-EXERCISE NUTRITION

During exercise, you use up water and fuel. You need to replenish them—in that order. Water, the recommended beverage, helps alleviate feelings of exhaustion. Give your body an opportunity to return to normal before eating.

Even if you are not consciously thirsty, drink an 8- to 10-ounce glass of water after exercising, and again at 20-minute intervals for the next hour. You cannot restore the water you lost in exercise simply by drinking a lot at one time. Your body's tissues, after all, can only absorb water at a certain rate; the rest is eliminated. The average water consumption per day for a healthy adult who exercises is eight 8- to 10-ounce glasses. What you do not use, the body will eliminate.

If you are ravenous after exercising, it may mean you have run out of fuel. You have depleted your supply of glucose and/or glycogen and your body wants to start replenishing it immediately. Pay attention to the amount of complex carbohydrates you are eating. You may want to start eating more as a part of your regular diet to build up glycogen levels.

While pre-exercise nutrition should consist of a high complex carbohydrate diet, post-exercise nutrition should include protein as well. Since you will need protein to rebuild or repair muscles and other tissues.

EXERCISE ALTERNATIVES

Doing the same exercises all the time develops certain of our muscles to the exclusion of others. Runners, for example, typically have very healthy internal body systems and well-developed legs, but they lack proportional upper-body strength. Combining different forms of exercise can help achieve a good balance of muscle activity throughout the body. Below are some aerobic alternatives to running.

Any aerobic exercise should be done three or four times a week for 20 to 30 minutes each time for maximum benefit. Start slowly, increasing the amount of time and intensity by about 10 percent every two weeks. Use good quality equipment, including proper foot gear. All sports require both pre- and post-game stretching.

After completing *any* aerobic exercise you should:
1.   Check your pulse. See if you have achieved your target heart rate. If you haven't, exercise a bit harder next time.
2.   Avoid hot showers, saunas, or whirlpools. Heat keeps the peripheral capillaries dilated, making it difficult for your blood to return to your heart right after exercise.
3.   Avoid strength exercises like weightlifting after doing aerobics. Weightlifting constricts blood capillaries so the blood does not return to your heart. Do them before the aerobic exercises or at another time.
4.   Rehydrate yourself, replacing body fluids lost doing exercise.

Cross-Country Skiing

Since weather or location may make this alternative difficult, indoor cross-country machines are available and can be used year round. Some experts even think that cross-country skiing is better aerobically than running, since in cross-country skiing you use more muscles than just those in your legs. The more muscles involved in exercise, the better the aerobic effect you get.

Swimming

Swimming is an outstanding cardiovascular exercise. It is rhythmic, uses all the major muscle groups, stretches the muscles and keeps you limber. The water's buoyancy reduces the pressure on bones and joints, pressure that can cause injuries in other sports. As a result, people unable to walk or jog because of a skeletal or structural problem often still can take up swimming.

If you are a nonswimmer, you can still take up a water sport. You can begin by taking your pulse while walking back and forth slowly in the waist-deep area of a pool. Swing your arms naturally when walking. Build up the intensity of this regimen to reach and maintain your target heart rate.

If you are a swimmer, take you pulse and do warm-up exercises. Once in the pool, start slowly and easily with a restful stroke, like the breast stroke or the side stroke. Build up slowly until you reach your target heart rate. You may eventually change to more intense strokes, such as the crawl or butterfly. Aim to swim for a full 20 minutes, even if you have to swim on your back for a while when you tire.

As with other aerobic exercises, swim for 20 to 30 minutes, three to four times a week. But be careful; daily swimming can lead to strained or pulled muscles. Skip a day to allow your body to recover. Periodically, try to increase your swimming speed by sprinting for up to 30 seconds at a time. As soon as you feel yourself winded, return to your normal pace. Repeat this three to five times in a row with a 30-second recovery interval between sprints. This type of interval training can enhance your cardiovascular conditioning.

Swimming builds powerful shoulders and arm muscles, as well as rear leg muscles. After swimming, stretch your rear leg muscles. And since the back stroke uses the anterior leg muscles more, they may also require additional stretching afterwards.

Wear a comfortable suit that will stay on without constant fuss and attention. The ideal pool water temperature is 77° to 81°F. Warmer water makes it difficult for the body to eliminate heat; colder water makes it difficult to warm up muscles.

There are some drawbacks to swimming. The biggest problem may be finding a pool. If you choose swimming, choose an alternate sport as well, for those times when a pool is not available.

Another disadvantage is the possibility of getting conjuctivitis or ear infections. You can protect yourself against both by wearing goggles and either a bathing cap or ear plugs. Select only good goggles—the cheap varieties are ineffective. Be sure not to use a nose plug if your nose is inflamed in any way, since that condition actually is better served by allowing the free circulation of moisture. Some people react badly to the chlorine in the water, especially, as is often the case, if the concentration is high.

Walking

Walking can be done by almost anyone, almost anywhere. For some, including the elderly, pregnant, arthritic, or those with heart disease, it is the only form of reasonable cardiovascular exercise. All you need is some comfortable old clothes, a good pair of running (walking) shoes, and a hat to protect you if the weather is hot and sunny or cold and windy.

Walking is a low-intensity exercise, so you have to do it for a longer time than a sport like running to get maximum cardiovascular conditioning. About 1¹/₂ hours of walking will give you the same aerobic effect as 30 minutes of running.

Walk with an even, rhythmic heel-to-toe gait; swing your arms from side to side in a natural way. Don't keep them pressed tightly against your body or in your pockets. Try not to carry anything since it will weigh you down and upset your balance.

Start by taking your pulse and doing the warm-up exercises. For the first two to three weeks, walk 20 to 30 minutes a day. Increase that to 1¹/₂ hours a day in 10 percent increments every two or three weeks. Begin each session by walking slowly, building up to your target heart rate, and then tapering off to a slow pace. Check your pulse every 10 minutes. If you feel tired, slow down or stop altogether until you recover. Then start slowly and build up your speed and heart rate again.

You can walk anywhere. First choice, and the most fun, is outdoors on a soft surface of grass or earth. If you walk in the street, be sure to face the traffic by walking on the left side. If the weather or your health do not permit you to go outdoors, walk indoors, up and down the hallway in your apartment building, or snake in and around the rooms in your home.

Cycling

Bicycle riding is excellent for the long distance runner. It works out the anterior leg muscles in the front of the leg, muscles that tend to weaken since running works the rear leg muscles more. By strengthening the anterior leg muscles, you can prevent knee and rear leg muscle injuries.

If you ride a bicycle very slowly, you need more time on it to gain proper cardiovascular conditioning. At the same time, if you sprint all the time you will lose any aerobic benefit as well, so never try to ride a bicycle to the point that you are exercising at over 80 percent of your maximum heart rate. However, you can do interval training, much like swimming, while you bike ride. Ride the bicycle as fast as you can for 30 seconds at a time.

Then rest for 30 seconds by riding at a normal pace. Do this three to five times in a row. Such interval training will help increase your aerobic capacity and stamina.

Remember to stretch out properly after bike riding. It is best to wear good biking shoes, since they transmit force to the pedals more efficiently. Walking and running shoes will do well, if you can't find biking shoes. You should use foot clips to secure your shoes to the pedals.

Bicycling causes less trauma to the joints and muscles than jogging or running. Still, problems can occur. In addition to collisions, the most common injuries are outer calf pain, knee pain, and chronic soreness of the hands.

Whether you use a 3-speed or 10-speed bicycle does not really matter. What does matter is that the bike is sturdy, that the frame is suited to your size and that it is kept in safe operating condition. Structurally, men's bikes are often sounder than women's, and for this reason many women buy them. Adjust the seat height so that you can pedal. Your knee should be almost straight when the pedal is closest to the ground, but even at that position, the leg should be slightly bent. Use pant clips or rubber bands to keep your pants from tangling in the chain. At night, dress so that you can be seen. A red leg light provides a moving signal of your presence on the road.

For exercising, you might want to use a bike with handlebars tilted upward, so you can sit up straight. Your bones will be in alignment, and such bikes are friendlier to your lower back than bikes with racing handles. For distance or racing, you will want to use downward tilted handlebars.

Riding indoors on a stationary bicycle is also beneficial. The same basic principles apply. The more interesting the exercise bicycle is, (for example, with built-in computers), the more the exercise will help hold your interest, reducing some of the boredom that you might otherwise experience.

Anybody who is able to ride a bicycle and at the same time read a novel or a magazine is not riding the bicycle hard enough to gain a cardiovascular benefit. Your concentration should always be on the sport itself.

Rope Jumping

Rope jumping, or jumping *without* a rope, gives you cardiovascular conditioning with a bonus: you can burn more calories per minute jumping rope than running, swimming, or bike riding. Jumping rope, however, can have a disastrous effect on the legs and lower back. Never start jumping for a *long* period of time. In the beginning, even a few minutes can be too long.

To begin properly, run in place, or walk in place, faster and faster, until your legs are coming off the ground at a very fast rate. Stay light on your feet. Avoid pounding them into the ground. Then, for a period of 10 to 20 seconds, start to jump very lightly on both feet at the same time. It is not necessary to jump high. Just keep jumping, and then after 30 seconds (with or without a rope), start walking or jogging in place again. Do this for a minute or two. As soon as you feel your breath return, start jumping again. Spend no more than 2 to 4 minutes jumping the first day. The older or heavier you are, the less you should do the first few times.

Never jump rope on a daily basis. It can lead to a lot of serious problems, since it can just be too stressful for the body. Increase your jumping time by about 10 percent every two weeks. This will allow your bones and musculature to develop proper stress build-up, as opposed to the overstress that would likely be caused by a too rapid increase, leading not only to calf pain and lower back pain, but to stress fractures of the bones in the leg and foot. Your ultimate aim is to jump for 20 to 30 minutes continuously. Interval training can be used with jumping rope, in much the same way described for swimming or bicycling.

Remember, duration is more important than intensity.

Rope jumping can be done in a small space, like a patio or small yard. In inclement weather, it can be done in a garage, basement or any room with a ceiling high enough for a rope to clear. A jump rope travels well; it packs easily and permits a workout almost anywhere.

To make a fine jump rope, you need a 3/8" nylon rope that measures double the length from the floor to your nipple, and two 6" PVC 1/2 pipes. You do not need bearings or digital counters. Simply monitoring your heart rate with a watch will tell you all you need to know.

Other Aerobic Alternatives

Other aerobic exercise alternatives include rowing (using a boat or rowing machine), roller skating, aerobic dancing, minitrampolining (or rebound jogging), and using a treadmill. You can also get aerobic effects from tennis, handball, racquet ball, squash, and basketball.

Chair stepping is an aerobic exercise, but we do not recommend it for *beginners*. It overstresses both your knees and heart.

POPULAR ANAEROBIC ALTERNATIVES

Each of the sports discussed below, as well as most others, actually fall somewhere between aerobic and anaerobic. They require explosive bursts of energy followed by longer periods of lower energy output or rest. They are anaerobic because they build one or all of the following in a concentrated effort: strength, power, endurance, or the skill of specific muscles or muscle groups.

Weight Training

Weight training can provide an excellent way for the runner to maintain strength and flexibility. By increasing the strength of all your muscles, not just those in your legs, you can increase your ability to withstand the stresses of long distance running. Also body parts that are weak tend to get injured much faster.

Arm, shoulder, and anterior leg muscle exercises should be emphasized in weight training. It is important, however, not to try to build up big muscles through weight training; this will only add to the weight and exercise burden you have to carry during running. While it is important to be strong, weight training can also tighten you up. Thus, flexibility and a range of motion programs as well as a good stretching program are needed to loosen you up.

Remember, allow a full 48 hours between weight-training sessions for the muscles to repair and heal since weight training breaks down muscle.

Start with low weights that are easy to lift. Do three sets of 8 to 12 repetitions. The last two repetitions should be difficult; your muscles strengthen only when they fatigue. The initial repetitions (or reps) result in muscle tone, the final reps give muscle strength. As soon as the last two reps become easy, it means it is time to increase the weights by a minimum of $2^1/_2$ pounds to a maximum of 10 pounds.

To build muscle mass, or "beach" muscles, use heavy weights and do fewer reps, about eight to ten. To improve tone, use light weights, and do more reps, about 12 to 15 per set.

As a rule, weight trainers think that athletes need to eat huge amounts of protein to rebuild and repair the muscle tissue broken down by exercise. In fact, athletes typically eat too much protein, and not enough complex carbohydrates (which are also excellent sources of protein).

Different forms of weight training will help increase general muscle strength. One involves the use of free weights. A second utilizes universal machines, and a third uses isokinetic, or Nautilus-type, training procedures. All three systems basically do the same thing. They help muscle become completely fatigued and so increase the size of the muscle fibers.

Free weights can be used at home as well as in an athletic club. But since it takes some time to prepare for each of the different exercises, it may seem to take a long time to get the effect you want. Free weights have to be used very carefully; they pose the most risks of all weight-training procedures.

They help develop better coordination, however, than other weight-training procedures.

Racket Sports

Tennis, racketball, squash, paddleball, and handball are basically discontinuous, stop-and-go sports. Players need power for explosive bursts of energy and stamina to run around the court. They come closest to aerobic activity when there are long volleys that result in the continuous use of large muscles.

Racket sports are very popular. Indoor and outdoor courts are abundant and many are accessible year round. To begin, find a place to play, and a good instructor who will guide you on proper technique, equipment and clothing.

Try to play with people who are at your level to avoid unnecessary tension and embarassment. Remember, exercise is supposed to benefit you—physically and spiritually.

Golf

Golfers need good neuromuscular coordination and focused concentration. The game is characterized by short bursts of energy interspersed with longer periods of slow activity or rest. Unfortunately, a good deal of stress builds up around each shot. Your caloric expenditure will depend totally on whether you walk (how far and how fast), or ride an electric cart around the five- or six-mile golf course. If you walk briskly between holes, you can approach some aerobic conditioning for brief periods of time.

To start, find a golf instructor who will guide you to appropriate equipment and clothing. It is best to learn proper stance and movement from the beginning, rather than later having to unlearn improper techniques.

If you are playing golf for exercise and pleasure, it can give you both. If you bring your business or social problems to the course, however, you lessen these benefits. Golfing in hot or humid weather can lead to dehydration. Drinking water before, during, and after play therefore becomes essential.

A 28-DAY EXERCISE PLAN

This comprehensive exercise program is designed for the runner or anyone serious about regular exercise who wants to develop and maintain good health. But for it to work, you must be willing to make a commitment to incorporate this gentle, realistic, exercise routine into your life-style. Exercise should be viewed in the same way as brushing your teeth, something to develop as a daily habit whose importance you recognize. Don't regard it as something extra you'll do if you have time after you do everything else. Exercise is part of everything else. Yet also understand you won't die if you miss a day.

The Basic 28-Day Exercise Plan calls for your choice of running or some other aerobic exercise on Days 1, 3, and 5. For the first 4 weeks, do the exercise for 20 minutes. Increase the duration by 10 percent every two weeks if you are under 35 years of age and have no history of heart disease. Increase the duration by 10 percent every 4 weeks if you are over 35 or have a history of heart disease.

These exercise plans are designed in one-week cycles, since most people plan their time that way. Day 1 of the exercise plan may be any day of the week. The sequence is what matters.

Your exercise program, to be viable, needs to reflect your goals, attitudes, strengths, weaknesses, and life-style. Use these suggested plans as guidelines; feel free to alter them to suit individual requirements.

When choosing aerobic alternatives, use both sides of your brain. Use the left side to choose activities that will enable you to get and keep your body functioning at your target heart rate for 20 to 30 minutes at least three days a week. Also be realistic in your expectations. So use the right side of your brain to evaluate activities that appeal to you.

Different exercises affect different muscles. You can combine two complementary exercises in your total program and rotate them according to whim or weather. You could have one indoor and one outdoor choice. For example, skiing and biking build up the anterior leg muscles while providing good aerobic conditioning. If you run outdoors and use a stationary bicycle indoors, you have come up with a set of complementary exercises good for all seasons. Either one could also be combined with swimming. There are outdoor and indoor pools. Weight training is a beneficial form of anaerobic exercise that augments any aerobic exercise. It can be done with free weights or an isokinetic machine, like the Nautilus.

When you purchase equipment, choose sturdy, safe, well-built, quality equipment. Junk breaks down quickly. Appropriate clothes and footgear are also important. Be particular about your running shoes. Perfect fit is critical.

Prior to starting any serious exercise or conditioning program, most people should have a complete physical exam, including a stress test. A cardiovascular stress test entails hooking you up to an electrocardiograph, which monitors your heart and blood pressure as you walk or run on a treadmill. The workload is increased at regular intervals. The results can indicate hidden or small conditions that could lead to trouble. Stress tests are done in various centers, hospitals, and some cardiologists' offices. If you are under 35 years of age, not overweight, and have no family history of heart disease, you probably do not need a stress test. A routine physical examination will do.

If for some reason you cannot or do not wish to have such an exam, the important point is to start and proceed very slowly. If any unusual signs manifest themselves, stop right away and check them out immediately with your doctor.

What time of day is best to exercise? If you guessed either morning, noon or night, you'd be right. There are three more facts to consider:

a. Most people are more flexible and looser (also more fatigued after a day's work) at about 6 P.M. So exercising in late afternoon takes advantage of the flexibility, pumps up energy to revitalize a tired body and reduces the tensions of the day. Exercising in early morning, on the other hand, takes advantage of a well-rested and fresh state of mind.

b. Each person needs to be in tune with his or her own body, following the monthly rhythms that seem to affect our intellect, mood, and physical energy levels. Do it when it feels good.

c. The right time for exercise is any time you manage to find in your busy schedule. It is best to plan your exercise.

If you feel exhausted, reduce the intensity and duration of any exercise by 50 percent. Your body is talking to you. Listen to it. That's good preventive sports medicine. The only legitimate reason for skipping your exercise is illness. Business is the worst excuse. You probably could use exercise most when you are under stress from work.

Relaxation, warm-ups and cool-down exercise should be used with all types of exercise: physical activity, aerobic, anaerobic, and all those in between. They maintain flexibility in muscles, tendons, ligaments, and joints, and help to prevent injury.

Too much, too fast, or too soon are the most common reasons for sport injuries. DO NOT OVERDO. Less is better—at the beginning—at least until your body adapts. Be in touch with your body to avoid injury and disillusionment because of some bad, though probably avoidable experience. Test yourself to see what affects your body. If you overdo, you will lose your sensitivity to the small clues your body will provide. So before beginning your Basic 28-Day Plan, review all cautions.

You are now ready to begin your Basic 28-Day Plan. It is a one-size-fits-all plan, and it is good for the rest of your life. The exercises will work for you as long as you do. There is a variation of the Basic Plan presented here if you wish to go beyond good health toward excellence, or have special fitness goals. Option A provides an opportunity for anaerobic exercise or sports. Option B adds interval training to aerobic exercise.

Steps 1 through 5 are the warm-up sequence: Relaxation, Nonspecific Warm-Up, Joint Warm-Up, Pre-sport Stretching, Specific Warm-Up. Together with Steps 7 and 8, the cool-down sequence (Post-sport Stretching and Cool-Down), they should be done every single day of your life to maintain good flexibility, circulation, balance, and a sense of well-being.

Step 6 is the slot in which you should put your running or chosen aerobic alternative. It is the one part of the sequence that will change from day to day, or from time to time, as your needs and goals change.

BASIC 28–DAY PLAN
(weeks 1–4)

DAY	STEPS	TIME
1	warm-ups (#1–5)	20 min.
	choice of aerobic exercise (#6)	
	cool-downs (#7–8)	
2	#1–5 & #7–8	
3	#1–8	
4	#1–5 & #7–8	
5	#1–8	
6	#1–5 & #7–8	
7	#1–5 & #7–8	

Repeat the 7–day sequence four times for a total of 28 days. Beginning on Day 1 of the fifth week (roughly the beginning of the second month), increase the time you exercise by 10 percent. Instead of 20 minutes, exercise aerobically for 22 minutes. Follow the increment schedule as described above until you reach the time limits listed below:

EXERCISE	TIME LIMIT
Walking	1½ hours
Running	30 minutes (unless you want to compete)
Swimming	45 minutes to 1 hour
Bicycling	30 minutes (unless you want to compete)
Jumping	30 minutes (due to high intensity of jumping, it is detrimental to go beyond this limit)

Monitor your pulse to be certain you are exercising within your target heart range. As you become more fit, and your body handles the stress of exercise more efficiently, you will have to work harder to get up to and stay at your target heart rate. Do this first by increasing duration until you reach the defined time limit, then by increasing intensity as measured by your heart rate.

This is a lifetime exercise plan. As such, it accomodates itself to you each year. On your birthday, recalculate your target heart range. The formula again is 220 minus your age times 70%.

If for reasons of your own you desire a more demanding schedule, do Step 6, your aerobic exercise, a fourth time during each week. A good choice is Day 6 or Day 7. If you decide to train for a marathon, you could train three days, rest one, train three days and rest one.

OPTION A

The 28-Day Plan's Option A suggests you choose an anaerobic exercise or sport to alternate with your aerobic exercise. Step 6 will be an aerobic exercise or sport one day a week. Option A is designed for persons who enjoy a particular sport, like tennis or golf, and want to incorporate it into their exercise regimen. It will also appeal to persons who want to develop stronger and more balanced musculature through weight training or calisthenics.

If you are enthusiastic about your sport and want to play twice a week, below is a suggested schedule to accomodate that. *Remember, you need to space bouts of anaerobic exercise at least 48 hours apart.* The intensity of such exercise breaks down tissue and it takes two full days to repair and recover from that stress.

The Basic Plan is sufficient to achieve and maintain optimal conditioning. Option A is only for those who want more.

Option A suggests an anaerobic exercise or sport on Days 2 and 5 (or only one day if you prefer). This allows you to include tennis or any other racket sport, golf, weight training, etc. You may choose to do calisthenics: 1) push-ups for the arms, shoulders, back, stomach and most of the body, 2) bent-knee sit-ups for the abdominal muscles, and 3) jumping jacks for the legs and shoulders. Start with a few of each and build up. Use proper form and technique with every repetition. If you get sloppy, you will get tired and then quit.

For the first four weeks of Option A, follow the Basic Plan. Begin here on Day 1 of week 5. Notice that on Days 2 and 5, Step 6 is anaerobic. On Days 1 and 3 continue your usual aerobic exercise—this time for 22 minutes each session.

Option A
(week 5)

DAY	STEPS	TIME
1	warm-ups (#1–5) choice of aerobic exercise (#6) cool-downs (#7–8)	22 min.
2	#1–8 #6 anaerobic	
3	#1–8 #6 aerobic	
4	#1–5 & 7–8	
5	#1–8 #6 anaerobic	
6	#1–5 & 7–8	
7	#1–5 & 7–8	

(week 6)

8	#1–8 aerobic	22 min.
9	#1–8 anaerobic	
10	#1–8 aerobic	
11	#1–5 & 7–8	
12	#1–8 anaerobic	
13	#1–5 & 7–8	
14	#1–5 & 7–8	

During weeks 7 and 8, increase the sessions by 10 percent if you are under 35 and have had no heart condition. The Step 6 aerobic exercises on Days 2, 5, 9, and 12 will be performed for 24 minutes. Repeat Days 1–14 for week 7 and 8 (Days 15–28).

At the beginning of week 9, increase the time again by 10 percent to:

a. 26 minutes of aerobic exercise if you are under 35 and do not have a heart condition;

b. 24 minutes of aerobic exercise if you are over 35 or have a history of heart problems.

If you feel like having a heavy workout, you may do your aerobic exercise AFTER your anaerobic exercise or sport. For example, you may want to swim after tennis. That's fine. *But do not do anaerobic after aerobic. It interferes with the body's ability to recover properly.*

If you reach a plateau, or a point in your regimen you cannot get past, yet you feel you have not reached your physiological limit, seek professional guidance. Something you are doing (or not doing properly) could be imposing a limitation. You could be getting in your own way. Or it may just be that your body can't work any harder.

OPTION B

This option adds interval training one or two days a week to the aerobic exercise in Step 6 of the Basic 28-Day Plan. This option is for those who strive for excellence in cardiovascular fitness, beyond what it takes to stay in good physical condition. This is not training for marathoners, but for those who want to do a bit more to improve their stamina, endurance and conditioning.

Interval training can be done with any aerobic exercise. For example, if you were running, you would run at your target heart rate for 10 minutes. Then run to get your pulse to beat as close to your maximum heart rate as possible (220 minus age times 85%) for 30 seconds. Then run at your target heart rate (220 minus age times 70%) for 30 seconds. Repeat 4 consecutive times during one exercise period. Increase by one repetition every month to a limit of 10 times.

There are cautions to be observed in interval training. The high-intensity nature of this kind of training can lead to injury, and *it is not recommended for persons who have heart desease or other serious medical problems unless they have a doctor's approval.*

Interval training is anaerobic, so the cautions regarding anaerobic exercise hold. A full 48 hours is required between anaerobic exercise periods to allow for recovery from the stress it causes.

Once a week for this kind of conditioning is recommended. If you have specific fitness goals, you may choose to do interval training twice a week. The plan schedules it twice to demonstrate the ideal spacing. Four sets are enough to fatigue most people. A set consists of a 30-second sprint plus a 30-second rest.

Do not attempt to *combine* the Basic Plan with Option A and Option B. It is too much to add both anaerobic and interval training to aerobic exercise without professional guidance.

Option B
(week 5)

DAY	STEPS	TIME
1	warm-ups (#1–5)	22 min.
	choice of aerobic exercise (#6)	
	cool-downs (#7–8)	
2	#1–5 & #7–8	
3	#1–8 with interval	
4	#1–5 & 7–8	
5	#1–8 without interval	
6	#1–8 without interval	
7	#1–5 & #7–8	

Repeat above for Days 8–14 (week 6).

Thereafter increase time by 10 percent every two weeks until you reach the time limit for that particular exercise as listed under the Basic Plan.

RUNNING A MARATHON

If you are really serious about exercise and about running in particular, you may someday go the final distance—like the ancient Greek Olympic athletes—and train to run a marathon. Here are a few sensible and practical tips for those who want to go that extra distance.

Top marathon runners seem to follow training routines in which they run 110-150 miles a week. This does not constitute normal training. If the average runner attempted this kind of regimen, it would probably end up totally wrecking his or her body.

The best way to train for a marathon is to do it gradually. Start with three miles, five days a week for the first month. Increase it one mile a day for the next three months, taking off one day and adding a longer run on Sunday. Increase until you are able to do six miles a day, let's say, Tuesday, Wednesday, Thursday, and Friday, rest Saturday, and do 12 miles on Sunday, for 36 miles a week. When you run 24 miles during the week and 22 miles on Sunday, you have a total of 46 miles a week. If one of the days during the week is for interval training (faster training), you will get both speed and endurance.

Consistency is very important when you train. So is getting enough rest. If you run seven days a week, your body never gets a chance to recuperate. If, on the other hand, you do a 20-mile run on Sunday, rest on Monday, loosen up with four miles on Tuesday, do eight miles on Wednesday, skip Thursday, run ten miles on Friday, and skip Saturday, you would be doing the same mileage with three day's rest. You should definitely rest the day before a marathon. Remember you will also need about approximately one day of rest for every mile after you race.

It's also important to keep a diary while you train. There are many factors that will impact your performance, including biorhythms and circadian rhythms, and keeping track of the way you feel can help you understand these subtle cycles.

Pacing

Try to focus in on your pacing. Keep a stopwatch so that you know, within two or three seconds every mile how well you're doing. Shifting pace throughout a long race can be very stressful on the body. If you start out slower and get faster in six-mile increments, you will be doing much better. Because of changes in blood and brain chemistry, proper pacing will improve the way you feel during a long run.

A marathon is tricky. You may feel like you have energy right up to the 23rd mile, and then suddenly, it's gone. Your muscles are tight, and you feel lucky even to be able to walk. Suddenly at the 24-mile mark, your legs might say, "I quit," and then you find yourself, with thousands of others, starting to walk. It happens because those people, in all likelihood, didn't do one or some of the following: They didn't eat properly; they didn't properly pace themselves in their training; they started their exercise program too vigorously, or they peaked weeks before the race.

Water

It is crucial to properly hydrate yourself before, during, and after a marathon. Drink at least a pint of water before the race. During a marathon, you need to have water *every* mile.

The best thing to do is have a plastic water container with a sipper in it. When you pick it up, you can sip it as you run for a mile. People who run races in areas where they have friends generally have two or three people throughout the course of the race helping them with water.

Diluted grape juice in your water gives you extra glucose, so that you're delaying the time that your body will have to rely upon the extra glycogen it has stored up. In effect, you're always keeping your reserve in reserve. When other people hit the 20-mile mark and their glycogen and glucose are gone, they're out of energy, not you.

Form

Keep your head high, breathe through your mouth, and keep your shoulders loose. Your hands and arms should not be swinging; the wristbone should be at the level of the hipbone. If you hold your arms higher, you'll cause a muscle contraction that will cause fatigue in that muscle group. When muscle fatigue in the shoulders causes the arms to be raised higher, the shoulders slump forward, the neck drops down, and you'll get less air and your cells will get less oxygen. Try to keep your feet close to the ground, almost in a shuffle motion, with your knees slightly bent. You don't want to be running stiff-legged because that can jar the knees. Your body should be slightly bent forward at the waist. When you're running uphill, elbows should be elevated slightly behind you; run more toward the ball of the foot and take shorter steps. Again, your knees should be bent. Your shoulders should be forward to take advantage of the momentum you'll get coming down.

Gear

Most runners tend to wear a pair of running shoes for a longer time than those shoes are able to provide good support. Run-down heels can lead to the displacement of musculo-skeletal structure and subsequent hip problems, tendonitis and strains. Yet they are not the only sign of the end of a shoe's serviceability. A good athletic supply store can help determine the condition of your running shoes.

Make sure that the back lip of the shoe, where the heel is, has been cut off. It serves no purpose, and it can actually dig into the Achilles tendon every time you move, bruising it.

Make sure you wear tight, thin socks. Heavy socks tend to bunch up because of sweat, giving you blisters. Improperly worn socks, more than anything else, also will give you blisters. Put vaseline around all your toes, around the ball of your foot, and around the heel. Also put vaseline in your crotch, around your breasts, under your armpits.

In cold weather, it's important to avoid overdressing, because trapped perspiration can lead to severe chills.

In warmer weather, wear clothes that permit free perspiration. Never wear sweat suits.

Diet

On the sixth, fifth, and fourth days before a marathon, you should eat only protein, three times a day. Animal protein is not recommended. You could have soybean powder, or protein powder, or tofu—in other words, a high-quality protein.

On the three days immediately prior to the race, you should have no protein, just complex carbohydrates. On the day before the race, cut out fruits and salads. Try to eat something that will be only partially through your intestines during the race.

That night, have something about an hour before you go to sleep. Try to retire around midnight. This will be a major meal because you want to really saturate your body with glycogen. You could have buckwheat pasta, or brown rice, and if you're not allergic to wheat, you could have whole grain pasta or whole grain bread. Avoid greasy, highly seasoned and sugary foods.

In the morning, if it's at least four hours before the race, you could blend two bananas with grape juice. This will give you additional carbohydrates that will help you through the race, digested in your system before the race. Eat no solid food before the race. Your body's system will be too nervous. When you're nervous and anxious, your body doesn't digest normally. Electrolyte replacers are very important. Try to have two of the electrolytes (like potassium or magnesium) prior to a marathon, one every five miles during the race, and two at the end.

Before and After

Try and get a full-body massage, a Shiatsu massage, or a reflexology massage the day before the marathon. It's also important to float, if possible. Do an isolation tank float one or two days during the week before the marathon, preferably the day before, along with guided imagery.

When you've finished your race, don't just stop running and walk. Take at least 12 minutes to cool down by going from your running pace to a jog, a slower jog, and then a brisk walk. *Never* go directly into a sauna, hot tub, hot bath, or hot shower.

Always enjoy what you're doing and what you've accomplished.

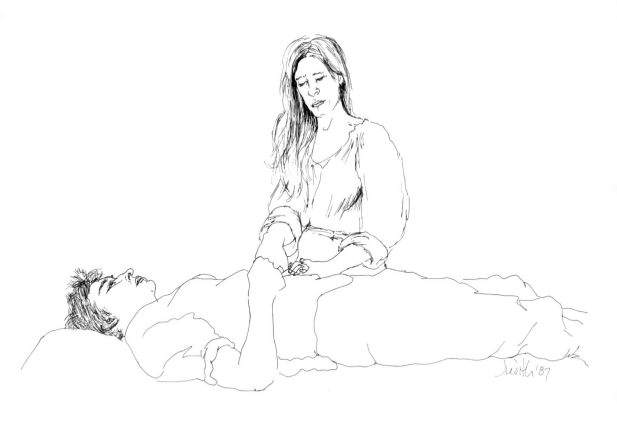

16 · SELECTING AN ALTERNATIVE HEALTH PRACTITIONER

"Frequent colds, recurring infections, and fatigue are all part of the warning mechanisms used by the body to signal an under-functioning immune system. But they are rarely recognized as such. The phenomenal sales of cold remedies, for example, reflect how little attention is paid to strengthening the immune system—an approach that would far more effectively reduce the incidence of these disorders."

ULTIMATELY, YOU ARE RESPONSIBLE for your own well-being, but having access to proper health care practitioners is an important element in health maintenance. Their educated guidance and treatment can be invaluable, both in times of uncertainty and crisis and for prevention and awareness building during times of complete well-being.

Alternative health practitioners can help define the weak links in your body's structure and function and then direct you toward optimal personal care. There are many different approaches, but some general guidelines are worth mentioning here.

A good holistic medical practitioner will perform at least these three basic types of analysis before prescribing any treatment plan:

1) Take a detailed medical history.

2) Perform a physical examination that goes beyond conventional methodologies.

3) Study carefully the results of appropriate laboratory tests taken at the time of the history taking and the physical examination.

In addition, you have the right to expect that the practitioner includes in his or her repertory, some or all of the following:

• as many noninvasive diagnostic techniques as possible;

• an awareness of the potential diagnostic value of even very minor signs and symptoms in the prevention of major dysfunction;

• a preference for noninvasive over invasive techniques (For example, substances will be administered orally rather than intravenously, except when a condition calls for the more direct route.);

• a recognition of the importance of strengthening the body's resistive capacities and an interest, wherever possible, in attempting to repair any malfunctioning organ or gland rather than to replace its function through the administering of its secretions;

• a tendency, whenever possible, to treat the primary weak link first if more than one has been discovered (For example, if the stomach is producing insufficient hydrochloric acid, resulting in the malabsorption of calcium, among other substances, the resulting calcium deficiency could lead to osteoarthritis, periodontal disease, or skin problems; by treating the hydrochloric acid insufficiency, the physician would be treating the primary weak link.);

• an approach that treats the person as a whole person, not just a collection of ailing parts;

• the demonstrated ability to listen carefully and to skillfully classify any relevant symptoms in order to arrive at the best possible diagnosis;

• an orientation toward optimal health and sensitivity to dysfunctions that signal an imbalance in the individual;

• familiarity with a combination of approaches to help the person regain balance (For example, in addition to orthodox treatments, the physician's recommendations may include advice about stress reduction and life-style changes to reduce or elminate causative factors in the environment.);

• a willingness to refer the individual, when the condition warrants, to other medical practitioners whose specialized knowledge in a given area may be necessary to provide the most valuable restorative program; and

• a demonstrated awareness of the importance of the individual's own attitudes toward health and disease, and a willingness to communicate openly with the individual.

The alternative health practitioner should expect you to be an active, committed participant in the process, and not a passive, disinterested patient who accepts everything the doctor recommends.

ASKING THE RIGHT KINDS OF QUESTIONS

One form of this active participation may be the questions you ask with a view to getting the important information you need to help you in your contributions to the healing process. Some examples are:

• What, specifically, is being treated?
• How do you know that that's the problem?
• What are some realistic goals in my situation?
• What is the time frame?
• Does every individual with this condition get exactly the same tests, the same treatments?
• What are my weak links?
• Are these tests and this treatment relevant to my body and my condition?

THE IMPORTANCE OF COMMONPLACE SYMPTOMS

Many people are living with symptoms that, because they are mild and do not constitute a full-blown disease state, are accepted, needlessly, as being an inevitable consequence of getting older. In fact, such people are often told by their conventional physicians: "Nothing is wrong with you. Everything is normal." And yet, the symptoms may be early warnings that something is out of balance.

Gas in the lower bowel (flatulence), belching, heaviness in the stomach, heartburn and bloating, for example, may all be indicators of a malfunctioning digestive system, depending on their frequency and severity. These conditions are not normal in a healthy state, and they are often correctable.

Similarly, many of the symptoms that accompany delayed allergic reactions (the masked, cyclical allergies) are widely accepted as normal, and therefore to be tolerated for no better reason than "that's the way it is." The failure to recognize a connection between these symptoms and allergies may be due to the fact that they do not appear for upwards of thirty hours after the ingestion of the offending food or chemical substance. Typical symptoms are headache, irritability, anxiety, sudden changes of mood, and excessive fatigue, as well as unexplained body aches and pains. These symptoms may not be severe enough to be labeled as disease states, so the underlying cause is repeatedly overlooked or denied by traditional practitioners. Even when the disorders are recognized, their true significance may still be missed by those who try to reverse the symptoms without addressing the underlying causes for their appearance. Thus frequent colds, recurring infections, and fatigue are all part of the warning mechanisms used by the body to signal an under-functioning immune system. But they are rarely recognized as such. The phenomenal sales of cold remedies, for example, reflect how little attention is paid to strengthening the immune system—an approach that would far more effectively reduce the incidence of these disorders.

TYPES OF PRACTITIONERS

It has never been my policy to make specific recommendations, to suggest to a person that a specific practitioner is the best doctor for them to see. The quality of a doctor's health care may depend on both the physician and the patient, as well as on their mutual compatibility. This is not something I, or anyone else, could predict in advance. But I still feel that people should be given some direction. So, what I have done here is supplied a directional guide. It is not meant to be a recommendation. Rather, I have offered some general guidelines. I have concentrated on modalities that the reader may not have easy access to. Chiropractors and osteopaths, for example, are not listed here. Nor are nutritionists listed here, although the experienced holistic nutritionist may be enormously helpful in helping you get the most from your diet.

Homeopathy, Chelation Therapy, Orthomolecular Medicine, Acupuncture, Clinical Ecology, and Naturopathy may be extremely useful when used properly, representing viable alternatives to conventional medical orthodoxies. Selecting the right health care professional can be an important decision that will benefit you for the rest of your life. In this chapter I have tried to provide the overview on how to go about finding and evaluating such a person. If I have succeeded in putting you on the right track, this may be one of the most important chapters in this book. Then go on to Part Five, where I go into more detail regarding some particularly difficult health topics, to help keep you on top of any lingering health problems you or a loved one may have.

HOMEOPATHY

Homeopathy is based on the principle that what causes illness may follow a law of similars, meaning that by giving a healthy person a dilute amount of that which is a causative agent can in fact help the body rebalance itself. If a person has a head cold, you would give the person a substance that would cause cold symptoms in a healthy person, but in a sick person it helps to cure them. Homeopathy is limited in scope at this time in the United States, although one hundred years ago it was the prevailing form of medicine—until allopathic medicine and the American Medical Association in particular launched an intensive drive against it, which culminated in its being virtually banned in this country. Very recently, there has been a renewed interest in homeopathy, and growing numbers of physicians are using its principles. The homeopath must be a medical doctor in addition to his or her homeopathic specialization. Homeopathy is particularly useful in the treatment of fevers, bacterial infections, toxicity, and the cumulative effects of alcohol, drugs, tobacco, caffeine, or sugar. It is not recommended for cancer, AIDS (acquired immune deficiency syndrome), or heart disease.

CHELATION THERAPY

Chelation Therapy is a relatively new medical science, having started only about a quarter of a century ago. There are at this time nearly 1,000 doctors, including many board-certified cardiologists, who are using chelation therapy. The modality involves an intravenous drip of a substance known as EDTA, a chelating agent. The agent helps stimulate the destruction of free radicals, which seem to be a primary causative agent of the aging process itself. By slowing down the destructive potential of these free radicals, it allows the cells to heal themselves. As the cells heal, they are more able to fight off whatever infection or disease affects us. Claims have been made that chelation therapy can open up the arteries. Moreover, objective data has substantiated this. Improvement of vascular circulation in people who had obstructed arteries, especially those to the brain and to the extremities, has been demonstrated following treatment with this modality.

Chelation therapy runs about $100 per visit and patients generally have from 20 to 40 visits, depending on the severity of the condition. People are also begun receiving chelation therapy as a preventative treatment to slow down the aging process, based on the view that free radicals are a primary factor of the aging process. The treatment may be problematic, however, for patients with kidney disease, and renal monitoring is crucial. A physician must be certified as a practicing chelating therapist to perform the therapy.

ORTHOMOLECULAR MEDICINE (See Ch. 19)

Orthomolecular physicians and orthomolecular psychiatrists are conventionally trained medical doctors with an additional specialization. The purpose of orthomolecular medicine is the establishment of the right balance of the chemicals naturally occurring in the body. They try to rebalance the chemicals within the body without using synthetic drugs that might interfere with natural processes. Their goal is homeostasis, or balance. Frequently, orthomolecular physicians use a high-dosage vitamin regimen, far higher than what the average physician would ever presume would be needed. But it is their experience that only with these very high amounts, these megadoses, do they see the best results. For example, orthomolecular psychiatrists have had striking success in the treatment of schizophrenics, putting the condition into remission by using massive doses of niacin (B_3), B_6, and vitamin C—amounts that you would never give a healthy person. Orthomolecular psychiatrists are also better able to treat depression, by examining possible chemical imbalances in the brain. Moreover, orthomolecular physicians have the benefit of being able to use psychoanalysis or psychotherapy if deemed necessary, but that would be as a last resort. The cost of treatment is comparable to that for conventional physicians.

ACUPUNCTURE

Acupuncturists work by opening up blocked energy pathways, or meridians, so that healing energy can go directly to a particular point in the body where it is needed, therefore stimulating the innate natural healing capacity of the body. The acupuncturist, in this country, must also be a medical doctor. Acupuncturists are particularly good for nerve problems, pain, musculo-skeletal problems, but not for cancer or heart disease. The cost of treatment may range from $75 to a $100 per visit.

CLINICAL ECOLOGY (See Ch. 20)

Clinical ecologists are unique in that they are able to closely examine the relationship between the elements of a person's diet and any symptoms they may be experiencing. For example, a person's irritable bowel may be due to consumption of milk. The clinical ecologist will be able to identify this causative factor. He or she examines all the different foods, inhalants, and liquids that a person consumes to see which one of these, or which combinations, may be causing a physical or mental reaction. This modality has been particularly successful, for example, in the treatment of symptoms of arthritis. One clinical ecologist, Dr. Marshall Mandell, has been able to eliminate all arthritic symptoms in about 80 percent of his patients using a four-day rotating and elimination diet, preceded by an initial five-day fast in a clinically controlled environment. Clinical ecologists tend to use a far broader arsenal of treatments than the traditional allergist. Outside of the initial visit, the cost of seeing a clinical ecologist is no more than for a conventional physician, ranging from $40 to $75, depending on the state. The initial visit may vary from $125 to $500, depending on which tests are performed and the time required.

NATUROPATHY

Naturopathic physicians can treat most conditions. They are not, however, allowed to perform major surgery (although they can perform minor surgery). Their very extensive background is centered in the botanical sciences, including the use of herbs and tinctures, with a wide variety of natural immune-stimulating properties. The naturopath practices a natural form of health care the traditions of which precede the advent of modern medicine, not unlike the traditional Tibetan physician who must be able to identify nearly a thousand different healing herbs, mineral sources, and animal sources. The naturopath has years of extensive study in the healing potential of such substances. He or she is also able to understand muscular and skeletal bodily adjustment. Naturopaths use a much broader basis for diagnosis than do conventional allopathic physicians. Finally, the naturopath is usually a very good teacher as well. Not only do you get a therapy, you also generally get an education about the nature of your condition and the rationale behind the therapy. Naturopaths tend to be relatively inexpensive, generally in the neighborhood of $40 to $60 per visit.

Part Five

Where Health

Fits In

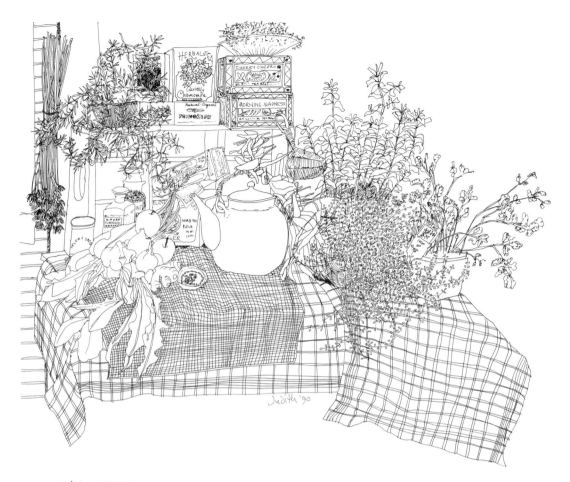

17 · BRINGING HERBS INTO YOUR DAILY LIFE

"Considered the master herb by the Chinese, ginseng is probably the most researched herb in the world. . . . Its powers to help the body cope with stress are so dramatic and far-ranging that a new term, "adaptogen," has been defined to describe it."

Some of the experts on herbs and herbal medicine who have contributed their knowledge to this chapter are: Dr. Paul Lee, director of the Platonic Academy in Santa Cruz, California; Jeanne Rose, author of Herbal Guides to Inner Health *and* The Herbal Body Book; *herbologist Ed Burke; Dr. David Festighi, author of* The End of Disease: Talking about Ginseng; *Dr. Ray Wunderlicht, Jr., an orthomolecular physician practicing in St. Petersburg, Florida; and Dr. Edward Alstadt, a Naturopathic physician.*

217

A BRIEF HISTORY
OF HERBALISM

HERBS HAVE BEEN USED for healing for as far back as we can trace the existence of man. In a Neanderthal grave in Iraq some 60,000 years old, scientists found pollens belonging to eight plants, seven of which are still used medicinally by the people in that area. The Chinese *Shennong Herbal* lists 365 herbal drugs; it has been historically dated back to 200 B.C., but legend credits it to the emperor Shennong, of around 2700 B.C. And herbalism was not limited to the East. It reached a peak in England in 1653, when Nicholas Culpeper published his *Complete Herbal*, the first and greatest herbal work in the English vernacular.

Yet soon after that time the pendulum swung away from the use of herbs, which had become inextricably tangled with magic, myth, and astrology. The Church of Rome objected to these pagan practices; the Swiss physician Paracelsus began to use inorganic cures like mercury and antimony instead of herbals in the sixteenth century, heralding the near-monopoly of chemical-based medicine which would last until today.

The first determined effort in the modern Western world to break this pharmaceutical monopoly came from America in the eighteenth century. Samuel Thomson, the son of a farmer, lived during a time of great yellow fever epidemics; the accepted medical practice in curing this (and almost any other) ailment was a liberal use of bleeding and mercury, which a healthy patient would be lucky to live through. Thomson instead used herbs and steaming—with great success—but was met with hostility from the orthodox medical establishment, and even imprisoned briefly.

In the nineteenth century herbal medicine made a popular comeback. So broad and exaggerated were the claims made for various tinctures, potions, "patent" medicines, and favorite cure-alls like mandrake root, however, that this popularity only contributed to a medical bias against herbal remedies. Modern science's success in synthesizing powerful drugs and the advent of highly rational double-blind testing procedures has confirmed this bias further.

Recently there has been another rebirth of popular interest in herbal remedies. A facsimile edition of Culpeper's *Complete Herbal* is one of a number of herbals that have been successfully published in the last decade. Yet the government has been indifferent or actively hostile to new studies which suggest that ancient beliefs about the healing powers of herbs have scientific foundation. The antipathy of the medical orthodoxy, the AMA, and government bodies like the FDA to herbs as medicine or even as nutrition has grounds in several factors. In the age of double-blind testing and standard doses herbs are difficult to quantify or analyze.

Sometimes a single chemical component can be isolated and purified or synthesized. Digitalin, used to treat heart disease, was isolated from the foxglove plant; quinine from the bark of the quinoa tree; salicylic acid (aspirin) from willow bark; and on and on. But herbal medicine is by nature an inexact, individualized science. Herbs may work differently on different people; the conditions under which a plant has grown, the time at which it is harvested, or the form which its preparation takes may all modify its effect. And despite successes such as aspirin and quinine, the "scientific" method of isolating, analyzing, and extracting the active ingredient in a plant often doesn't work very well. A chemical which might be isolated as *the* active component in an herb may in fact be modified by other, less obvious constituents which make it more powerful or moderate its side effects. And sometimes, even with rigorous research, the ways in which a plant affects the body can remain stubbornly mysterious; though there are many theories about ginseng, for example, it is not clear exactly how it boosts resistance to stess.

A second, no less powerful reason for the hostility of the AMA, particularly, toward herbal remedies is the threat which they present to the vastly powerful, multibillion-dollar pharmaceutical industry. Herbal remedies cannot be standardized, packaged, and marketed like drugs; they can usually be grown and prepared by anyone and cannot be patented; in many cases they cut into the consumption of over-the-counter and prescription medicines. The pharmaceutical companies underwrite the very existence of the AMA. The pressure of the AMA and the pharmaceutical industry has dictated that herbs may be treated as food additives but not in any way as medications; the law forbids labeling any herb in connection with a specific affliction.

Other modern countries have no such hostility to the complementary use of herbal remedies within an orthodox medical framework. In 1958 Chairman Mao urged that China's traditional sciences of herbal medicine and acupuncture should not be abandoned; China's goal now is to develop a medicine which combines both the ancient and the new. For instance, herbal tonics are often used to strengthen a patient's ability to cope with modern chemotherapy. Russia has been committed to research on herbs, carrying out hundreds on Siberian ginseng alone, which has even been used to combat stress on Russian cosmonauts. Even in Britain, the National Institute of Medical Herbalists (created in 1864 as the National Association of Medical Herbalists) is a flourishing—and scientifically respected—body.

THE PRACTICAL USE OF HERBS

You don't have to be a herbalist, know complicated formulas, study the chemistry of plants, or learn the Chinese philosophies of herbal medicine to enjoy the benefits that herbs can bring into your life. If you are a novice in the world of herbs, go to a bookstore or library for books in their health and diet sections. Start small, with perhaps five herbs—some good ones to try first might be garlic, rosemary, comfrey, echinacea, and thyme. (Some herbs and their benefits, along with recommendations for the forms and quantities that they can be taken in, are listed below.) The best way to begin to use herbs is the simplest; incorporate them into your cooking in progressively increasing amounts, or make a tea of one or more herbs. Cookbooks already often recommend the kinds of herbs that go well with different foods, but make your own experiments. Just put a few pinches in the stew pot, sprinkle them over a salad, or mix a little with a sandwich spread. Also, start reading the labels on the herbal tea boxes at the supermarket. Pick out a tea you think would taste good. Add an herbal tincture to your shampoo, your skin lotion or massage oil, or your bath tub. Within a short period of time, you will have incorporated a number of different herbs into your life. And you should start feeling better naturally.

Remember, though, not all herbs are equal. How they are grown, harvested, stored, and prepared will effect their potency and usefulness. Fresh and homegrown is always best, because you know the conditions under which herbs have been planted, monitored, fertilized, and cared for. Many nurseries sell not only herb seedlings but kits that can be used to conveniently grow herbs on the windowsills of city apartments. Investment in a full-spectrum light tube will even allow you to grow herbs on the kitchen counter. If you live in the country and you really know which plants you are looking for, some herbs can be collected wild. Be careful, though; some toxic plants can look very like useful herbs. It would be best to have someone with an expert knowledge of wild plants in your area along at first. A city dweller should not pick herbs that are just growing in the streets. With people, animals, and traffic circulating around them, such herbs can actually become quite toxic.

When buying herbs from a store, especially in bulk, make sure you use your senses of smell and sight. The herb shouldn't seem dusty or have a moldy aroma. If it looks more brown than green, then it will definitely have reduced effectiveness. Consumers ought to insist on fresh herbs if they're buying in bulk in herbal stores. The more information you can get about where the herb was grown, how it was cultivated, and when it was harvested, the better. Stay away from potent dried herbs in powder or capsule form. They generally have not been tested for safety or efficacy and are all too often a rip-off. It is almost impossible to determine what the actual ingredients of a powder inside a capsule are; you have no way of telling the age of such a preparation or even if it is made from the herb it claims to be.

Also, some people may have allergic reactions or other problems with specific herbs. To test those sensitivities, use one herb at a time at first. Try them out, see what they're like, see which plants are for you, taste and smell them. If one causes no problem, add another.

As well as fresh herbs and dried herbs, there are several other forms in which herbal medicines can be taken. Often the form in which an herbal remedy is prepared is as important in therapeutic terms as which herb is used. *Infusions* and *decoctions*, two of the simpler forms, are both made with boiling water. Infusions are made by pouring boiling water over dried or fresh herbs, while roots and barks are boiled in water and left to steep as they cool. Distilled or spring water is preferable; the traditional proportion is about one ounce of dried herb to a pint of water. The pot or cup should be covered to prevent the escape of volatile oils; it should not be made of aluminum, which can enter the preparation in minute amounts.

Tinctures are made by macerating herbs in a mixture of water and alcohol for at least two weeks. Water extracts many constituents of plants, but oils, gums, and resins are most efficiently extracted in alcohol, which also preserves the preparation. The strength of the alcohol varies; vodka or brandy can be used to make tinctures at home. Some herb liqueurs, such as Chartreuse, were originally a kind of therapeutic remedy in the tradition of the monks who made them, although they no longer have these properties. *Ointments*, which are useful to treat some skin conditions, can be made with herbs and oils.

HERBS AND THE IMMUNE SYSTEM

One area in which herbs can play a vital role in our day-to-day lives is by stimulating our immune systems. Many people find that their health seems to be sapped by recurring or chronic colds and viruses; synthetic drugs, far from being a solution, seem to be merely encouraging new, more resistant strains of bacteria and viruses. Those people with more serious immune problems, like AIDS and cancer, too, can help their systems to fight back as much as possible by using herbs to stimulate a healthy immune system.

Dr. Paul Lee, the founder of the Platonic Academy in Santa Cruz, California, is one of America's leading authorities on the use of herbs for immune health and overall well-being. Dr. Lee links herbology, immunology, and molecular biology together in his theory that there is an herb code in our immune memory which is carried by our DNA. One of the most phenomenal aspects of our immune system is this immune memory, genetically transmitted from our ancestors, which records their own struggle against illness and disease. When the Spanish conquistadors brought smallpox into Mexico, three and a half million Mexican Indians died; they had no immune memory to ward it off.

No one in the world dies from smallpox today, because the World Health Organization has effectively eliminated it. But despite all our triumphs in conquering diseases, it seems that cancer and other immune diseases have taken their place. Dr. Lee believes that our generation is suffering from a kind of immune amnesia. We have become detached from the botanical basis of health care and the medicinal herbs which are the natural agents of our immunity.

The body's ancient natural response to herbs is evident to anyone who has grown them. The aroma of specific herbs brings a unique and clear reaction. Anyone with any familiarity with herb gardening would never mistake thyme for oregano or oregano for rosemary, even with their eyes closed. The recent development of aromatherapy is a recognition of the power of our genetic memory of certain herbal substances, which responds to just the smell of them.

Most humans in the modern world have lost the ancient talent for "intuitive herbalism" that ancient cultures recognized, and that animals still possess. Dogs and cats will nibble certain grasses when they feel ill. More startling is an observation of African chimpanzees recorded in the *International Herald Tribune* in 1986, showing that sick chimps methodically seek out the leaves from a bush called Aspilia, keep them in their mouths for about fifteen seconds, and then swallow them whole. Analysis showed that the Aspilia leaves contain a powerful antibiotic chemical. Humans, however, have largely forgotten how to select herbs that they need to keep their immune responses healthy. Certain herbs can augment immunity because we're coded or programmed for them; this needs to be reactivated in our generation because one of the worst health problems that faces Americans today is a collective deterioration of the immune system. If we could restore a botanical emphasis to health care in a widespread way, it would make a great contribution to public health.

Rather than just concentrating on a better immune system, however, look at your system as a whole. As much as possible, consider the elements which contribute to your condition: lifestyle, stress, clinical and subclinical infection, toxins, and anything else that would divert the immune system from functioning properly. Then, with all this in mind, examine the herbs that can help you in these areas.

Although it is important to try to treat the body as a whole for almost any disorder, some herbs can be suggested as specifics for weakness or disorder in one system or organ. (More information on each herb is contained in the Glossary of Herbs below.) A few suggestions follow:

Antibiotics: Dandelion, garlic, goldenseal, marigold, myrrh, and thyme.

Arthritic disorders: Alfalfa, cayenne and feverfew for pain relief, and sarsaparilla.

Blood-clotting: Cinnamon helps mild passive hemorrhaging.

Circulation/Heart tonics: Barberry, blackberry, and, especially, hawthorn.

Cholesterol reduction: Cayenne, ginger, and garlic.

Cleansing and detoxification: Barberry, blackberry leaves and fruit, celery, chaparral, goldenseal, rosemary, and seaweeds.

Colds and flus: Cayenne, chaparral, garlic, osha, and thyme.

Digestive system: Alfalfa, barberry, celery, chamomile, cinnamon, comfrey, and marigold.

Diuretics: Dandelion and celery.

Immune enhancement: Astragalus, echinacea, garlic, ginseng, goldenseal, marigold, pau d'arco, suma, turmeric (especially for allergies), and wild indigo root.

Liver tonics: Dandelion and milk thistle.

Nervous system/Brain tonics: Avena, chamomile, ginseng, and rosemary.

Pain reduction: Cayenne and feverfew.

Respiratory tract: Cayenne, garlic, and milk thistle.

A GLOSSARY OF HERBS

Alfalfa (*Medicago sativa*), used as a tea or eaten whole as sprouts in a salad, is rich in a variety of vitamins and minerals, as its roots can reach as far as thirty feet into the ground to gather up essential minerals. Alfalfa is also plentifully stocked with enzymes that can help in the digestive process. Alfalfa is used as a tonic to increase vitality, appetite, and weight—interestingly, it is fed to horses for the same reason. The root of tooth-leaved clover, a close relative of alfalfa (which, in fact, is given the same name—*mu xu*—as alfalfa by the Chinese), was found to be very successful in curing night blindness in a 1960 study in China. Alfalfa also has a reputation for healing peptic ulcers and is an old folk remedy for arthritic conditions. It may work by cleansing the bowels.

Alfalfa grows wild throughout America and is also cultivated as livestock food and other commercial purposes; it is a major raw source in the manufacture of chorophyll. Extracts of alfalfa are used commercially to flavor beverages and food products. It is easy to grow alfalfa sprouts at home for use in salads. Some caution should be observed in using alfalfa, however. Some individuals may be allergic to alfalfa; in addition, it is difficult to tell if powdered alfalfa sold in health foods in capsule form is pure, or, indeed, if it is really alfalfa at all.

Astragalus, a Chinese herb, is only now gaining popularity in this country although it has been used for thousands of years in China as the basis of a immune enhancing therapy called *fuchang therapy*. The immune system is basic to the Chinese approach to health, which is concerned with bringing the body back into balance. Dr. Sun Yan, who came from China to a research program at the University of Texas Medical School, Houston, works with astragalus and ligustrum, another traditional Chinese remedy, which are routinely used in China to protect the immune systems of cancer patients undergoing chemotherapy and radiation treatment.

This root is a staple of traditional Chinese medicine and can be found easily at herbal markets. It is best prepared in a decoction, simmering the root for ten to fifteen minutes, then straining while still hot.

Avena, The fresh, undried oat plant—*Avena sativa*—harvested at the milky stage (a seed will give off a drop of milky juice when squeezed) has been a folk remedy for several hundred years as a general nerve tonic, for nervous exhaustion and certain kinds of mental disease. Ayurvedic medicine in India uses avena—oat plant extract—for opium addiction, as did the eclectic physicians in the U.S. at the turn of the century. Evidence from studies in Scotland suggests that avena also helps with nicotine addiction, and it may prove effective in treating such addictions as alcoholism or even heroin addiction. Several companies have now come out with commercial oat extracts.

This extract from the oat plant can be mixed into porridge or baked into cakes or cookies.

Barberry, a common shrub, is of interest to the herbalist primarily because of its bark, although the Japanese barberry's berries were once used to make jellies and relishes. Like goldenseal and yellow dock, barberry bark is yellow because it contains berberine, an antibacterial and antiviral alkyloid. Barberry bark is a tonic to almost every organ in the body. It has excellent bitters, much preferable to those of the marigold, which makes it a good digestive. It stimulates the liver and the gall bladder, aiding not only digestion but the cleansing of toxins from the body through the eliminative functions. It is also a tonic to the spleen, which strengthens the immune system. As a laxative, it again plays a role in detoxification. Finally, it increases the circulation.

The bark can be infused into teas or tinctures. To make a tincture, crush about eight ounces of the bark and add it to a screw-top jar filled with six to eight cups of a clear spirit, such as gin or vodka. Store the tincture in a warm, dark place and shake the jar twice a day to thoroughly mix. After two weeks, strain the tincture through a cheesecloth, draining well. Keep in tightly sealed bottles. Instead of alcohol, you could use a sweet cider vinegar.

Blackberry leaves are astringent; an infusion is considered an effective blood cleanser and may be useful for improving the circulation of the blood. Blackberry fruit is useful as a cleansing food to help correct diarrhea. It can also be used as a gargle for throat inflammation or in douching to help with vaginal discharges.

A tablespoon or two of dried leaves can be brewed in tea.

Cayenne shares with ginger an ability to help the body metabolize cholesterol. Studies in Mysore, India, in 1985 found that it depresses the liver's production of cholesterol and triglycerides, countering the effect of cholesterol-rich foods. It also seems to have a host of other benefits. Chili peppers and other spicy foods act as expectorants in the bronchial passages, benefiting patients with chronic bronchitis and emphysema. Swedish research has indicated that capsaicin—the ingredient that makes a chili hot—desensitizes the lungs to irritants like cigarette smoke. A common cold can be temporarily relieved with a gargle of a little chili sauce in water.

Surprisingly enough, the capsaicum that stings your mouth in food is also an effective pain suppressant, inhibiting the relay of pain signals to the central nervous system. Thomas Burks, Ph.D., of the University of Arizona, has been studying this effect on guinea pigs and believes capsaicum may eventually be useful in combating arthritis pain.

In 1965 German researchers discovered that chili peppers seemed to dissolve blood clots. Further research in Thailand has confirmed this finding; after eating hot peppers the blood-clot–dissolving activity increases almost immediately. The effect is short-term, lasting about half an hour, but frequent consumption of chilis in food can prevent clots from building up.

Finally, chili peppers have an effect on the brain; the burning they cause in the mouth provokes the release of endorphin, a natural morphine which blocks pain and induces a sensation of pleasure related to the "runner's high" which also results from endorphins.

A pinch of finely chopped fresh cayenne peppers added to a curry or in chili is perfect for the most benefits. Cayenne is the active ingredient in Tabasco sauce and a few dashes in anything from tomato juice to brown rice adds a healthy jolt.

Celery has a cleansing diuretic effect, whether it is taken as a tea or as juice, which can be combined with the juice of other vegetables like carrots. Carrot juice is a good complement to celery as it contains a different kind of pectin from that in apples. Celery's alkalinity also makes it soothing to the digestive system.

A handful of chopped celery can be added to salads, but it is best when a few stalks are juiced along with carrots or other vegetables. An aromatic tea can be made from steeping a tablespoon of seeds in a cup of boiling water for three to five minutes.

Chamomile is an herb that can be used as a tea or a tincture. Chamomile has a slight alkalinizing effect on the blood; it helps to stimulate digestion and acts as a nerve tonic. Folk wisdom has aptly given chamomile a reputation as a calming herb. It can be taken at night as a mild sedative. In a bath or as a decoction chamomile soothes the skin, and it brightens blond hair when added to shampoo. It is antispasmodic when taken internally.

Tea made from a tablespoon of dried leaves should be taken before bedtime to help fall asleep. For swelling or pain in the joints chamomile oil can be applied. To make the oil, use about one ounce of fresh or dried flowers and combine with a half cup of olive oil. Crush the flowers in the oil and let them steep for twenty-four hours. Strain the flowers out and rub the oil on the affected areas.

Cinnamon is a very effective diarrhea remedy. It can be made into a tea, with just a pinch or two in a cup of hot water; an old-time variant is apple sauce with cinnamon, doubly effective since apple pectin is very soothing to the intestinal tract, as well as delicious.

Cinnamon was also used by the Eclectics—a school of nineteenth-century American herbalists devoted to the specific, proven use of herbal remedies—as a first aid remedy to treate mild passive hemmorhaging, such as blood in the urine or sputum. Many midwives swear by cinnamon for postpartum hemmorhaging. Of course, never attempt to treat any serious bleeding in this way without consulting a doctor first.

Comfrey (*Symphytum officinale*) is an ancient healing herb. It has a soothing effect on the stomach lining. A 1983 British study showed that comfrey activates local hormones called prostaglandins, which protect the stomach lining from inflammation. Comfrey root contains mucilage—a slimy or gelatinous form of sugar which is soothing to digestive tract mucous membranes. Comfrey also contains allantoin, a natural cell healer; it is one of the few plant sources of vitamin B_{12}.

A tablespoon of dried leaves steeped in hot water for three to five minutes makes a gentle tea. Fresh leaves can be chopped and added to salad.

Dandelion is an unlikely healer to most of us who know it as a lawn pest, but in fact the entire dandelion plant is a valuable herbal resource.

Dandelion is rich in potassium, which makes it an ideal diuretic as it does not leach potassium from the body as diuretics tend to do. Dandelion greens are also very rich in Vitamin A, and are an excellent salad ingredient. Dandelion root has been used for centuries as a laxative, tonic, and diuretic, and in treating liver, gallbladder, and kidney conditions. Its extracts are used in modern pharmaceutical preparations for these properties. Recent Chinese research has shown that the juice of the dandelion fights certain bacteria; it is particularly efficient in treating upper respiratory tract infections, bronchitis, pneumonia, appendicitis, mastitis, and dermatitis. It creates fewer side effects than modern antibiotics, and these disappear as soon as treatment is discontinued.

A handful of tender, fresh leaves can be a delicious addition to a salad. Dandelion juice can be easily extracted by putting a few leaves in the juicer with carrots or other vegetables.

Echinacea, commonly known as the purple cornflower, is the most popular herbal immune stimulant in America today, although serious research of its properties in this country only began in recent years. Dr. Edward Alstadt, a Naturopathic physician in Portland, Oregon, is one of the leading experts on echinacea. Echinacea is indigenous to the United States alone, where the American Indians have used it for over a recorded one hundred and fifty years. In the 1930s the German scientific community began to research this herb. It was a New York doctor who provided the first written documentation of it, however; he reported that it caused an increase in leukocyte formation, resulting in a greater ability to attack bacteria and a general immune system stimulation. Nevertheless, echinacea was relegated to the realms of folk medicine until the 1960s, when renewed in-vitro studies focused on its stimulation of leukocytes. It was found that echinacea also inhibits *hyaluronadase*, an enzyme which pathogenic organisms use to break down our body tissues to make way for their own spread, and strengthens the tissues against this enzyme by stimulating the production of *hyaluronic acid*, the base of the cell membrane in most body tissues. Finally, echinacea helps the body to regenerate new tissue by stimulating fibrocytes.

Many researchers see a similarity between echinacea and cortisone; a 1953 study by Koch and Heugel demonstrated that echinacea was more effective than cortisone in stopping streptococcus in rats. Echinacea stimulates the adrenal cortex, the area where the *corticosteriods*—which have a cortisone-like action—are released within our own body.

The most prominent researcher on echinacea is Dr. Wagner, at the University of Munich Institute for Pharmaceutical Biology. His studies have indicated that echinacea's effect is due to polysaccharides, or sugar molecules, which fool the body into believing that they're pathogens even though they're perfectly benign and non-toxic. Thus, they boost the body's natural immune reaction, giving it a jump start on fighting colds and infections.

At the first symptoms of cold or flu, echinacea taken immediately, and regularly, every two or three hours for about ten days, will stop the cold or flu before it has a chance to get hold.

Only the root of echinacea is used. There are two kinds of echinacea: *Echinacea angustifolia* and *Echinacea purpurea*. Most research has involved the *angustifolia*, which seems much more effective. Because echinacea is expensive, the consumer should be aware of forms which have been adulterated or substituted for by *purpurea*.

The root of Echinacea can be steeped in boiling water for fifteen minutes. The tea should be taken every two or three hours up to six cups a day until symptoms of cold or flu have begun to subside.

Feverfew (*Chrysanthemum parthenium*) is an immune enhancer that lowers inflammation. Its name is due to its ability to reduce fever. It's good for arthritis because of its anti-inflammatory properties.

Attention was first focused on feverfew in England when a miner gave the wife of a medical officer of the National Coal Board a cutting of the plant to cure her migraines. Dr. Stuart Johnson, intrigued by this report, carried out clinical trials in which feverfew completely cured the migraines of a third of migraine patients; seven out of ten noticed some improvement.

The dried or fresh leaves can be steeped in boiling water for a therapeutic tea.

Garlic has always had a down-home folk reputation as a restorative; how many grandmothers swear by chicken soup with plenty of garlic for a cold? And this reputation has a history almost as long as written history itself, as Jean Carper notes in her recent best seller, *The Food Pharmacy*: "An Egyptian medical papyrus dating from around 1500 B.C. listed twenty-two garlic prescriptions for such complaints as headache, throat disorders, and physical weakness." The confidence the Egyptians had in garlic is demonstrated by the fact that they reportedly used it to strengthen the workers who built the pyramids. Pliny recommended garlic for sixty-one maladies in his *Historia Naturalis*; Hippocrates recommended it as a laxative, diuretic, and cure for tumors of the uterus. Garlic has been used to treat high blood pressure for centuries in China and Japan. In first-century India, garlic and onion were thought to prevent heart disease and rheumatism. Garlic even had a reputation as an aphrodisiac in Shakespearean England. It is probable that only the smell of garlic has prevented it from becoming as omnipresent a cure-all as aspirin.

Garlic's distinctive odor is due to its sulfur-containing compounds—the most important being allicin—which also are responsible for many of its therapeutic effects. Allicin is a powerful inhibitor of bacterial growth with an extremely broad spectrum; hundreds of studies have confirmed its effectiveness over as many as 72 separate infectious agents. Not only does garlic directly attack microbes, but it also seems to boost the body's own immune powers. A 1987 study found that the immune system's killer cells from people who had consumed large quantities of garlic destroyed half again as many cancer cells in a culture.

Studies also show that garlic lowers cholesterol and thins the blood, lowering the chances of dangerous blood clots. If this was not enough, it is a hypertensive; Bulgarian studies have demonstrated that it produces dramatic blood pressure drops in humans. Finally, garlic is an effective decongestant for common colds and can prevent or ease chronic bronchitis.

The best way to get garlic is to grow your own or buy bulbs that are as fresh as possible. Raw garlic is most effective, especially in antibacterial activity; but garlic in cooking retains many of its therapeutic benefits. The garlic sold in health stores as capsules, pills, and deodorized preparations, however, may have relatively little power. It is the smelly part of garlic that is the most therapeutic. Japanese Kyolic paste in one commercial garlic preparation that may approach the value of fresh garlic, but certainly is no better. The best approach is the most simple and natural. If you can't stomach eating garlic cloves raw, cook with it; use it in salad dressings, soups, and garlic bread.

A teaspoon or two of freshly chopped garlic is a healthful addition to all menus. An infusion of two cloves of mashed garlic to an 1/8 cup of room temperature water can be dripped into each nostril to clear sinuses.

Ginger is useful for upset stomachs or motion sickness. A double-blind study published in the *Journal of the American Medical Association* compared the effects of ginger and Dramamine, a common over-the-counter motion sickness drug, and found that ginger was actually more effective. In addition, ginger had none of the side effects—such as drowsiness—of the commercial drug.

Ginger is an even more effective anticoagulant than garlic or onions; gingerol, one of its compounds, has a structure very much like that of aspirin, which also thins the blood. Ginger is a folk remedy for menstrual cramps. It reduces blood pressure and cholesterol, stimulates the heart, and has blocked mutations leading to cancer in mice.

Ginger can be taken in capsules, fresh in cooking, or as a tea. Caution should be taken, especially with powdered ginger, which can burn the esophagus.

A slice of fresh ginger should be taken to avoid motion sickness. A few tablespoons of grated fresh or powdered ginger can be used in cooking to add some excitement to your meal.

Ginseng (*Panax ginseng* is the Latin for the Chinese variety; the species native to North America is *Panax qinquefolium*), considered the master herb by the Chinese, is probably the most researched herb in the world. It is highly valued in China; in fact, the first diplomatic liaison between the U.S. and China was a trade agreement for selling ginseng. Ginseng was used as far back as 3100 B.C. in China; around 2597 B.C. it was discussed as a medicine in a scroll. At one time only the imperial family was allowed to grow or own ginseng.

Wild ginseng, which has been left to grow for thirty, forty, or even up to a hundred years, is extremely expensive, if it can be obtained at all, and is highly prized. Cultivated ginseng may be uprooted anywhere from the age of two to six years. Preferably it should be at least six years old for optimum pharmacological quality. Interestingly, the soil from which a six-year-old ginseng root has been pulled is permitted to lie fallow for ten years to recover its nutrients—an indication of ginseng's ability to pull nutrients into itself. In America, ginseng is grown extensively in the Wisconsin-Michigan area of the midwest, but most of this crop is exported to the Orient.

Ginseng does not only improve physical efficiency and stamina. Experiments with proofreaders found a 12 to 54 percent reduction in misreadings when ginseng was used. It is thought that this results from an improvement of oxygenation of the brain cells. One of the elements found in ginseng, germanium, is a *chelator*—that is, it can pull heavy metals, such as mercury, lead, or cadmium, out of tissues. Experiments in animals have found that the concentration of mercury in tissue was reduced after the administration of ginseng. Germanium also seems to rid the cells of excess hydrogen; in consequence there is a higher proportion of oxygen, and more efficient energy production.

One of the most fascinating properties of ginseng is its apparent ability to protect the bone marrow against radioactivity. A study given at the Third International Symposium on Ginseng in Seoul, Korea, showed that mice pretreated with ginseng survived intensive x-ray irradiation at a rate some 82.5 percent better than the control group. The damage done to the bone marrow—an important factor, because this is where the red blood cells are synthesized—was significantly less in these mice.

Siberian ginseng (*Eleutherococcus senticosus*) has been the subject of more than 400 studies in Russia. Discovered as a result of a search for an indigenous substitute for Chinese ginseng, it was found to make mice able to swim half again as far as those without it before becoming exhausted. Another study was done on several thousand carefully monitored telegraph operators, a group in which it was easy to quantify efficiency, for two decades. Not only was the work efficiency of those who had taken the ginseng greater, but they also had fewer sick days, less cancer, less heart disease, and less diabetes. In 1962 Siberian ginseng was added to the official Russian pharmacopoeia. So convinced are the Russians of the therapeutic value of *Eleutherococcus* that it is used by their athletes and cosmonauts.

Ginseng's powers to help the body cope with stress are so dramatic and far-ranging that a new term, "adaptogen," has been defined by Dr. I. I. Brekhman, a Russian physician who oversaw many of the studies on Siberian ginseng, to describe it. Both *Panax* and Siberian ginseng function as adaptogens. An adaptogen works as a balancing mechanism: it raises low blood pressure but brings high blood pressure down, for example. An adaptogen has nonspecific properties that enable animals to cope with both physical and mental stress more efficiently, to be more resilient, and to maintain a balance, or homeostasis, under widely varying conditions. As an adaptogen, ginseng helps the body to balance itself under a wide variety of stress factors.

Steep one ounce of the macerated root in boiling water for fifteen minutes and strain. Also try concocting a tincture of two ounces of ginseng with two pints of rice wine.

Goldenseal (*Hydrastis canadensis*) has been much misunderstood, and used as a panacea for many ailments. This root is quite powerful, and should be used sparingly and for limited periods of time; the consumer should also be wary, as goldenseal is expensive and may be sold in adulterated preparations.

Goldenseal contains alkyloids which are strong antiseptic and antiviral compounds. One of these, berberine, has been used to treat malaria when quinine is not available; berberine gives goldenseal its yellow color. Goldenseal is effective on the mucous membranes of the gastrointestinal tract, activating the stationary immune system through a cleansing of the lymphatic tissue of the gastrointestinal system. It reduces inflammation throughout the body. Goldenseal also indirectly stimulates the immune system by helping to build up the glandular system, rather than directly attacking microbes as its alkyloids do. Goldenseal also acts as a mild laxative and, as such, detoxifies the system.

It is best to chew goldenseal, or, if preferred, drink it as a tea with one tenth to one quarter of a teaspoon per cup. If it is self-prescribed, begin with a very small amount, perhaps one-tenth of a teaspoon, slowly increasing to a quarter teaspoon.

An infusion made with 1/4 ounce of golden seal has been shown to help sinusitis. Also a gargle prepared with a tincture of goldenseal in warm water can soothe a sore throat.

Hawthorn (*Crataegus oxyacanthoides*), the familiar red-berried tree, is used extensively throughout Europe as a heart tonic. In this country digitalis, or foxglove, is used for this purpose, but it is highly toxic; hawthorn, on the other hand, has none of this toxicity. Hawthorn berries, leaves, and flowers are all excellent for the arterial and peripheral circulation.

Use the leaves to brew a stimulating tea. The berries can be preserved in a tincture and used as needed

Marigold especially the flowerhead, is a very effective herb. The marigold flowerhead is antibacterial, antiviral, and antiseptic. It also enhances the function of the lymphatic system, which in turn aids both the acquired and the fixed immune system. The flowerhead is useful in treating superficial wounds.

Most of the benefits of the marigold flowerhead come from its volatile oil. This oil, when extracted, has been shown to promote blood clotting and the formation of granulomatous tissue, the first stage of healing in wounds. It also contains salicylic acid, which in itself is helpful in reducing the inflammation.

Both the leaves and flowerhead of the marigold contain bitters, which trigger beneficial gastrointestinal responses, boosting the production of hydrochloric acid and enzymes in the stomach. Chefs often use marigold flowers in salads for color, as well as the greens. Do not underestimate the marigold; it is not only beneficial but very gentle. The flowerheads are so light that there is no need to worry about dosage.

Sprinkle a few freshly chopped leaves in a mixed green salad.

Milk thistle (*Salybum marianum*), a noxious weed to farmers, is effective in treating liver disorders, helping the liver properly process toxins and poisons. Milk thistle contains tyramine, which stimulates mucous secretions. Thus, milk thistle tea can be used to help stimulate congested lungs to discharge their excess fluids and mucous, especially in the winter.

Milk thistle is available in tinctures.

Myrrh, a resin extracted from the myrrh tree, is packaged in its solid form, looking somewhat like rock candy. Myrrh is used in a number of consumer products because of its antiseptic qualities; for example, it is often an ingredient in natural toothpaste. Myrrh is also antifungal and antiviral. Clinical tests have shown it to fight *Staphylococcus* and *E. coli* bacteria, for which reason it has been used clinically in hospitals in Egypt and India. Myrrh seems most effective in local application, but should not be ruled out for systemic use.

Myrrh is not easily used because of its market preparation; it must first be caramelized—liquefied with water over heat—and tends to become a gummy mass when stored in water. The recommended internal dosage is about one-half teaspoon.

Dissolve a small portion, about an ounce, of the gummy resin in warm water and use as a refreshing mouthwash. Also, sip the liquid as a cure for a stomach ache.

Osha, a herb native to the Rocky Mountain area of the United States, is used extensively in that area for colds, flus, coughs, sore throats and urinary tract infections.

Pau d'arco (as it is known in Brazil; known as **la pacho** in Argentina), is a native of South America that has attracted a lot of attention with evidence of its strong antiviral, antitumor, antifungal and antibacterial action since it was introduced here in 1980.

Grind the root into a powder, then fill gelatin capsules. Take one capsule twice a day.

Pectin is not a herb, but rather a substance found in some plants. The most well-known source of pectins is apples; carrots contain a different variety. Pectin is soluble fiber; it is used commercially to make Jello. It is a well-known depressor of cholesterol levels. A more recent discovery is that pectin helps to absorb and remove some toxic metals that can accumulate in our tissues, and may increase our ability to withstand irradiation.

Increase your apple consumption for the best quality pectin. Try apple sauce or baked apples for variety.

Rosemary has been gaining publicity recently as an antioxidant, helping to counter the destructive effects of modern industrial toxins and pollutants in the air. Traditionally it has been used as a preservative, especially to keep meats and fats from going rancid; chemicals extracted from rosemary are used in the modern food industry for this purpose. The folk history of rosemary has been as a brain or memory tonic; this may have something to do with its antioxidant properties. Scientists have found that rosemary promotes menstrual discharge in women and hair growth.

Rosemary oil is used widely in cosmetics such as soaps, creams, and lotions. Infusions of rosemary are used externally for wounds, sores, bruises, eczema, and rheumatism.

Crush the dried leaves and sprinkle in soups or salads.

Sarsaparilla root (*Smilax ornata*) is an adaptogen (see the entry for **ginseng** for a definition of adaptogens) which has been around for centuries. It was first introduced to Europe in the Middle Ages as a treatment for syphilis—though there is no evidence that it can cure syphilis, it may relieve its symptoms. Chemically, sarsaparilla falls into the class of phytosterols. Phyto is from the Latin for "plant," and sterol is related to the adrenal hormones called steroids, so phytosterols are plant analogues of steroid hormones. Claims have been made that sarsaparilla contains testosterone, the male sex hormone. There is no evidence for this, and the related claim that sarsaparilla increases the production of male testosterone, especially in older men, has been suggested by new evidence but not proven. However, sarsaparilla has been touted as a male sex tonic for centuries, all over the world. Interestingly, it is also used as an anti-inflammatory; and it is chemically similar to the clinical steroids used in modern medicine to treat inflammation.

Several major pharmaceutical companies in Germany make a product for psoriasis using sarsaparilla extract; it is also effective in alleviating eczema and other skin diseases, as well as arthritis.

Steep the leaves and berries in hot water for an aromatic tea. The root was once used with wintergreen and sassafras to flavor root beer.

Seaweeds contain virtually all the vitamins and minerals needed in a diet. Algae and the sea plants such as hijiki, kombu, wakame, nori, and arame combine with toxins in the body, enabling them to be more easily excreted. Seaweeds also contain above-average amounts of iodine, which helps stimulate the thyroid gland.

Sprinkle steamed hijiki on salads. Roll your own vegetable sushi with sheets of nori and steamed rice.

Thyme (*Thymus vulgaris*) is mentioned here together with oregano because they are both high in a chemical known as thymol. Thymol is used throughout the pharmaceutical industry; in fact, it's a main ingredient in Listerine. It is a strong antiseptic, effective as an antibacterial and antifungal. Interestingly, thyme's Latin name is the same as that of the thymus gland, the central organ of the immune system.

Thyme can be used to make a mouthwash, a bath oil, or a deodorant. I strongly recommend oregano and thyme tea for the common cold and mild infections—most people have it around and like the taste of it. As a strong tea it is a good wash for minor cuts and scratches. Also use to flavor soups or salads. Crush the dried leaves and sprinkle on.

Turmeric, a vivid yellow spice made of ground roots, gives curry powder (and mustard) its classic color. Studies in China and Russia in recent decades have found that in tests on animals turmeric promotes bile secretion, lowers blood pressure, stimulates the appetite, alleviates pain, and reduces inflammation. A recent study in China showed extracts of turmeric to prevent 100 percent of pregnancies in rats. It also seems to have antibiotic properties.

This powdered spice has a subtle taste, but helps support the stronger spices in curries, and prepared mustard. Use a teaspoon along with other aromatic spices.

Turmeric has been getting a lot of attention lately from evidence of its ability to stabilize mast cells, which line our trachea and intestinal tract and serve as a first line of defense for the immune system. Healthy mast cells have a tight weave that can keep out deviant material from our bloodstream—bacteria, pollen, protein which has not been property broken down. Turmeric contains corsitin, a bioflavenoid which can strengthen the mast cells over time.

Many doctors use turmeric for allergies. You might think of the lining of your trachea or sinuses as fabric; tears or holes in this fabric, or a loose weave, allows things like pollen to enter the bloodstream, where they trigger an exaggerated response from the immune system, leading to inflammation and all the symptoms of allergy. Turmeric heals the crack and tightens the weave, providing greater resistance to allergens. In the same way, food allergies can be lessened by strengthening the mast cell tissue in the intestinal tract.

Although it should not be taken as a panacea, turmeric is very safe and is already used in many foods. It can also be taken in capsule form or made as a tea.

Wild indigo root is not a very popular herb, but it is valuable for its direct antimicrobial activity, which helps infections throughout the body and particularly upper respiratory infections. More importantly, wild indigo root is a gastrointestinal tract stimulant, maintaining its levels of hydrochloric acid. This is the first line of defense in the immune system; without an adequate level of hydrochloric acid in the stomach, microorganisms which enter with the ingestion of food may pass through the stomach and enter the lymphatic or blood systems. Wild indigo root is also a liver tonic, helping to detoxify the body.

The strength of wild indigo root lies somewhere between that of echinacea and goldenseal. A self-prescribed dose should be not more than half a teaspoon in a daily cup of tea, and should not be continued for more than a month.

The root can also be used in prepared ointments to help soothe the inflammation of arthritis. Macerate about two ounces of the root and leave for twenty-four hours in a well sealed jar filled with two cups of olive oil. Shake frequently. Then strain and apply as needed.

HERBS, REGULATION, AND THE GOVERNMENT

In recent years millions of Americans have been trying the herbal remedies commonly found in health food stores as cures for specific diseases. People take them with the expectation of being cured of their condition, often at great expense. I have contacted a number of the companies producing and marketing these herbal remedies and could not find one that had performed scientific tests to confirm the efficacy or safety of the cure as proclaimed on the labels. In my opinion, this is clearly an unethical policy.

As Dr. Lee notes, the problem of regulatory control is a burden to the herbal industry. Because herbs are neither food nor drugs, they are extremely difficult to define and hence hard to regulate. When the use is medicinal, they can be considered as drugs; when the use is culinary, they can be considered as spices; but it is not always easy to draw the line. The regulations of the Food and Drug Administration stipulate that a product that is being sold as a food or a nutritional supplement is limited as to the health benefits that can be claimed to result from its use. On the other hand, the cost of testing drugs, which tends to be in the millions or tens of millions of dollars, is prohibitive for herb companies, which tend to be relatively small as compared to the huge pharmaceutical conglomerates. This puts herb companies in a bind. Some, aware that the FDA usually takes several years before they will catch up with a company, choose to go ahead without scientific proof of the efficacy of their product.

If the mainstream health industry were to consider the health properties of herbs more seriously, there would not be this problem. Traditional Western medicine in this country has long been prejudiced against herbs. In no other country is this the case to such an extreme. In one recent case, for example, an internationally renowned scientist, Dr. Bruce Halstead, M.D., was sentenced to eight years in prison for prescribing an unapproved drug when he recommended herbal teas that enhance the immune system to his cancer patients. In less industrialized, less wealthy nations, there tends to be a greater acceptance of medicinal herbs. In part, this is due simply to economics. In many countries, if you are poor, your health care will depend largely on medicinal herbs because industrial medicine is only for those who can afford it. Recently, one of China's leading cancer researchers, Dr. Sun Yan, was invited to the University of Texas to perform a three-year study of two prominent Chinese herbs that enhance the immune system. Both are used in China to help bolster the immune systems of patients that have undergone chemotherapy and radiation therapy. Perhaps the willingness to test the herbs is a sign that the attitude in this country is changing. But there are few other signs. And it is all too characteristic that while America is one of the world's foremost producers of the renowned herb ginseng, 98 percent of the American crop is exported to the orient, and in this country its properties remain relatively unknown.

Were conventional health practitioners to include herbal medicine in their training and the delivery of health care, a significant improvement could occur almost immediately in the quality of medicine available to patients. In particular, the problem of iatrogenic (doctor-induced) illness, would be substantially reduced. The side effects of synthetic drugs are often substantial: the medicines we take frequently make us sicker. In many patient care situations, if medicinal herbs were used, there would be little or no side effects.

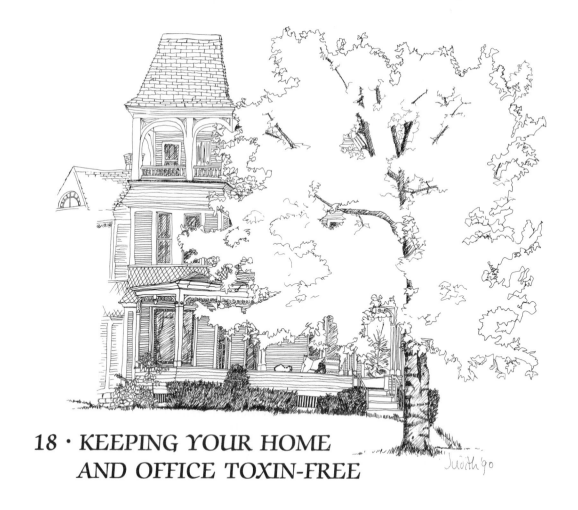

18 · KEEPING YOUR HOME
AND OFFICE TOXIN-FREE

"Ammonia is very toxic, and will stay in your blood for hours. . . . There are alternatives to chemical cleaners in the kitchen. Apple cider vinegar and hydrogen peroxide, mixed half and half in cold water, do the same job as ammonia. After you've finished with the floor, this preparation will clean windows and glassware perfectly, too."

IT IS NO LONGER enough to watch what we eat or the medicines that we take; in the twentieth century environmental toxins have become an unavoidable reality, especially for those living in densely populated urban areas. The very air that we breathe, on the streets or in our homes and offices, can attack our health; noise pollution and artificial lighting add to the physical and mental stress of urban life.

The myth is that you should look for the big toxin. But it's the chronic, day-in, day-out, exposure to small toxins that does you in. It may take decades—none of these environmental toxins, even asbestos, will knock you out right away—but you will pay for your lack of awareness with lung cancer, leukemia, arthritis, or heart disease down the line. Perhaps worst are the subtle symptoms of fatigue, anxiety, and minor nagging physical problems which you come to accept as a normal part of life.

Elimination of the unseen substances that attack your system stealthily, over time, is half of health. If you never used any supplementary vitamin, mineral, or herb, but simply eliminated those factors which depreciate your health, you should be able to live to a hundred years of age in a healthy way. One group of people nearly 70,000 in number, in the north of Pakistan at the base of the Himalayas, often live to 115 or 120, putting in full days of work daily until they die. It may not be possible for all of us to live in the pure atmosphere of the Himalayas—not to mention emulating the diet, activities, and social structure of these people—but we can alter our environment, realistically and functionally. A good place to start is where we live. Dr. Alfred Zann, a Fellow of the American College of Allergists and the American College of Physicians, has written a book, *Why Your House May Endanger Your Health*, which explores the relation between our homes and our well-being more thoroughly than we can here; much of the following discussion is indebted to information which he shared on the Gary Null show, as well as to Dr. Richard Podell.

THE SICK BUILDING SYNDROME

The "sick house" is a relatively new development. Materials and methods used to construct houses have changed considerably since World War II; an extreme example is the energy-efficient office buildings built during the energy crisis of the seventies, about which we'll have more to say later in this chapter. But not only are houses built with more of an emphasis on energy efficiency—which means heavy insulation and minimum ventilation to the outside—but the materials of the construction itself, as well as the furnishings—carpeting, fabrics, furniture—are new, often more convenient, cheaper, lighter man-made compounds unheard of in prewar houses. The particle board which is so useful in modern house and furniture construction exacts a price for this convenience; it is a silent time bomb, giving off invisible, odorless—but no less dangerous—vapors years after it is installed.

Formaldehyde is a major culprit in the modern house or office building. Particle board, new synthetic carpets, insulation, many interior paints, and even permanent-press fabrics can give off formaldehyde. It is invisible and odorless except in high concentrations, but even quite low chronic levels can cause symptoms ranging from burning eyes and headaches to asthma or depression. New houses may be largely built of materials which vaporize formaldehyde for years; the worst culprits are mobile homes, which are, in addition, often poorly ventilated.

Another important factor in a house's potential toxicity is its source of heat. Combustion-heating appliances using natural gas, oil, coal, kerosene, or wood can all create afterburn byproducts, even if you can't see or smell them. Good ventilation can help, but makes it harder to keep a house warm. Electrical heat, though expensive, is the safest source.

What can be done about a toxic house? Some changes can be made in the furnishings, floor coverings, and ventilation and heating systems—below we'll go through a typical house room by room—but often much of the problem lies in structural components which would be expensive and difficult, if not impossible, to alter. Building your own house or having it built, with attention to all material used, is one solution if you can afford it or have the time and skill. If you are looking for a place to live, consider an older home. Prewar houses are often constructed of bricks, plaster, and hardwood, not the chemical-treated plywood, composite board, and other synthetic materials used almost universally now. If synthetic materials were used in an older house they will have had years to emit their toxins. Often a house built before the energy crisis will allow more air circulation. Ceilings are often higher, allowing fumes to rise away from the inhabitants. There may be disadvantages in an old house, however; molds and mildews may have accumulated over the years. Old carpet is a fertile ground for mold as well as accumulated dust, animal hair, and whatever toxins have been tracked in or sprayed over the years, but it can often be pulled up to reveal a hardwood floor. Outdated heating systems can usually be replaced without too much trouble.

If moving or rebuilding your house are not options, you can still do a lot to detoxify your home. We'll go room by room, identifying weak spots. It might be best to start outside the living area.

THE GARAGE AND GARDEN

An attached garage is like a toxic waste dump stuck to the side of your house. Many garages have heating and cooling systems which lead directly into the house—anything that can be absorbed through any crack or ventilation system will end up in the house. What's in the garage? The car, of course—and gasoline. Gasoline vaporizes. The afterburn fumes caused by inefficient burning of gasoline are mostly carbon dioxide, which has no odor and is invisible. Breathing these fumes results in headache, dizziness, and mood swings. (Think of people stuck in traffic jams, breathing the afterburn of all the cars around them for hours at a time.) When you park a hot car in the garage and close the door behind it, the hot oil in the engine is volatile and gets into the air. Park the car outside and wait for it to cool off before you bring it into the garage.

Other things you may keep in the garage—paint thinners and removers, and turpentine—also vaporize easily, and stay in the air for months at a time. If you smell a rag that has been used for paint thinner three months ago, you will see that it is still giving off these fumes. Try to keep down the number of these substances in your garage. If you must keep them, use a small shed or garbage can outside the garage to store them. And the garage should be ventilated out, not into the house, with a suction fan. There should be no ducts from the garage into the house.

Your garage is probably where you keep chemicals you use on your lawn and garden—pesticides, fungicides, or herbicides, for instance. In the first place, do you really need them? Look at it this way. If it's going to kill an insect, a plant, or a mouse, it's a toxin and it can affect you, your pets, and your children. If you spray a weed killer on your lawn and then walk around on it, you will repeatedly be bringing it inside on your feet. Where do you think it goes? It doesn't just go away. Think of all the things you bring in on your feet—and think, for instance, of your kids playing on the carpet, perhaps putting things into their mouth that have been on it. You wouldn't let your kid rub his hand over a New York pavement and lick it, would you?

These are things we seldom think about. And, taken individually, none of them is going to kill you. But be aware that everything you spray outside is likely to be in the air you breathe or will make its way back into your house and settle there. There's no real need to run this risk: we can use diatomaceous earth, natural biological controls, or just weed without spraying.

THE BASEMENT

A typical basement in a private home is often damp. People like their lawns unencumbered by debris that might wash down from the gutters of the roof through the downspout, so the downspout is kept close to the house. Thus the water runs off the roof, down the downspout, and into the ground directly by the foundation of the house. They might just as well run this water directly into the basement, since its walls are rarely waterproof. A little dampness in the basement is enough to support a healthy growth of mold, which can then permeate the house. A forced air system of ventilation in the house, which has ducts running to the basement, will create a vacuum-like effect—known as the Bernoulli effect—that will suck particles of mold into the system, to be dispersed around the house.

Many patients react to mold, whether it is eaten or inhaled—a point made obvious to anyone who begins to sneeze as soon as he or she walks into a damp basement. More insidiously, though, mold which is inhaled even in small quantities cross-reacts with mold which is ingested in food. This effect, known as concomitancy, means that a small quantity of mold inhaled—which would hardly in itself cause a noticeable reaction—will enhance sensitivity to foods which contain mold.

Any food which is made by fermentation can induce this reaction. Wine and vinegar are fermented fruit juice; cheese is fermented milk; yeast in bread ferments; and even mushrooms are in the mold family. Thus, it is easy to ingest mold three times a day, exacerbating our inability to tolerate the mold which has circulated upward from a damp basement. Obvious symptoms are sneezing and watering eyes; but allergic symptoms can also be systemic, making them harder to pin down to a specific trigger reaction. Fatigue, headaches, depression, even arthritis, can have a basis in chronic allergic irritation.

As well as water coming into the basement from the downspout, groundwater can roll down a hill toward the house, which then serves as a dam. Here it can be diverted by raising the earth around the house to encourage it to flow away from the house. If a high water table is the problem, a sump pump is needed. Thoroseal, a dense cementous material, can be applied to the outside block foundation as caulking to keep water out.

If the basement is still damp, a dehumidifier can help, but these work well only above a temperature of 50 to 60 degrees Fahrenheit. Chemicals like baking soda only serve as temporary measures. The best way to remove the mold itself is to scrub the area down with sulfur water. The basement can be hosed down and the water removed with an industrial vacuum.

THE KITCHEN

What's the most dangerous toxin in most kitchens? Gas. You should always have a vent in the kitchen; it has been shown that cerebral allergies are often directly attributable to the gas burnoff of pilot lights on stoves, which leak constantly. If you often have headaches and you suspect that they are more common when you're spending time in the kitchen, try disconnecting your stove when you're not using it. If this makes a difference, you should consider replacing the gas stove with an electric one. Not only gas ovens are a health risk, though. Microwave ovens can leak; a defective microwave creates a very unhealthy environment within about eight feet of it.

What else? Freon in the condenser of the refrigerator. Freon is a highly volatile, dangerous chemical. It is a very good idea to replace refrigerators that are more than ten years old.

The refrigerator contributes to another seldom-considered form of pollution found especially in the kitchen: noise pollution. You should be able to tolerate background noise of about 30 to 35 decibels. Higher than 50 decibels becomes uncomfortable. Above 80, you become substantially irritated and above 100 may cause ear damage or central nervous system overstimulation. A compressor in most refrigerators is up to 60 decibels. You don't appreciate this until you turn on a refrigerator when everything else is totally quiet. But think of a kitchen with a television or a radio on, things cooking, telephone conversations—you can't even hear the refrigerator, and the noise level may be up around 100 decibels. The kitchen is one of the most stressful places because of this level of background noise. Even if you are unable to replace appliances like refrigerators and air conditioners with less noisy ones, you can cut down on the number of noisemakers you are using at the same time—for example, avoid trying to cook and listen to the news at the same time.

Not only the kitchen suffers from noise—street noise can be irritating in any room. This can be helped with noise-buffering double-fold drapes that keep noise down as well as insulate.

Mold and mildew are common invisible toxins in a kitchen. When was the last time you changed the water drip area of your refrigerator? There's a condenser coil and a tray under it to collect water—but it can also collect all kinds of mold. Mold spores are in the air all the time and you're inhaling them. If you're sensitive and your immune system is low, you'll feel it—your eyes will get puffy, your nose will clog, your throat will get sore. Keeping this area clean and dry could make a big difference.

Look under the sink in your kitchen; you'll be amazed at the range of toxic chemicals you keep there, so close to your food. Cleansers, for instance, especially ammonia-based products, often vaporize easily. Ammonia is very toxic, and will stay in your blood for hours when you've smelled it. When you wax the kitchen floor, the floor wax will evaporate and you will be breathing it in. Try, if you can, to install floors that will not need waxing—but if you don't want to tear up your present floors you might want to settle for a matte finish rather than a high sheen, if you have to constantly apply volatile chemicals to get that sheen. And, as with the weed-killers and insecticides in your garage, there are alternatives to chemical cleaners in the kitchen. Apple cider vinegar and hydrogen peroxide, mixed half and half in cold water, do the same job as ammonia. After you've finished with the floor, this preparation will clean windows and glassware perfectly, too.

Roach sprays are very stable. They can last for months, and vaporize constantly. A dog or cat licking the floor can pick them up directly. A safer alternative is to use boric acid—you can mix it with sugar as a bait but be sure pets and children can't reach it—and line all the counters and fittings underneath with a strip of this no thicker than a pencil. This mixture is not volatile and is safe as long as it's only put in inaccessible places. Diatomaceous earth is safe to use and works well too. Or, use the roach motels which use resin that roaches get stuck on instead of poisons.

Aluminum-based cookware, when the aluminum can come into contact with the food, should not be used. Aluminum has been implicated in Alzheimer's disease. It is a heavy metal that lodges itself in the blood, brain tissue, and central nervous system where it can cause motor problems. Aluminum foil is alright for storage of cooked food but should not be used while you're cooking, when it can oxidize in microscopic amounts. You can't see this, but it can get into your food and your body. Teflon, or any of the nonstick coatings, should also be avoided. They easily scratch or flake off with age, getting into food as well as exposing it to the often inferior metal underneath.

Next time you fill up a glass with water from the kitchen tap, consider that it may contain over a thousand chemicals—those that the government puts in, like fluoride, traces of herbicides and pesticides that have leached down into the water supply from fields, and traces of metal, rust, and molds from the inside of your pipes. Most water filtration systems can only remove a portion of these; the finer particles, including toxic chemicals like pesticides, come through. If you live in a polluted area and your water supply is from underground streams, buy bottled water. I would buy plain distilled water—you get minerals from food, you don't need them from water. Since 72 to 74 percent of our bodies is water, we should be sure it is the purest possible.

THE BATHROOM

One of the most common causes of allergy is what we put on our bodies—soaps, deodorants, cosmetics. We use these things day in and day out, rarely thinking about their effect on us. For example, women who wear lipstick every day and lick their lips are absorbing chemicals never meant to be eaten. Perfumes vaporize and get breathed in. Read the ingredients of your antiperspirant; most likely it contains an aluminum-based compound which can be absorbed through your skin and carries the risks of aluminum outlined above. You can minimize these sources of toxins by using natural soaps and shampoos made out of vegetable ingredients, a non-fluoride toothpaste like Dr. Bronner's or Tom's, mouthwash which you can make yourself with a little ascorbic acid in water, and natural loofa pads to scrub yourself.

The bathroom is one of the wettest rooms in the house and is a likely site for mold. It's important to air out the bathroom after a shower or bath and let it dry out. A window fan to evacuate the moist air is a good idea, but keeping the window open works almost as well. Even in the winter, give the bathroom time to air and dry out. Bathrooms are too often closed up most of the time, and can be like little poison chambers trapping the perfumes, deodorants, and cleaning fluid fumes in a small space. Odor disguisers like pine- or lemon-scented aerosol sprays are worse than useless; the odor is a molecule floating around in the air that can only be removed by letting the air escape. Products that claim to take away odors only cover them up with a chemical which probably smells worse and is certainly worse for you.

The "disinfectant" cleaners so popular for bathroom tiles and tubs are virtually useless. To disinfect something you have to boil it for twenty minutes, but within one minute it will be covered with germs again. And those germs are not going to kill anyone, despite the fear tactics used to market these floor cleaners. Their heavy aromatic odors are often more of a problem than the germs; pine, for example, is a resinous material that is quite troublesome to allergic or sensitive people.

Never store medications in the medicine chest; it's hot and humid in the bathroom and can cause them to go bad. Store medicine and vitamins in the refrigerator.

As with the kitchen, look around the bathroom and think about potential toxins—cleaners for the tiles and sink, toilet fresheners, and so on—do you need all those things? Can they be substituted by natural, non-toxic products? Awareness of your environment and what you put in it is the key.

THE BEDROOM

We spend a third of our lives in the bedroom; if you live 72 years, that means 23 years in bed. An ecologically ideal, safe place to spend all this time should be as free of dust as possible. Many bedrooms have wall-to-wall carpeting, which is an ecological disaster. Carpeting is toxic in your home in several ways. New synthetic-fiber carpeting contains chemicals like formaldehyde which will vaporize for a year or more. Old carpet collects dirt, yeast, fungus, and mold. Dust mites live in it. Through an electron microscope these mites look like tiny dinosaurs; their diet is chiefly composed of the shed human skin cells which are another large component of dust. House dust mites can be wafted into the air by currents and breathed into the lungs. People who are allergic to them react as if to cat or dog dander. Like dander, they can get into your eyes and make them red and puffy.

How many of you have thought about ripping up your old carpet and putting in nice hardwood floors? They're easy to maintain and non-toxic. The Japanese have never had polyvinyl flouride or no-wax floors; they use natural resins on wood, and some of these floors are five hundred years old. If you feel you must have carpets, buy wool or natural fiber, with natural dyes. Stay away from synthetic carpets. And learn to vacuum efficiently. Most people just zip the vacuum over the carpet; by the time the dust has had a chance to get up through the nap into the air the vacuum has moved on, and has only raised the dust. You've actually increased the pollution in the air. So run the vacuum very slowly over the carpet—give the dust you raise time to get into the vacuum.

You may be sleeping on foam-filled synthetic pillows, with synthetic-fiber pillowcases and sheets. Replace them with down-filled pillows and comforters and pure cotton sheets. Also be aware of what you're putting in your sheets when you wash them—bleaches and fabric softeners can be potential irritants. Many manufacturers of bedding use chemicals to fire-proof the material, which many people are allergic to. The way to test for this is to sleep on bedding which is not treated to be fireproof and see if your symptoms disappear. Again, if you feel better when you are sleeping away from your house on vacation, it should alert you to the fact that something in the bedroom is causing trouble.

Sleeping on clean sheets changed frequently reduces possible reactions to dust and dust mites. When you wash bedding, it's best to keep things simple. Don't use perfumed detergents, avoid antistatics and softeners, and look for biodegradable brands. Bleach should be oxygen bleach, not chlorine, which leaves an irritating residue. Miracle White, made by Beatrice Food Company, works well. If you suspect that a pillowcase, for example, is bothering you, wash it with a simple unscented detergent, rinse it three or four times, and try it again to see if the problem goes away.

Electric blankets can affect the electromagnetic field around the body and should be avoided. It's also best not to sleep near a digital clock, which can affect the body's electromagnetic system from three feet away.

Even your closets can affect your health; moth balls emit a poisonous gas. Chicago weavers use a mixture of rosemary, mint, thyme, ginseng, and cloves instead, which has the additional advantage of smelling good.

AIR QUALITY

If you ever see the sun slant into a room at a certain angle, you know how much dust and smoke is in what you thought was clear air. It's there all the time. An air purifier with a negative ionizer is the best way to eliminate airborne toxins—spores, dust, cigarette smoke, hydrocarbons and pollutants from the street, cat hairs, positive ions. A Bionaire 2000 with a negative ionizer will circulate the air about every eight minutes. The ionizer bombards the room with negative ions which attach themselves to the positive ions of pollutants, which then drop to the ground and can be filtered out by the filtration system.

Humidifiers are fine for improving air quality as well, as long as you use distilled water in them. Otherwise mineral deposits from the water will end up all over your carpet, floor, and furniture.

PLANTS

One efficient and natural air-quality improver is living greenery in your house. The more plants in your environment, the better. A large number and variety of houseplants will increase the oxygen level in the air. Green, non-flowering varieties are best, as they will not issue pollen. Plants are also a great natural air pollution filtration system. New York City would hardly be bearable if it were not for Central Park. Plants help maintain humidity levels and a proper electricity balance in the air.

Plants are calming to the mind as well as good for air quality. As living things, they create an energy of their own. Not only are plants alive, but many people believe that they have a consciousness. If you've ever noticed how some people seem to have great luck with plants and others can never keep them alive, you may have thought about this. Plants don't just function as air purifiers; they create a living energy field which we can share and be invigorated and calmed by.

LIGHT

Your visual environment is more important than you might realize. If you feel tired, ill, or depressed inside in the winter, especially if you live at a high latitude where the days are very short, and if you spend most of your day indoors, you may be suffering from *seasonal affective disorder*. In this condition the hypothalamus of your brain is deprived of full-spectrum natural sunlight—most artificial lights use only a part of the spectrum. The best solution is to allow plenty of natural light into your house; use double-glazing rather than small windows or heavy drapes if insulation is a concern. Try to spend time outdoors or arrange your activities so that you're near a window. If getting more daylight is beyond your control— the days are short, your house is dark, and you must stay indoors—the situation can be improved with full-spectrum lightbulbs. Full-spectrum incandescent lighting works on a completely different priniciple from that of flourescent lighting (discussed in the section on the office below) and is more natural for the eyes. These bulbs are available in health stores in all sizes; using them in your office as well as in your home can make a big difference in your energy level and mental state.

HEAT

In cold areas, we shut down for the winter, closing and sealing the windows to avoid ventilation from outside. These methods contribute to the toxic state of the air inside. The air in many New York apartments in the winter would generate an official air pollution alert outside.

Oil heaters often burn inefficiently and release unburned oil fumes into the house. An after-burner catalyst, available on the market now, can recycle these, creating a clean air burn. Electric stoves are not a problem. Gas or oil space heaters are one of the worst offenders. Dry radiated heat can dry up your nose and skin. Wood-burning stoves may seem rustic and natural but can be one of the worst sources of indoor pollution.

One major problem can develop in forced air combustion heating systems, using either gas or oil; a little pin hole not infrequently develops between the heat exchanger, which is next to the combustion chamber, and the air going past it to be heated. As the air that we're going to breathe goes around that heated chamber, it sucks in the partially combusted gases. You may not even perceive this in the air, because it's at a very low level, but over a six-month period this air can produce severe illness. Therefore you must have your forced air system checked out electronically for these pinholes every year. The smell test is not satisfactory. If you don't do this, you're at risk.

THE WORKPLACE

The energy crisis of the seventies has led to a generation of very well insulated, but poorly ventilated, office buildings. People who work in these buildings often complain of fatigue, nasal congestion, dizziness, and a host of other mysterious symptoms. Yet there has been clear-cut documentation of toxic levels of pollutants in very few cases. The levels of toxins in these buildings are rarely high enough to provoke official alarm, but they are enough to cause fatigue and illness through long-term, chronic exposure. Even low levels of organic chemicals, pesticides, formaldehyde, carpet cleaners, and tobacco smoke can effect those exposed to them for long enough.

The individual pollutants can be located and reduced, but the single most important factor is ventilation. Monday is the worst day for headaches and stress, and that's at least partially because the ventilation systems have often been shut down over the weekend; you're breathing old, stale air. The ducts of your office air venting system probably haven't been cleaned in years. Dust and molds have built up inside them and are coming out into the air you breathe when the system is restarted. Ask the maintenance people to clean them; if they won't, get a heavy-duty charcoal filter and put it in the vent, with a thick white insulation pad over it. These can be bought inexpensively at any hardware store. In one week, if you look at the insulation pad it will be covered with black particles large enough to see.

If it's noisy where you work, wear ear plugs. You can also make your desk more pleasant with a small portable ionizer. This can actually fit in your pocket, and is also useful in airplanes or on the dashboard of your car.

The fluorescent lighting often used in offices flashes on and off rapidly and constantly, creating great stress on your central nervous system. Although you are not consciously aware of this very rapid flickering, your eye and nervous system are overstimulated by it—two or three hours of work under fluorescent light can have the effect of three or four cups of coffee. At a certain level of overstimulation the central nervous system will start to shut down, and you will find yourself deeply fatigued. Replace the fluorescent lighting at your desk with a lamp which uses incandescent bulbs, and use the natural full-spectrum lightbulbs which we described earlier. It's best to have an office with a window or skylight for true natural lighting; if you don't and can't arrange it, it's especially important to have natural—and sufficiently bright—lighting.

Stay away from the photocopier at the office as much as possible; it uses very volatile chemicals. Don't leave typewriter ink or corrector ribbons lying around open; put them in a sealed plastic bag when not in use. An exhaust fan on the ceiling will help draw away vaporizing fluids.

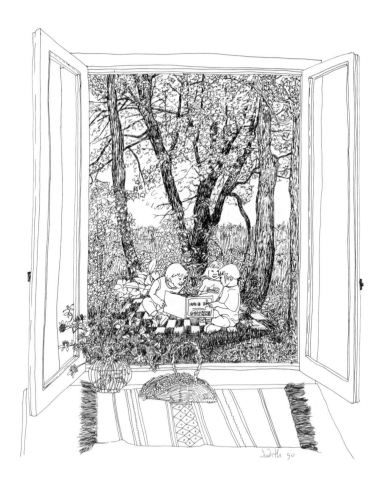

19 · NUTRITION AND MENTAL ILLNESS (ORTHOMOLECULAR PSYCHIATRY)

"Sometimes we have to use Lithium and other drugs, but when a person uses the orthomolecular approach, it is amazing how you can get by with only small quantities of the drugs, enabling you to avoid most of the dangerous side effects which are so devastating to patients when the drugs are the primary therapy."

WE HAVE BEEN LED to believe that we are a nation with a mental illness epidemic. The National Institute of Mental Illness estimates that upwards of forty million Americans may be suffering from emotional problems severe enough to restrict or limit the quality of their lives. We are told that the illnesses are sociologically or psychologically induced, and therefore that the appropriate therapies are psychiatry or some other form of psychotherapy. Most cases fall into the categories of depression or anxiety. Both are often treated with toxic, noncurative, psychotropic drugs. Or worse: lobotomy, electric-convulsive therapy, and thorazine, or some other equally powerful mood-alterators that turn the person into a virtual vegetable.

With no major improvement in our mental health outlook in more than fifty years, there is now a feeling that these approaches are off the mark, and that a new direction must be taken. Filling this void for the past thirty years has been a group of psychiatrists and mental health workers, collectively known as orthomolecular psychiatrists. Their approach is, first, to do no harm. They try to rebalance the body's chemistry and work within a system of medicine that acknowledges that we are affected by our environment, by what we eat, breathe, drink, and think.

What follows are samplings from the practices of three orthomolecular psychiatrists: Dr. Ray Wonderlick, M.D., whose work emphasizes the special needs of children; Dr. Richard Cunin, M.D., who has been a leading researcher of the impact of pesticides on our health; and Dr. Abraham Hoffer, M.D., Ph.D., one of the founders of the orthomolecular psychiatric movement.

TREATING CHILDREN

Dr. Wonderlick, who has a background in pediatrics, explains his approach to treating children with learning disorders or behavior problems: "We try not to give them Riddilin or amphetemines when they have hyperactivity or attention-deficit disorders. Instead we look at their basic quality of life and their lifestyle. Are they troubled by any infections? Do they have allergies? Do they have nutritional deficiencies? Do they have chemical toxicities? Are they having some kind of nutritional disorder that is underlying the problem? We are directly opposed to the conventional approach, which relies primarily on just treating the symptom by the use of medication. We've determined that very rarely is it necessary to use prescription drugs for these children. The drugs may be needed on a temporary basis while you're testing the patient or while the family is discovering how to reform the diet, for example, or deciding which vitamin and mineral supplements to use. However, in the vast majority of cases—ninety percent, I would say—we were able to manage the problem, whether behavioral or academic, without the use of drugs."

Five million children are now using Riddilin, which does nothing to cure the child, and may actually mask the real nature of the problem. Dr. Wonderlick feels that if you use the drug, and you get a "good" response, everybody thinks everything's okay. They couldn't be more wrong. The kid sails along, but without growing well, without eating well, and the actual nutritional problem may be compounded. His approach, by contrast, utilizes amino acids, herbs and other nutrients: "We assess the child's amino acid pattern through a plasma amino acid test or a 24-hour urine test to spot the amino acid deficiencies and imbalances. We often find that the essential amino acids are not being received by the child. It could be because the diet is so poor, or it could be that the child's digestion and absorption are inadequate, so that the child, while eating well, isn't achieving the amino acid levels that he needs. We address that issue with supplements to correct either the inadequate input of food or the digestive, malabsorption problem.

"We use herbs in the detoxification process initially. Many of these children are toxic—their bodies react adversely to other elements to which they're exposed. Sometimes, if you give these children vitamins for example, they are unable to take them. The same applies to adults. And when you see that, you know that there is a high level of toxicity in the body and you have to go to some kind of detoxification process. Herbs are very safe and a very convenient way to do that. You get a good response and the family often will see the difference in the child and will then listen more openly to the nutritional message.

"These herbs are given under professional guidance. It is not something that individuals should do themselves. Some of the herbs we use are Red Clover, Goldenseal, Black Walnut, and Acansosyanicide—acansosyans come from blueberries and from pine bark. They strengthen the blood/brain barrier and that enables us to protect the child whose brain is more or less on fire—hyper-reactive because of reactions to foods, indogenous chemicals or exogenous toxins. These herbs have been a great help in protecting that brain until we can get the diet changed or the environment cleared up so that it isn't suffering such a toxic assault.

"As far as amino acids are concerned, in some children you have to use just a general, across-the-board supplement including all eight or ten of the essential amino acids. In others, we use tyracine, cellalonine, triptophane, cistyne—particularly the sulphur bearing amino acids—glutamic acids and, of course, the branch chain of amino acids, particularly in individuals who have an absorption problem.

"Typically we see the most dramatic improvement in the child's use of his or her intellectual ability. It's like putting an engine into gear. The child is better able to listen in class, respond in a communicative way, participate in a dialogue, handle visual tasks—this is enormously important because auditory/visual functioning are linked in learning and control of eye movement in focusing is a big factor in how well one learns. In many cases, the special lenses which optometrists sometimes prescribe for children with learning difficulties can be discarded several months after these nutrients have been added."

THE PROBLEM OF PESTICIDES

Dr. Richard Cunin has produced volumes of research on pesticides and how they impact upon our well-being: "In 1983–1985 I learned that the so-called organophosphate pesticides and herb gas pesticides, which are supposed to be the safest ones in common use today, weren't necessarily safe as far as my patients were concerned. I won't dispute entirely the good work and good intentions of our predecessors in science who were trying to contribute to the common good by increasing crop yields, making life a little more sanitized, and eradicating some forms of disease. But, as a clinician with my background as a certified M.D. and psychiatrist, I have an obligation to respond to the needs of my patients. Some of them have incurable diseases whose symptoms mimic those of psychiatric diseases—anxiety, depression, concentration difficulties and a host of psychosomatic-type disorders—due to the organophosphate nerve gas pesticides. The pesticides seem to over-stimulate most of the autononic nerves in the body, thus producing an overreaction emotionally and of nearly every gland in the body. The initial symptom might be nasal congestion, tightness in the chest, increased activity of the stomach similar to a pre-ulcer syndrome, or bloating and diarrhea with no parasites and no particular abnormality of the bowel flori such as yeast. Or you might have sweating, moist hands. Such problems as these are common and sometimes intractable. Doctors tear their hair out because the simple solution patients are looking for may not be easy to find.

"I test my patients for a universal substance called colonesterase. I found, to my surprise, that a large number of my patients were actually pathologically low or borderline in their colonesterase level, an abnormality that is almost always induced by environmental exposure to these nerve gases—the poisonous enzyme having produced an over-reaction of the nerves in the body.

"I first reported these findings to our orthomolecular medical society under the title 'Was Governor Brown right about Melathione?' If you recall, Jerry Brown more or less lost a Senate race because at first he resisted using Melathione to fight the fruit fly down in the peninsula—

over an area of two million people. He resisted it at the advice of his Health and Hazards chief, Mark Lampay, the husband of Francis Moore Lampay who is very well known in ecological, literary and political circles. So he gave good advice: Don't spray two million people with Melothione to kill off a few fruit flies when you could perhaps use dummy fruit flies and breed them out, instead, as they did thirty years ago in Florida. Brown lost the Senate office over this issue, and as I went through my records and found three dozen related cases in about two years, just among my own patients, I realized that Brown had probably been right in the first place.

"Since then, I've been looking at organochlorine pesticides, the descendants of DDT, and with them the nonpesticide but related compound called PCB. These chlorine compounds seem to degrade in the body in the nerve cells where they destroy vitamins among other things, and create peroxides and other compounds that are damaging to the nerve cells. Ultimately, as they accumulate over a lifetime, they are very likely to do serious harm—if not obvious harm, at least enough to impair the quality of life for many patients."

As Dr. Cunin is well aware, many of the pesticides he has studied are commonly used in some form around people's homes, in parks—in other words, where tens of millions of Americans are exposed. And also on the foods that we eat. The pesticide may damage an enzyme in the nervous system that affects our vitamin absorption and how we feel.

Dr. Cunin explains, "there are two major classes of pesticides: one of these is called the nerve gas type which is in common use because it is shortlived and therefore believed to be safe. However, because it's so common, people get repeated low-level exposure which lasts anywhere from one week to eight weeks at a time, depending on your own level of resistance. In these little steps, the poison may build up until you have major damage, discomfort, distress or illness—enough, at least, to make you think you're a neurotic and keep you in analysis for quite a while! Nerve gas—aptly named.

"The other type is the chlorine type, which is more dangerous in the sense that it accumulates and stays in your tissues for a lifetime, getting worse and worse.

"I reviewed the last one hundred patients that I measured and grouped them into a high and a low group. Those in the high group were running twenty to forty parts per billion of DDT and as high as ten parts per billion of PCB. In total chlorines, they were averaging about twenty-five parts per billion. In that group, taking the top ten, we had five with cancer. By the way, this group was older because, as these were organochlorines, they accumulated. That is their danger; the longer you live, the more you get. They stay in your system unless you take a positive action to get rid of them. Cancer proved to be one of the major symptoms. A second major symptom was Alzheimer's.

"The low pesticide group, meaning those under two parts per billion—how little that is, yet enough to impact on the functioning of the nervous system!—did not show specific symptoms. Instead, they had a hodgepodge of hard-to-diagnose symptoms."

TREATMENT

"Over the course of a few years of trying things, I found empirically that an amino acid named Torine seemed to contribute to people's comfort levels—they just felt better. We added in niacinimide and they slept better, probably due to the anti-oxidant action of the niacinimide. Thirdly, there is the remarkable effect of Vitamin B_{12}. It turns out that these chlorinated byproducts or intermediates of these chlorine molecules respond to Vitamin B_{12}. We do not yet fully understand the process at the cellular level. But we do know that people are responsive to megadoses of Vitamin B_{12} administered by injection. I've found that oral B_{12} will also suffice, in larger doses to equate the large dose effect achieved with muscular injection.

"Torine deactivates chlorine—rendering a chlorine radical neutral; niacinimide aids the insomnia accompanying the disorder; and B_{12} helps to restore cognitive functions.

"Of course, the first line of treatment for any toxin is to avoid exposure to the toxin in the first place. If you can avoid it, it is most important to do that. That's why I am convinced that it is worthwhile for clinical doctors, when they see patients presenting nervous symptoms, to respond immediately. Check early, because the nervous symptoms always precede the late symptoms of cancer. If people come in with otherwise unresponsive anxieties, depressions, numbness, or lingering psychosomatic symptoms, check for the pesticides. If they're there, look for the source and then help the patient to avoid it. That comes first.

"Also, a high fiber diet can absorb many of these pesticides and help pass them out of the system. Without the fiber, they can reabsorb and accumulate in your body tissues."

THE CAUSES OF MOOD DISORDERS

Dr. Abraham Hoffer, one of the world's most distinguished orthomolecular psychiatrists and research scientists, pioneered the use of nutrition-based therapies for schizophrenic patients as early as 1952. He relates that today there is an increased acceptance of the ideas and therapies of orthomolecular psychiatry. Many orthodox physicians are beginning to react favorably, something which occurred only rarely ten years ago. There are probably between five hundred and one thousand orthomolecular physicians currently practicing in the United States and Canada. That's approximately five hundred out of five hundred thousand—one-tenth of one percent—of practicing physicians, so there's a lot more that needs to be done to get more doctors aware of this approach.

But this small group of psychiatrists has an extraordinary influence. For example, there is a tremendous amount of interest today in using niacin to lower cholesterol. That was an orthomolecular discovery. In order to introduce new doctors to the field, Dr. Hoffer has recently published a book called *Orthomolecular Medicine for Physicians.*

On the subject of mood disorders, anxiety, fatigue, depression and tension, Dr. Hoffer estimates that twenty to thirty percent of our population will at one time or another, if not all the time, suffer from manifestations of these disorders. "There are a number of factors which I think lead to these difficulties with moods. In my judgment, the most common causes of depression and anxiety are nutritional deficiencies. In fact, the first symptom of almost any vitamin deficiency is depression. Second, we have allergies, and one of the most common villains is sugar. You would be amazed at how many people are depressed because they consume huge quantities of sugar. Some of my best recoveries have occurred when a patient has agreed to go off sugar. This can also apply to common foods which generally are okay, but which can cause depression if you happen to be allergic to them. I've estimated that at least sixty-five percent of all depression is probably caused by food allergies.

"Third, there are the additives, toxic sprays, and toxic minerals like lead and mercury. We must not forget that often the first symptom of physical illness is depression. Then there are a large number of psychiatric depressions where we really can't pin down for certain what has brought them about."

TREATMENT

"So we have a large variety of factors which lead to people becoming depressed. Depression and other mood disorders are very common problems. As for treatment, if the causes are nutritional, the cure may be as well. It is simply not good enough to put people on anti-depressants, or lithium, or tranquilizers, and hope that these, by themselves, will be the answer in every case. It is impossible to get well while taking tranquilizers because they only ameliorate some of the symptoms; they never cure.

"My approach is, first of all, to determine whether or not there's a problem with nutrition. If there is, one corrects this by taking the junk out of one's diet and also determining what foods the patient is allergic to and how to get rid of them. We also have to use vitamins because the neuro-receptors, which have a lot to do with the way we see, think and feel, have to have vitamins in adequate quantities before they can perform properly. So we find that many of the vitamins are helpful, not just one. It could be Vitamin C, B_6, niacin, B_3, B_1, folic acid, B_{12}—any one of these vitamins may be needed in quantities which are a lot larger than the generally recommended RDA.

"We have also begun to explore the healing properties of the amino acids. Some extremely interesting work is being done currently showing that the use of pyracine in the morning and triptophane at night can be a very fine substitute for some of the common antidepressants. And triptophane is also coming in as a treatment for manic depression or bipolar psychoses. I have several patients taking two grams three times a day of triptophane instead of Lithium because they became very ill while they were taking Lithium.

"Sometimes we have to use lithium and other drugs, but when a person uses the orthomolecular approach, it is amazing how you can get by with only small quantities of the drugs, enabling you to avoid most of the dangerous side effects which are so devastating to patients when the drugs are the primary therapy.

"The orthomolecular approach to mood disorders consists of a comprehensive program. Of course, the treatment has to be administered by a physician who understands what these patients are going through, who can deal with them and provide support, because there is nothing worse than a deep depression. I don't know of any condition that's more devastating than this. And unless the doctor understands what is going on, he will not help his patients sufficiently."

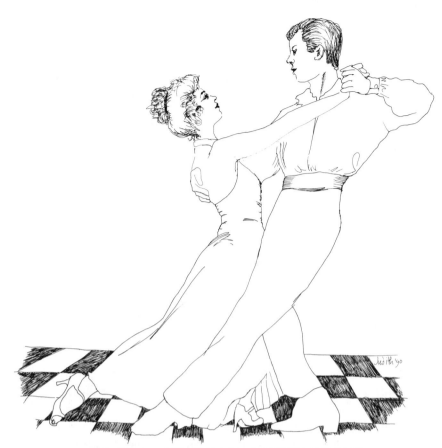

20 · ENVIRONMENTAL MEDICINE (CLINICAL ECOLOGY)

"The conventional practitioner is concerned primarily with two things, the symptoms and the suppression of those symptoms. By contrast, the environmental medicine specialist will use the symptom as a clue and then embark on a course of inquiry aimed at finding the underlying cause or causes."

CLINICAL ECOLOGY, ALSO KNOWN as environmental medicine, may be the fastest-growing and most exciting new field in modern medicine. This is at least in part because it represents a return to common sense. One early pioneer in environmental medicine was Dr. Walter Alvarez, a Harvard Medical School graduate, chief physician at the distinguished Mayo Clinic, medical columnist and book author in the period between the world wars. In order to complete his diagnosis, Alvarez used to listen carefully to the patient. If that didn't provide him with the necessary insight, he would talk to the patient's family. And if he still wasn't sure, he'd go to the home to observe the environment there, including things like noise levels and exposure to chemical toxins. Very often it was in the character of the patient's daily life that Dr. Alvarez found what he was looking for, in the form of immunologically or toxically driven symptoms including everything from flu-like symptoms to cerebral reactions, behavioral disorders, cardiac arrhythmias or gastro-intestinal disorders.

DIVERGING PHILOSOPHIES

Fundamentally, environmental medicine is an empirical science (meaning that it is based on direct observation and experiment), which puts it at odds with traditional Western medicine, which long ago diverged from its empirical roots. Thus, in 1973, according to clinical ecologist Russell Jaffe, the Rand Corporation reported that up to eighty percent of the complaints which send people to their physician cannot be properly assessed or treated by the means at his or her disposal.

Using as an example the symptom of postnasal drip, here is the difference between the diagnostic approaches of a traditional physician and an environment medicine specialist, or clinical ecologist. The conventional practitioner will prescribe an antihistamine, along with a cautionary mention of possible side effects. In other words, this doctor, whether an internist or a traditional allergist, is concerned primarily with two things, the symptoms and the suppression of those symptoms. Little in his education or in his practice will have taught him to go beyond this narrow minded way of seeing.

By contrast, the environmental medicine specialist will wonder why his patient's nasal mucous membranes have become more reactive. Is there a nutritional deficiency at cause, or a decrease in the ongoing repair processes of these nasal tissues due to an overload of immunologic responsiveness? A decision may be made to perform testing of delayed food and chemical sensitivity. The environmental medicine specialist in this case may also want to rule out an occupational exposure to petroleum solvent, formaldehyde or other aromatics including tobacco. If he or she finds any such factors to be present, a decision may be made to mitigate exposure to the toxin or irritant by introducing an electrostatic precipitator or ionizer into the patient's home or work environment. In other words, the clinical ecologist will not simply try to identify and then suppress the symptom. He or she will use the symptom as a clue and will then embark on a course of inquiry aimed at finding the underlying cause or causes. If the cause can be identified, then a program aimed directly at it can be inaugurated: e.g., providing nutritional supplementation that will help nasal tissue repair, ridding the work or home environment of a toxic chemical, improving ventilation in a work space, etc.

DIVERGING APPROACHES TO CHANGE

Chapters 8 and 9 of this book examine the role of allergies and allergy testing from the point of view of environmental medicine. Environmental medicine specialists define allergies much more broadly than do conventional physicians. For example, according to environmental medicine specialist Dr. Marshall Mandell, central nervous system diseases such as multiple sclerosis may have a significant relationship to food sensitivities. Mental illness is another example where allergies may play an important role. According to Dr. Mandell, as many as eighty percent of those hospitalized for mental illness could be helped by adjustments in their nutritional intake or other changes in their environment. Another example is arthritis. Dr. Mandell refers to one patient with osteoarthritis who was told by his conventional physician that he would have to have both knees replaced. The environmental medicine specialist demonstrated this simply was not the case.

There are several other areas where this approach will shed light where conventional medicine remains in the dark, especially those involving other forms of testing. In America too many x-rays and intravenous pyleograms (IVPs)—both potentially harmful to patients—are performed, for example, simply because these tests are more familiar to practitioners entrenched in their ways than are the far less risky, newer technologies, such as nuclear magnetic resonance imaging (NMR) or ultrasound. Although environmental medicine specialists are holistic, that does not mean necessarily that they are always against the newest technologies.

While we are used to considering an allergy as a very limited factor affecting our overall sense of well-being, environmental medicine specialists tend to view chemical or food sensitivities as a primary suspect in the presence of any symptoms of a wide range of illnesses and complaints, including: fatigue, headache, insomnia, confusion, rapid mood swings, depression, anxiety, hyperactivity and schizophrenia; Tourette's Syndrome; heart palpitations, muscle aches, bedwetting, hayfever, hives, shortness of breath, joint disorders, including osteoarthritis and rheumatoid arthritis; muscle problems such as polymyalgia and myocytis; gastrointestinal disorders such as colitis, irritable bowel syndrome, nervous bladders, diarrhea and constipation, among other symptoms. Environmental specialists (clinical ecologists) also recognize heredity as a major factor. Children in families where both parents share a common allergy have a seventy-five percent chance of inheriting it. If only one parent is allergic, the risk that the child will have the same or a different allergy is reduced to roughly fifty percent. Psychological stress at work or at home is another predisposing factor which the environmental medicine specialist may consider important.

IMPORTANCE OF GOOD DIGESTION

Equally important is the healthiness of a person's digestive system. The stomach must secrete sufficient hydrochloric acid, and sufficient enzymes must be released through pancreatic secretions, for protein to be broken down into much smaller units, to enable thorough absorption eventually in the blood stream. If the digestive process is impaired anywhere along the digestive tract, any food or substance sensitivities will be intensified. Here lies one key to why the high-protein diet favored by Americans is so unhealthy. Since it takes so much longer to digest, it effectively sabotages, by means of a slow-down, the digestive process, greatly increasing the likelihood of an allergic reaction. Many types of illness prevalent in our country, such as peptic ulcers and heart disease to name just two, are relatively rare in certain less-developed countries in Africa and the Far East, which rely on a diet low in protein and high in complex carbohydrates.

BACK TO NUTRITION

As high as seventy percent of cases which conventional physicians will diagnose as "psychosomatic," will be diagnosed by environmental medicine specialists as reactions to inhaled or ingested foods or chemicals. In other cases, as Dr. Mandell notes, clinical ecology can assist even when it cannot cure. This may be the case with individuals suffering from epileptic seizures or in patients who have multiple sclerosis (MS). Severe cases of arthritis also fall into this category. In many cases, according to Dr. Mandell, these people have nutritional needs that are not being met. And in his opinion, that goes for eighty percent of the people in mental institutions as well. Not to mention many of those among us who suffer from standard allergies like hives, eczema, or hay fever.

FASTING

In many cases the clinical ecologist will begin by putting the patient on a fast which includes pure spring water and an environment completely free of cleaning agents, cigarette smoke, cosmetics, etc. In many cases, the patients symptoms will disappear after three to four days. Then it is a matter of tracking back to find what it was in the patient's daily life that had been triggering the allergic sensitivity.

PURE WATER

According to Dr. Mandell, about ten percent of his patients react adversely to chlorine. Although chlorine is necessary as a preventative measure for waterborne illness, you can buy a simple and relatively inexpensive purification system for your home that will draw out the chlorine after it comes through the faucet. It is important to be drinking pure water that is free of agricultural run-off, free of manufacturing waste, free of fluoride and free of chlorine. All of these chemicals may be affecting people adversely without their ever suspecting. Purifying the water can be an easy way to upgrade the feeling of well-being among those around you.

Just because an environmental factor did not cause a disease, that doesn't mean it isn't important to the subsequent course of the disease and recovery. As Dr. Mandell said on my radio program in September of 1989, "There is absolutely no question that environmental factors play a major part in many diseases; where they do not actually start the disease, they can complicate them. Anything that makes your illness worse is important for you to know about."

In the same way that cocaine goes right from the nose of the user to the nervous system in a matter of seconds, producing a wide variety of effects, so do toxins in the food or air produce a range of effects in the systems of highly sensitive individuals. Conventional physicians and traditional allergists simply miss out on this phenomenon by recognizing only a very limited range of symptoms. If their patients aren't sneezing or itching, they will not recognize the possibility that an allergy may be present. But, logically, once a doctor recognizes that minute flecks of animal dander or pollen in the air can produce marked symptoms, is it so difficult to see that chemical toxins in meat or milk, or air pollution, among a host of other possible causes, might also have an adverse effect? Simply put, the human race has evolved over millions of years and adapted to most of the conditions on this planet. But many of the pollutants and toxins we are dealing with have arisen over the last thirty to fifty years. Our bodies just haven't had time to evolve in response to these changes in our environment. Unless we act sensibly, by at least recognizing this discrepancy, we may cause great damage to ourselves and our environment.

Whatever you breathe in enters your body along with the oxygen. If your home, work or school environment is polluted, the pollutants will travel through the walls of the lungs, into the blood vessels of the lungs and ultimately reach the heart through the pulmonary circulation. Similarly, chemicals, additives and contaminants in our food and beverages will pass through the digestive system and reach the heart. Once there, they will be pumped through the blood stream. Every tissue in your body is exposed to what you eat, drink and breathe. That is why so many people are sick today.

Food addiction allergies are often misdiagnosed as hypoglycemia. The patient may find that each time he or she eats the particular food, say chocolate, he or she feels fine. But what is actually happening is that the patient is having a delayed allergic reaction to the food. Ingesting the offending food is causing an allergic reaction, but only after a time delay, so that the patient never connects the food with the symptoms. Or in another case, an individual may feel better immediately after eating. He or she does not connect the foods in the meal to any chronic symptoms which may occur much later, and yet they may indeed be the cause. Dr. Mandell claims to have seen thousands of patients, previously diagnosed as having low blood sugar, who actually suffer from some form of food addiction. In extreme cases, the patients may have been diagnosed as being mentally retarded or learning disabled. According to Dr. Mandell, fasting can free them of abnormal symptoms within two weeks. Once the culprit is found and removed from the diet, the improved behavior can be permanently established.

PERSONAL ACCOUNTS

Patty B. was diagnosed twelve years ago as having multiple sclerosis. She heard about Dr. Mandell and decided to try the environmental medicine approach.

"On the very first day, I had responses on some of the tests he [Dr. Mandell] performed which were exactly the same as my neurological MS symptoms. I couldn't lift my arms, my legs got heavy and my feet would drag. I felt very tired. And with each test I reminded myself, 'this is how I feel all the time at home.' After the tests wore off and I felt better, all I could think was, 'If only I could stay in this stable condition all of the time.' The next step was a nine-day fast under supervision."

Dr. Mandell explains, "We don't fast everyone for that length of time, but since we had already seen the difference foods made in this patient, we wanted to maximize the effects of the detoxification period. Of course, this patient did have MS and we weren't going to take that away from her. But her allergies were making her symptoms much worse than they had to be, and that we were going to change. We wanted her to be as well as she could be, so we fasted her one day at a time to see what changes would occur."

After the fasting period, Dr. Mandell was able to identify which foods did not produce an allergic reaction. Here's how the patient describes the difference:

"Before the treatment, there were days when I couldn't go up or down the three steps on the stoop of my house. I had to sit in a chair in order to bathe and couldn't wash my own hair. After altering my diet to contain only the food which we found to be nonreactive, I can go up and down a flight of stairs four or five times without trouble. On good days, I can do it ten times. I'm also able to hold a pencil under my right hand in order to write. I had previously lost use of that hand for three or four years."

Another patient of Dr. Mandell's is Debbie B., a 38-year-old teacher. Debbie teaches handicapped children who have the same disease she herself has, cerebral palsy.

Debbie describes the experience of going through the testing procedure: "In [Dr. Mandell's] office, I had the most bizarre reactions to the substances that were being tested. The uncontrollable involuntary movements I was producing made me feel like I was leading an orchestra. Then on my right side, which is my CP-infected side, the muscles of my right leg moved of their own accord in reaction to substances being tested. In response to one substance in particular I was literally unable to walk."

Dr. Mandell says, "We were able to bring on CP symptoms by having her eat beef or pork. Within an hour or so, her calf muscles tightened up so that her ankle came up off the floor, the muscles in her foot curled, and Debbie was walking with her ankle up and the back of her toes dragging on the ground behind her. By fasting her, and then spacing out meals, we could increase her tolerance. But with beef and pork in her diet on a daily basis, it took only four and a half days to bring back the symptoms. Now Debbie has it in her power to be completely crippled or not. She knows what brings on symptoms and how to avoid making her CP worse. We haven't cured one brain cell from among those that were damaged by the time she was born. But we have given her an awareness that enables her to make her life so much better than it was. Her neurologist had told her only that she had CP and there was nothing she could do about it. Our approach can make a difference in most CP patients, and yet, so far, UCP (United Cerebral Palsy) has shown little or no interest.

Fred J. had severe osteoarthritis. His orthopedic surgeon told him he needed knee replacement surgery on both sides at a projected cost of $30,000 per knee, or $60,000. Dr. Mandell describes their first meeting:

"During his first consultation with me, Fred mentioned that he had recently had a bout of flu during which he had involuntarily fasted for three days. During that period he noticed substantial improvement in his symptoms. Another thing Fred had noticed was that small doses of alcohol had the effect of alleviating the pain of his arthritis. We know that very often persons who have problems with alcohol are reacting not to the alcohol but to the food from which the alcohol is made. From the pioneering work of Dr. Randolph as early as 1956 we know further that the food residues in alcohol are rapidly absorbed. Since tiny doses of substances to which one is allergic can provide relief, in this case the malt, rye, corn, etc., the fact that he felt relief from symptoms in association with alcohol consumption gave us an important clue. These are some of the things which, as clinical ecologists, we are trained to recognize. Instead of discarding this vital information under the throw-away rubrics of terms like 'spontaneous,' and 'coincidence,' we used these clues to help us delve deeper. In the end we found what Fred's chemical sensitivities were. He never had to have that knee replacement surgery. Today, instead of needing the help of a cane or artificial joints, he walks on his own two legs."

In Fred's own words, "I only wish I had known about this thirty or forty years earlier, before the deterioration had started in my joints. I might have avoided all those years of feeling helpless."

Tim O. was a hyperkinetic child. The public school principle urged his mother to put him on Ridalin three days after he entered kindergarten because he was disruptive and inattentive. Year after year he stayed on increasing doses of the drug and Tim remained a problem child.

Tim's mother explains, "Whenever I asked doctors about my concerns that food might be affecting him, they always responded that diet was not a factor. Then I found Dr. Mandell. He identified sensitivities. One year and three months ago we put into effect a new diet based on chemical avoidance, using the information provided by the tests. Today, Tim is off his medication, an 'A' student and no longer a behavior problem."

Dr. Mandell comments, "Mothers usually aren't believed, even though they're the experts who live with their child's condition and know it best. It's not unusual for the child's behavior to be blamed silently on the mother, and this is one of the reasons why the doctor doesn't search deeper—he feels as if he already knows the real problem. But he is invariably wrong, since he has not considered the possibility of unrecognized allergies, unmet nutritional requirements, and so forth.

FOUR CLUES TO PROPER TREATMENT

Dr. Michael Schachter, also a clinical ecologist, or environmental medicine specialist, who received his medical training from the Columbia University College of Physicians and Surgeons, identifies four contributory factors which he considers to be the key in his examination and in determining a course of therapy. First, the quality of nutrition generally and the identification of any nutritional deficiencies; second, infections; third, psychological stresses; fourth, toxicity. According to Dr. Schachter, the course of therapy should be determined by the condition of the patient according to these four criteria. Nutrition must be complete, after being adjusted to remove any allergic reactions; infections must be treated; the causes of psychological stress should be removed or lessened; electromagnetic imbalances can be corrected; a detoxification program can be initiated to cleanse the body of toxins.

Dr. Schacter is also concerned with improving the oxygenation and energy utilization of the body at the cellular level. Anything we can do to improve that process is going to strengthen the immune system and thereby help reduce a person's tendency toward sensitivity and reaction. Thus Dr. Schacter encourages the use of oxidant therapies, but only up to a point, since oxygen in too high quantities can have a damaging effect. The key here, as in virtually every area of health, is balance.

Vitamins and minerals are another key component in Dr. Schacter's approach. Vitamin A is seen to be a major protective factor, guarding against both chemical sensitivities and infections. Thus cod liver oil, which parents once gave automatically to children, is indeed an excellent preventive medicine, with its high concentrations of vitamins A and D. Treating children with recurrent ear infections, Dr. Schacter has found that by simply enhancing their diet, removing most of the sugar and refined foods, and adding a spoonful of cod liver oil, the ear infections can be controlled and prevented in many cases. Other useful vitamins include vitamin C, vitamin B_{12}, and vitamin E, which is an anti-oxidant. Selenium and beta carotene are also important antioxidants. Vitamin B_{12} can help counteract the adverse effects in the body of pesticides in the environment. Moreover, while conventional physicians may test for B_{12} levels in the blood stream, normal levels may be present in the blood while there are deficiencies at the cellular level.

As for oxidant therapies, the first and foremost must be aerobic exercise. Keeping in mind that oxygen is the main nutrient of the body, it is easy to understand that as we improve oxygenation, we improve the body's ability to detoxify and we enhance the immune system. Beyond exercise, a number of new nutrients are available to enhance oxygenation, such as germanium and ubiquinome, as well as a variety of traditional oxygenation techniques.

According to Dr. Schachter, infections are a key factor in going from troubled to good health. Frequently, he says, infections will yield to non-toxic treatments.

Take candida, for example. There is a tendency for patients who have been exposed to repeated use of antibiotics, who include a lot of refined carbohydrates in their diet and who may have been exposed to steroids or birth control pills, to develop a chronic overgrowth of candida, a yeast-like, fungus-like organism which we all have in our bodies. In certain cases, the infection will give off toxins which may impair the immune system and produce a variety of symptoms. Some of these will be the result of food and chemical sensitivities which have been aggravated by the infection.

Dr. Schachter has found that starting the patient on special diets which exclude refined carbohydrates, especially sugars and alcohol, and include various nutrients, including certain fatty acids which inhibit candida growth, will go a long way towards controlling the infection in many cases. He also notes that garlic is a strong anti-candida property.

Chronic viral syndromes are another key problem. A previously healthy individual suddenly gets a flu and instead of recovering completely, the flu is followed by frequent complaints of fatigue, exhaustion, swollen glands, sore throat, night sweats, anxiety, and loss of appetite. And yet conventional testing shows nothing definite. More sophisticated testing may show exposure to various viruses. But the main problem here may be that the person's immune system just isn't responding as it should. Dr. Schacter has obtained excellent results in patients with this kind of profile by using nutrients to bolster the immune system. Intravenous vitamin C may be used, along with germanium and a variety of other vitamins and minerals given orally. In cases of herpes virus, for example, he may use high doses of the amino acid lysine, which has anti-viral effects for the herpes virus and certain other viruses. For short treatment periods, he may administer as much as ten to fifteen grams of lysine per day in these patients.

Psychological stress is another key factor, according to Dr. Schacter. Environmental medicine specialists, he warns, must be careful that in emphasizing the importance of the physical environment they do not underestimate the importance of psychological factors in determining the strength of an individual's immune system.

As for toxicity, Dr. Schacter feels that hydrocarbons and other chemicals are already playing a major role by damaging our immune systems. Heavy metals are also playing a role, in his opinion. He sees chelation therapy as a valid treatment to detoxify our systems of the effects of heavy metals, as well as for cardiovascular disease, where chelation therapy has shown impressive results.

In sum, in treating the allergic or chemically sensitive patient, Dr. Schacter believes it is important to look at the specific kinds of food allergens and chemical sensitivities that may be involved, employing rotation diets and neutralization diets, but also to go beyond these issues to seek any underlying factors which could be important as well, like infections, chemical pesticide poisoning, heavy metal poisoning, and stress. It is important to deal with each aspect independently and it is equally important that the program be synergistic, one which will make the patient less sensitive to his environment, more resilient and healthier overall.

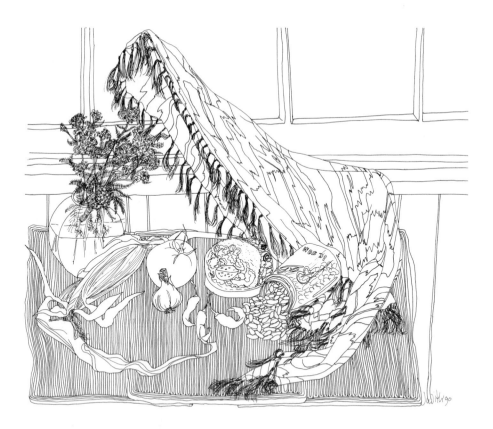

21 · CANDIDA

"If candida is suspected, an experimental regimen of antifungal medications and the corresponding nutritional treatment can be implemented; if the symptoms clear up with treatment, the diagnosis is confirmed."

CANDIDA ALBICANS IS A yeast-like fungus that lives in the mucous membranes of warm-blooded animals, including humans. Usually it co-exists with its host in perfect harmony and does no damage. However, in individuals whose immune system is depressed, the balance between candida and our body can become skewed and the condition can become pathogenic, creating a variety of non-specific symptoms that affect entire body systems. Japanese research about fifteen years ago found that a toxin could be isolated from candida, which created the range of systemic systems associated with yeast infections in humans when it was injected into mice. Dr. Orien Truss first described the candida syndrome at a meeting in Canada ten years ago; his research shows that candida affects the body's metabolic processes.

Candida can attack the nervous system, resulting in fatigue, headaches, irritability, memory loss, and depression; the hormonal functions, especially in women, causing premenstrual syndrome, menstrual irregularities, and loss of sexual interest; and the digestive system, causing bloating, constipation, or diarrhea. Yet often a general medical examination will fail to reveal the cause of all these symptoms.

Several factors can create the imbalance between candida and its human host which makes it toxic. One is the prolonged use of broad-spectrum antibiotics, especially tetracyclines. This use is quite common; low doses of tetracyline are frequently used for months, even years, to treat acne patients, or bladder or ear infections, for example. Cortisone, too, can be at fault; cortisone decreases the T-helper cells, an important component of the immune system.

It's not necessary to have taken a long course of antibiotics to be at risk for candida, however. We must not forget that our foods can contain any of 2,700 different preservatives which are approved by the FDA. Our food also contains low-grade doses of antibiotics and hormones commonly fed to animals before slaughter. Our environment, too, can affect our immune system; pesticides, weed-killers, and industrial wastes find their way into our air and water supply, where they are almost impossible to avoid.

Another factor in candida is the hormonal fluctuation which occurs in women in the third trimester of pregnancy, as well as in the week before the beginning of the menstrual cycle. At these times hormonal changes alter the vaginal secretions and elevate their glycogen content, favoring *Candida albicans* growth. The birth control pill also changes the lining of the vaginal membrane, making it more apt to develop a vaginal yeast infection.

The diet also affects the growth of yeast in the body. Sugar—and maple syrup, honey, fructose, and other simple carbohydrates—triggers a yeast imbalance.

FOOD ALLERGIES AND CANDIDA

There is a great overlap between food allergies and the candida problem. In a survey which Dr. William Crooks recently made of twenty-five doctors who treat candida, every one indicated that these patients also have food allergies. Yeast, wheat, milk, and corn are some of the worst culprits. Part of this overlap may have to do with cross-reactions taking place between the candida yeast organism and yeasts or molds in food; in addition, patients who have had their immune system weakened by antibiotics or some other factor tend to have both food allergy and candida problems.

DIAGNOSING A CANDIDA PROBLEM

A total clinical history is most important in identifying a patient likely to suffer from a candida imbalance. Because of the systemic nature of candida symptoms—that is, the disease manifests itself in a wide variety of ways and affects the whole body, rather than creating clearcut and unique symptoms—it is difficult to diagnose from an examination and description of symptoms alone. A medical history should include records of the use of antibiotics, cortisone, and radiation or chemical therapy for tumors. Any of these are a warning sign that the immune system has been tampered with and suppressed, a major factor in yeast infections.

Symptoms which tend to be worse on damp days, or in moldy areas, also point to a candida problem; the person who has a candida problem will have a cross-sensitivity to yeast and mold in the air. Symptoms that are triggered by eating sweets or simple carbohydrates are also an indication, since candida affects the body's metabolizing of carbohydrates. These patients will often crave the very sweets that set off their symptoms.

There are laboratory tests available which measure antibody formation. Their value for candida diagnosis is limited, however, since candida patients are often just those who are already immune-suppressed. For an antibody test, the patient's system must be able to form antibodies toward the pathogen, which is the yeast factor. Many patients, especially cancer patients and candida patients at certain stages, will not be able to form enough antibodies to show on these tests; as a result, their antibody tests might be perfectly normal. Research has shown that there is a false negative of as high as 25 percent with these tests in those who have a definite candida infection.

Antigen tests, however, bypass the formation of antibodies, as they look for the presence of the candida organism itself—the antigen—in the bloodstream. The mere presence of the candida cell in the bloodstream—not in the gastrointestinal tract where it normally belongs, along with friendly bacteria—indicates a candida problem more accurately than is possible with the antibody tests.

Stool tests and vaginal smears can detect candida but, again, have several caveats associated with them. First, even healthy people will have some candida cells in the vagina or intestines. Someone who has been on a long antibiotic regime may have considerably more yeast cells. To make matters more complex, though, there are two forms of the candida organism. One is a little round cell, or bud; the other has branches, or mycelia, which can dig into the mucous membrane. This second type may stay in the deeper tissues and not show up in the stool.

Finally, if candida is suspected, an experimental regimen of antifungal medications and the corresponding nutritional treatment, as outlined below, can be implemented; if the symptoms clear up with treatment, the diagnosis is confirmed.

A CAUTION

The diagnosis of candida infection as a catch-all for chronically ill patients should be treated with caution and some skepticism. Candida has become in vogue recently, especially among some cosmopolitan, health-conscious groups. Doctors should be especially alert; patients often enter the office wanting a diagnosis of candida. The hope of a "magic-bullet" cure for a yeast infection may appeal to chronically ill people who are suffering from more significant diseases. Before anyone who is ill jumps onto the candida bandwagon, it is a good idea for them to get a thorough medical examination to rule out the possibility of tuberculosis, diabetes, cancer, and other serious conditions which can also cause wide systemic disfunctioning.

TREATMENT

Many doctors will treat candida with Nystatin, an oral antifungal medication. Long-term use of this—or any other—drug will tend to become less and less effective, however; the underlying conditions that caused the misbalance in the first plalce must be addressed in any truly effective regimen.

Dr. Luke diSchepper, author of *Candida: The Symptoms, the Causes, the Cure,* outlines a seven-step therapy. First, look at the diet. At the mention of the word "diet," people tend to ask how long they will have to keep on it. This diet cannot be a temporary "fix," though; it must be a transformation of a person's eating lifestyle. Simple carbohydrates—sugar, maple syrup, honey, fructose, processed white bread—should be avoided, but the diet should provide plenty of complex carbohydrates. For the first few weeks fruits are cut out of the diet, but reintroduced gradually after that. It is vital to keep away from all yeasts, molds, and fungus at first, as well. It is almost impossible to keep all of these foods out of the diet indefinitely; Dr. William Crooks, in his book *The Yeast Connection*, advises patients to try some brewer's yeast after a week of total elimination of yeasty foods, to see if it causes trouble. If there is no reaction, the patient may be able to take foods containing yeast and molds, including mushrooms, in moderation.

Diet will starve the candida cells, but they should be replaced with friendly bacteria—lactobacilli, bifidia bacteria, and vulgaricus—which are normally present in our gastrointestinal tract and which help to suppress yeast cells and maintain a natural balance. Unless these organisms are encouraged, it's like leaving a door open for yeast cells to return. Acidophilus milk, supplied as soon as the diet is begun, will be very useful in supplying these friendly bacteria. This should be taken before the introduction of any antifungal drug.

Drug therapy, the third step, should be used carefully, and not by itself as an easy cure. Nystatin, which has been prescribed routinely by many physicians, is outdated for several reasons. It is expensive for what it is, and it doesn't kill all the strains of candida. Some patients stay on Nystatin for two years without result. At first, it kills many of the candida organisms, but over time the strains which it doesn't affect assert themselves. The patient reaches a plateau and keeps taking the drug with less and less effect. In addition, people can easily become allergic to Nystatin, and may suffer withdrawal symptoms if the dosage is decreased or discontinued after a long time, when the candida will increase dramatically. Nystatin is only really useful for short-term and local use: vaginal or rectal, or as a post-nasal drip.

Caprylic acid is more effective, especially when candida is found in the blood. Other products are only available in Europe, not having been approved for use in the United States. Fungizone, for example, is available in America only in the intravenous form, which can have some unpleasant side effects. The oral form, which has been on the market in Europe for fifteen years, has almost no side effects. Intensive research has shown that three- to four-gram doses are needed to kill the candida, rather than the one gram that has habitually been used.

Caprylic acid, Fungizone, and Nystatin to some extent provide relief from the effects of candida, but they all have the shortcoming that they only address the candida, and not the weak immune system which allowed it to get out of control in the first place. The most important steps in therapy for candida are aimed at reinforcing the immune system.

Acupuncturists faced with the symptoms of the candida syndrome five hundred years ago would have called it "Deficient Spleen Pancreas Energy." The spleen pancreas organ plays an important role in the metabolizing of food into energy, and it is also the main organ in producing T-helper cells, a vital component of our immune system. Thus the immune system can be strengthened through acupuncture points on the spleen-pancreas meridian.

Many supplements can be used to boost the immune system. Antioxidants are especially important. These are: vitamin C, at least 10,000 mg. per day; vitamin E, 400 IU a day; selenium, 100 micrograms; beta carotene, 25,000 units; and zinc—for instance, 50 mg. of zinc oratate a day. People with a candida problem tend to lose magnesium, which can also be supplemented. The essential fatty acids, found in fish oils, linseed oil, and evening primrose oil, play an important role in maintaining the immune system and metabolism.

Staying fit both physically and mentally is vital to an efficient immune system. Exercise and support from doctors, family members, and, if necessary, a counselor, are the sixth and seventh steps in candida therapy; they will boost resistance to candida and the ability to deal with it.

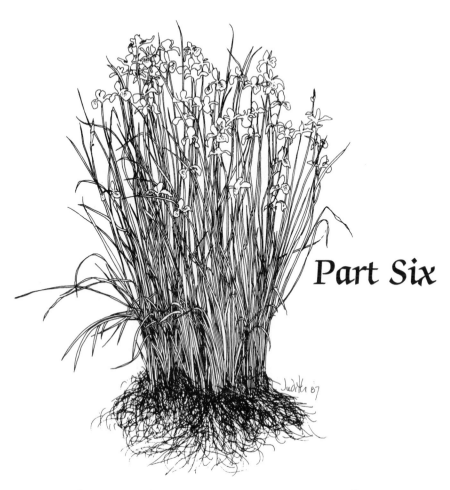

Part Six

Alternative Approaches
to Illness

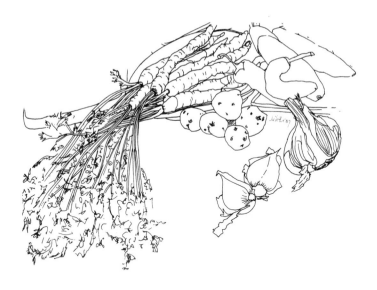

22 · PAIN MANAGEMENT

"Many people are strong in many areas of their life, in career, in forming relationships, in playing sports, but when it comes to their own health, they cede all control to a doctor. To really escape pain, the patient must take a big part in the recovery process."

EVERY DAY TENS OF MILLIONS of Americans wake up knowing they are going to contend with pain, whether it be from arthritis, migraine, muscular skeletal problems or other aches. Many do not realize that there are varied ways of treating pain naturally.

In this country we need a different approach to acute and chronic pain. We need to go from treating just the symptoms to treating the sufferer holistically through a mind/body approach.

Getting the proper nutrition through sensible eating and ingesting natural supplements, such as minerals and herbs, are key ways of treating pain, though other methods, such as the Trager technique, shiatsu and acupuncture also have a part to play. In this chapter, we survey a broad range of healing strategies that can be used by anyone suffering from chronic or occasional pain.

NUTRITIONAL THERAPIES

Herbs

Herbs eliminate pain by dealing with the underlying causes. In Chapter 17, we spoke at length on the way herbs can be used to deal with different health problems. We stressed how herbs help stimulate the immune system. We mentioned the theory that our DNA may carry an immunological memory, grounded in our inherited knowledge of the efficacy of plants. In this section, we will add a little to what we have said so far by suggesting some uses of herbs to lessen or do away with pain, specifically the pain of menstruation.

There are different types of pain. Some are inflammatory, hot and pounding. Some are due to toxins in the body that need to be cleansed. Proper herbal treatment can assist the body to do away with both the pain and the causes of this pain.

Herbalist Letha Hadady says we must approach the pain of PMS (premenstrual syndrome) from both the emotional and physical sides. Emotionally, there are two types of PMS. One is the angry type. Aloe root is recommended for this. It cleans the system and cleanses the liver. It may taste a little bitter, but it is easy to take when added to a little apple juice.

A stronger gall bladder and liver cleanser that lessens the impact of menstrual pains is the Chinese preparation Lung Tanxieganwan—20% ginseng, it aids digestion and reduces anger. It also calms and quiets headaches and other pains.

The second type of PMS is weepy. It comes from sadness and excess phlegm, brought on by eating foods that are too rich, too sweet, and too oily, or by drinking too much milk. Eating radishes, parsley, or barley soup will cut down on the phlegm. A remedy for this type of period is homeopathic Pulsatilla.

To treat the pain of both types of menstruation, warming herbs like cinnamon and myrrh are invaluable. Capsules or drops taken in tea will increase blood circulation and clean the uterus, inducing a more complete period; one that does not start too early, stay too long, or finish early only to begin prematurely. A warming and cooling remedy for the pain is as follows:

1/2 cup aloe vera gel,
10 drops or one capsule myrrh,
apple juice

This combines the cleaning action of myrrh with the cooling of aloe.

VITAMINS, MINERALS AND OTHER SUPPLEMENTS

In Chapter 5, we saw how minerals are essential for building up the body, maintaining the body's fluid balance and helping with many chemical reactions. Now, we look more narrowly at how minerals and vitamins have proved effective in treating pain.

Dr. Luke Bucci states that for handling spinal column disorder, Carpal Tunnel Syndrome, or arthritis, an antidepressant may prove helpful. Carpal Tunnel Syndrome occurs when, because of repetitive tasks, the tendons in the wrist are inflamed, which squeezes the nerves, which then tingle and go numb. About one third of the cases of this syndrome can be cured by the administration of B_6 (100 mg/day) to which can be added B_2 (50 mg/day). To deal with the pain of the condition, one should take St. John's Wort (hypericum perforatum). This substance has a molecule that works like a pharmaceutical drug without any of the drawbacks or side effects.

TMJ (Temporal Mandibular Joint Syndrome) is a condition of the jaw that can cause acute, long-term suffering. TMJ is of two types. It either derives from muscle spasms or degenerative joint disease. The spasm type can be treated with Feverfew or magnesium (citrate), also effective for migraines. With the degenerative type (recognizable by clicking and popping joints) where it will be necessary to rebuild cartilage, one should take glucosamine (1,500 mg), chondroltin sulfate (1,000 mg), magnesium, manganese, and vitamin C (2-4g/day, in divided dosages).

Magnesium salts are also useful for those facing pain from torso or joint aches. Many people are already deficient in magnesium. It is a calmative mineral, obtained from nuts and seeds that are raw and unroasted. Nuts are also beneficial in that they contain essential oils, including the Omega 3 fatty acids, which also have mild anti-inflammatory properties that help reduce pain.

For torso and joint problems, the dosage of magnesium (citrate) salts should be 400 mg/day, divided into doses of 100 to 200 mg each. (See pages 52-53, for a more general profile of magnesium and its sources.)

Sound sleep is an essential part of good health. For those people who have trouble sleeping due to headaches or other pains, there are a number of useful supplements. Valerian can be used or Hops (the same element found in beer), skullcap, or passion flower. These supplements, which can be mixed, should be taken one half hour before sleep, in either capsule or tincture form, in a dosage of 1 or 2 capsules. One might also try taking 1mg of melatonin before sleep.

For the pain arising from PMS, GLA (Gamma Linolenic Acid) is valuable. It can be obtained from Evening Primrose Oil, Black Currant Seed Oil, or Borrage Oil. The sufferer should take 3 to 6 pills per day. As an adjunct to GLA, vitamin E is helpful. Also to be taken is B_6 (100 mg/day) and magnesium, which smoothes muscle contractions.

Here, as with all vitamin therapy, the patient must be consistent, following through on taking the supplements for two or three months to be assured of the effects.

The pain of sciatica, or pinched nerve, can be reduced by lowering the inflammation at the nerve root. Here one should try a proteolytic enzyme, such as Bromolone, Papain, Trypsin, or Chymotrypsin to support the body's natural healing properties.

Muscular skeletal pain, which may be due to too much lactic acid, can be removed by a number of substances. L-Carnitine allows the body to burn fats and soak up excess lactate. Also helpful with muscles are the methyl donors, such as DMG (di-methyl glycine) and TMG (tri-methyl glycerin), taken at a rate of 100 mg/day.

To reduce the soreness after exercise, one should take vitamin E (400-800 I.U./day), which prevents the leakage of enzymes from the muscles.

A final way to approach pain is to modify the way the brain perceives it. DLPA (D.L. Phenylalanine), which is a synthetic form of amino acid, slows down endorphins, making the ones you have work better. Taken in a dosage of 500 mg/three times a day, it reduces chronic pain while getting the sufferer off analgesics.

Thus, there are many ways to nutritionally enhance the body without using pharmaceuticals that overwhelm the receptors.

TOUCH THERAPIES

Beside eating herbs and supplements so as to give the body additives that assist it in reducing or eliminating pain, another set of natural therapies applies pressure to the body to stimulate energy flows or tonify the organism. These strategies, which are often derived from Oriental medical practices, include shiatsu, rolfing, Trager technique, acupuncture, and cranio sacral therapy.

Shiatsu

Shiatsu is based on the principle that a vital energy, called *qi* (*chi*), flows through the body. The primary cause of pain is imbalance of this energy. The goal of the healer is to balance the client's energy so pain and discomfort do not manifest or, if they do appear, will be relieved.

As Thomas Claire, a body work practitioner, explains, in performing shiatsu, he use thumbs, fingers, palms, forearms, elbows, and even knees to apply pressure to specified points in the body to modulate the flow of energy. During a shiatsu treatment, the client lies on the floor on a comfortable padded surface, such as a futon, fully clothed or undressed to his or her level of comfort. What the client feels is pressure, which can be gentle or deeper at the places where the practitioner is working. As the pressure continues, the patient will generally feel relaxed and energized at the same time.

Shiatsu is good for treating a variety of different pains. It is especially beneficial in combating chronic pain that may be found in the back, neck, or shoulders but it has also proved effective in treating whiplash, herniated disk, and nervous problems, such as Bell's palsy.

The shiatsu healer concentrates work on certain pressure points that have metaphoric names that tell us something of what they do or how they are to be worked with.

The first point of interest is on the ankle and called Spleen 6. It is at the meeting of three yin meridians and is the most powerful point for tonifying the feminine energy in the body. It can be located by placing the little finger on the border of your inside ankle and counting up four fingers. At the very top of these fingers and at the center is Spleen 6. To modulate the energy, you can put pressure on this point with your thumb, pushing three times in succession for 7 to 10 seconds each time. This pressure will stimulate the feminine energy, helping a woman control PMS and irregular cycles. Moreover, since all of us have feminine and masculine sides, use of this point can also be beneficial to men and can help with sexual problems such as impotence.

The corresponding point for male tonification is called Stomach 36. To locate this point, find the indentation just outside the kneecap. Put one finger at this indentation and go down four fingers. There you'll find Stomach 36, which is also known as Leg 3 Mile. This second name is given since, it is said, if you have a strong Stomach 36, you can walk three miles with no trouble due to your strong stamina. Manipulation of this point can lead to a tonification of masculine energy as well as the whole body. For women, this point can be used to ease childbirth and labor pains.

A third important point, located at the middle of the web of the hand, is Large Intestine 4, also called Meeting Mountains. This latter denomination comes from the mountain of flesh found jutting up between the thumb and index finger when you close your hand. To locate this point, find the highest point on that protruding flesh, then open your hand. This point should also be pressed three times running for 7 to 10 seconds in order to tonify the upper body. Pressing this point can also help with nausea, vomiting, colds, and constipation.

Pericardium 6, or the Inner Gate, is found on the forearm. If you flex your hand, you'll find two tendons that pop up on the inside of your wrist. You go up these tendons and press. This point is particularly good for controlling nausea (such as that from morning sickness or motion sickness).

Another valuable point is found right in the middle of the palm. Pressing it can relieve tension like that arising from a stressful work environment or relationship.

Runny nose, allergy, colds, and sinus infections can be treated by pressure on the point called Welcome Smell, so named since nearly any smell is welcome to a person whose nasal passages have been blocked. To approach this point, take the index finger and bring it in at a 45 degree angle to the crease under the nose. This pressure can be applied on either side of the nose though it is not recommended that both sides be touched simultaneously, which might block breathing.

In fact, all these pressures can be applied to either side of the body, since the meridians are bilateral and bring the same energies to each side of the body.

Acupuncture

In a brief note in Chapter 16, we mentioned acupuncture as a means of releasing blocked energy pathways. Like shiatsu, acupuncture sees pain as derived from this blocked energy or *qi* (*chi*). In treating this blockage, the practitioner has to determine whether it stems from an overabundance or deficiency in energy, so the treatment can be adjusted depending on whether it is necessary to strengthen or decrease *qi*.

The acupuncturist first records the patient's medical history in the manner of a conventional doctor. Then, with the patient lying down or seated, depending on the area to be treated, fine-gauge, stainless steel needles are inserted into significant points and meridians to exert different physiological effects on the body and induce both relaxation and energization. The patient will remain in this position from 20 to 30 minutes, though an appointment with an acupuncturist may last up to an hour, since part of the time will be spent consulting about the employment of other traditional and herbal treatments that might be recommended. Body work and massage might also be included in the session.

Dr. Christopher Trahan notes the treatment will have analgesic and anesthetic effects, will block pain, and accelerate recovery from motor nerve injury. Moreover, it enhances the immune system, can have a sedative effect, help with muscular spasms or neurological problems, have a homeostatic effect so as to balance blood pressure, and have psychological effects, acting directly on brain chemistry.

If we look specifically at what acupuncture treats we would have to mention muscular, skeletal and structural problems of the body, arthritis, TMJ, Carpal Tunnel Syndrome, insomnia, asthma, headaches, digestive problems, such as ulcers and irritable bowels, menstrual cramps, and pleurisy.

Trager Technique

The Trager technique is a way of working with the mind and body simultaneously. According to the philosophy backing up this technique, pain comes from the accumulated action of the patient frequently tightening his or her movements and posture. To correct it, the practitioner uses gentle motions to increase the patient's pleasure in the quality of the tissues and decrease the restriction and the sense of holding. The practice works by reaching into the functional subconscious with particular qualities of movement, posture, and sensation. Gentleness is emphasized so that no message will be sent to the body alerting it that pain is on the way or causing the patient to tighten in on him or herself. The movement reaches into the central nervous system with a motion at once pleasurable, lengthening, softening and opening, conveying this sensation to the tissues and joints. The movements can be very small and internal or at the peripheries of the body in the limbs. In the latter case, the limbs are used as handles to reach the core.

Roger Tolle, Trager practitioner, says some clients will feel results immediately as the touching allows them to release pain. In other cases, it takes a repetition of the information into the body/mind, which will gradually allow the client to re-learn how to go about daily activity with a different quality of motion.

The Trager method works with the kind of pain we see in the neck and upper back, in migraines and sciatica, in holding patterns in the lower back, in the pelvic rotation muscles, in TMJ, and Carpal Tunnel Syndrome, also with pains due to repetitive motion of a constrictive kind.

Rolfing

According to the practitioners of rolfing, pain is due to chronic shortenings in the tissue. Correction of this pain can be accomplished by soft tissue manipulation. This manipulation acts to create order in the body so the client stands tall and free of restriction.

David Frome, a physical therapist, states rolfing is done in a ten-session series, designed to address all the shortenings in the structure systematically. Each session works in a different area. In the first hour, for instance, concentration is on the trunk, shoulders, and hips. The second hour works on the back and lower leg. Going through the complete series allows the therapist to work through all the body's shortenings. During a session, a patient may experience a tingling sensation and a sense of release. The patient should strive to draw the deepest possible breath to aid in the treatment.

The major goal of the treatment is not pain relief per se but it has been found to help with TMJ, frozen shoulder, tennis elbow, Carpal Tunnel Syndrome, chronic hip problems, sciatica, cervical neuropathies, and knee, foot, and ankle problems.

Cranio Sacral Therapy

The sacral region is that at the top of the spine. Between it and the head there should be a balanced rhythmic motion maintained for the health of the organism. When pain arises, it may be due to a restriction that disturbs the harmony between these two regions or between them and the rest of the body.

In cranio sacral therapy, the practitioner places his or her hands on the client's body in such a way as to try and bring the cranium and sacrum back into alignment with a natural rhythm re-established. Charles A. Kaplan, the founder and director of the Center for Pain Management, points out that this hands-on technique is usually centered on touching the head or lower back but can be done anywhere, such as on the fingers or toes. Some patients will go through a first treatment and not feel anything, but most will leave the treatment table feeling very relaxed and stress free.

Cranio sacral therapy is recommended for dealing with muscular and skeletal pain, headaches, pains in the back and neck, sports injuries, sciatica, and nerve pain. It can also be beneficial to those recovering from pneumonia or bronchitis, helping by loosening the ribcage. This treatment is a tremendous stress reducer, while it can eliminate back pain and improve the immune system.

OTHER THERAPIES

Magnet Therapy

With an ancestry as old as that of acupuncture and shiatsu, magnet therapy, like them, acts to influence the body's energy.

Dr. Jim Joseph mentions that the healing power of magnets was known in 2200 B.C. China. Such ancient fathers of medicine as Galen and Aristotle discussed magnets as did Paracelsus, one of the founders of chemistry. Magnet therapy was believed in by Mesmer and others in the nineteenth century and is still being developed and practiced today.

Down through history, magnets have been used to deal with the causes of various ills. As Joseph remarked, "Pain is a messenger. We don't want to kill the messenger but find the cause."

When there is pain in the body, it can be because positive energy is being drawn to the site of injury. To bring about this transfer, the brain sends out a negative signal. Using the negative side of a magnet can augment and assist that reaction. Furthermore, around an injury there will be an acidic buildup. The negative side of the magnet is an alkalizing force that can help alleviate the pain accompanying this acidity.

A second source of pain arises when a person is overworked or suffering from undue stress. The individual cells of the person become distorted, overly positively charged. Putting a negative magnet on a weakened area will repolarize the cells, bringing them back to balance.

The distortion of the cells' polarity and resultant pain may also be caused by our technological environment. We are swamped with positive electromagnetic pulses coming from TVs, radios, electric clocks, and all the other electrical devices around us. The pulses of their fields are not congruent with the one found in our body and so can throw us into disharmony and disease.

Magnets can be obtained in a plastiform that can be molded and shaped for a particular area. They last indefinitely and are low priced. A medium-sized magnet may cost $20. Available healing magnets are color coded with the negative pole green and the positive red. The positive side of the magnet is active, sun oriented; while the negative side is relaxing, and earth oriented. All of the treatments to be discussed utilize the negative pole. One must be careful with the positive pole since positive magnetism causes growth to any biological system, even the growth of cancer when it is present. Treatment should last from 20 minutes to overnight. The magnet's power should be from 1,000 to 6,000 gauss.

A magnet can be wrapped on the area to be covered with Velcro. Special wraps in which the magnets are inlaid in the Velcro are available. These wraps can be placed on most parts of the body though they should not be used on the eyes. Since negative magnetism pulls fluids and gases, placed near the eyes, the magnet would draw out its fluids. If work is to be done on the eyes, the magnet can be placed off to the side. From this position, magnetism can be exerted on cataracts to reduce oxidation and free radical development. The magnet's value in reducing oxidation is due to the fact that oxygen is para-magnetic. When you breathe, you are pulling negative energy from the earth into your body.

To deal with edema, a magnet is placed on the body, not at the site of the problem, but near it and directed toward the heart so as to pull the edema away from its place of occurrence. If you have edema in the calf, for instance, place the magnet above the knee to draw the fluid up from the site of the disturbance to the kidney from which it can be excreted.

For the pain of menstrual cramps, a magnet should be placed on the lower abdomen, two inches below the belly button. This placement should not be used, though, for one or one-and-a-half hours after eating since it will interfere with peristalsis. Also, a magnet should never be used by a person using a Pacemaker or implants of any metal.

The negative side of the magnet is also good against parasites, who will stop eating when hit by the negative energy.

At night, it is useful to lie on a magnetic bed pad and put magnets behind the head where they will bathe the pineal gland in energy. This usage will induce a restful night's sleep. By using a magnet, one could sleep less than one's normal night's sleep and feel even more rested than one did with the greater time. The magnet has also been known to increase sexual abilities.

The magnet can help with shoulder pain, that of the rotator cup, as with aches in the back and lumbar regions. Magnets can be attached to the head or neck to deal with hypo-thyroidism, depression, migraine headaches, and problems with the vestibular system. For depression, the magnet should be placed near the occipital lobe.

MIND/BODY CONNECTION

Lastly, some therapists have recommended a more eclectic approach, one that looks for and relies on the often overlooked synergies that flow between the mind and body. One physician, Ron Dushkins, brings up a number of points to consider when dealing with pain. He notes, first, the importance of relaxation, which will quiet and calm the nervous system. Remember that when we feel pain, we also are feeling a layer of stress on top of that pain. If the layer of stress is relieved, then the pain will diminish significantly.

Human touch can also play a part in relieving pain. As babies we like to be touched and as adults we still find this important.

A third overlooked factor in healing is humor. The writer Norman Cousins tells the story of how he was hospitalized with a critical health problem. As he saw it, a lot of his physical deterioration was due to stress and negative thoughts from that stress. He reasoned if we can create disease by stress than by alleviating stress, through means such as humor, we can cure disease. He had a movie projector brought into his hospital room and began showing Marx Brothers' films and other comedies. Soon his room became a place of congregation for other patients who wanted to enjoy the shows. It got rather chaotic because so many people were coming into this room and laughing. You're not supposed to do that, not supposed to laugh in a hospital. Some people were scandalized. Cousins said doctors would give him blood tests before and after he had been laughing at a humorous film and they would find an improvement. He had less pain after laughing.

Guided imagery is also an element of the mind/body connection. With this technique, a sufferer will place a hand over the injured area and invite the other cells in the body to go to the aid of this damaged area. After all, the body's cells always work together and this is one way to encourage their interplay.

All of the methods mentioned as part of the mind/body connection get the patient to take charge of personal recovery. Many people are strong in many areas of their life, in career, in forming relationships, in playing sports, but when it comes to their own health, they cede all control to a doctor. To really escape pain, the patient must take a big part in the recovery process.

This could be said to inform all the strategies for dealing with pain we have encountered in this chapter. Whether you are taking appropriate herbs or mineral supplements to reduce suffering or selecting a non-traditional, natural healer to help you redirect your energy or re-polarize your cell, in each case, you have studied, meditated, and selected the natural way to diminish pain.

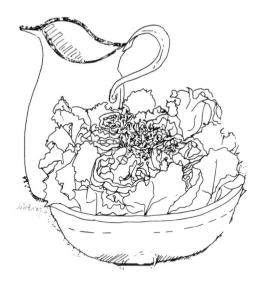

23 · ARTHRITIS

"The way I treat arthritis is probably quite different from the approach of most physicians. As a naturopath, I was taught we should not always think about treating a disease, but about treating a person. Arthritis is a very good example of a disease which is highly individualized. Not only are there different types of arthritis, but people get it and express it in different manners."

—Dr. Peter D'Adano

IT IS ESTIMATED THAT 40 MILLION Americans suffer from some form of arthritis, whether rheumatoid, osteo arthritis, or lupus. We know the kind of discomfort this can mean: swollen joints and excruciating pain. It can be so bad it prevents a person from having a quality life. The mainstream medical community has done the best it can, giving immediate relief but seldom sustaining it or, even less often, offering a cure. But are there techniques that have a different view of cure and treatment? Is it possible, by radical modification of lifestyle and by acquiring knowledge of detoxification, perhaps by working with acupuncture, reconstructive therapy, herbs, physical therapy, chiropractic and other alternative methodologies, to actually prevent and reverse all the different forms of arthritis? Let us look at the natural approach.

WHAT IS ARTHRITIS?

The word arthritis means pain and swelling of the joints. A joint is the place where two bones meet. Cartilage covers the end of each bone and prevents the bones from rubbing together. The joint capsule surrounds the joint and protects it. Special membranes surround the joint and make a fluid that lubricates. Muscles and ligaments around the joint provide support and make it move. When all these parts are working right, the joint moves smoothly and easily, but when something is wrong with the joint, arthritis may develop. In osteo arthritis, the cartilage is worn away so the joints rub against each other. When the cartilage breaks down, the joint may lose it shape. The ends of the bone may thicken and form spurs. In rheumatoid arthritis, the lining of the joint becomes inflamed, swells, and feels warm, tender, and puffy. Eventually the bone and cartilage may be destroyed.

Besides these two types of arthritis, there are over 100 diseases that affect the area around the joint, including lupus, fibromyalgia, polymyalgia, gout, sclerderma, juvenile arthritis, and ankylosing spondylitis.

TRADITIONAL TREATMENTS

Dr. Warren Levin, of Physicians for Complementary Medicine, emphasizes blending alternative and traditional medicine, except in the case of rheumatology, where there is very little good to say about conventional treatment.

Peter D'Adano, N.D. (a naturopath physician), mentions that the Latin word 'arthritis' actually means inflammation of the joint. The problem is that physicians' treatment of this disease is nothing more than the long-term use of something that is best used to briefly treat an acute case of chronic inflammation rather than be applied over a period of time for a less severe inflammation.

Michael Schachter, M.D., at Physicians for Complementary Medicine, states, "For the most part, conventional physicians use a variety of over-the-counter anti-inflammatory drugs like Motrin or Advil which, although they give temporary relief from pain and inflammation, over the long run, seem to make the disease worse. They inhibit the formation of cartilage, which is one of the root causes of the osteo arthritis. Also they damage the internal lining of the intestines, which results in 'leaky gut,' whereby large molecules of food get into the bloodstream, causing antibody formation, which can bring on faster damage to the joints."

According to Morton Teich, M.D., the orthodox approach works well at times, but it treats the symptoms and does not get to the cause and, moreover, has deleterious side effects. To look at the cause is very important because if you do that, in many cases you can abate the cause and not have to deal with the side effects.

AMA

Dr. Levin recalls that a couple of years ago the AMA put out a series of videotapes instructing physicians on how to take care of and diagnose rheumatoid arthritis. The lecturer on the tape was adamant that nutrition had nothing to do with arthritis. "His whole face filled the screen and he said, 'Nutrition has no place in the treatment of arthritis. We can use drugs.' That is the AMA way. They have not come to Physicians for Complementary Medicine to see what success we have with our methods and how the vast majority of our patients dramatically improve without the use of the toxic drugs that characterize American medicine's treatment of arthritis."

Dr. Teich points out, "The problem is the people who insist there is no relation between nutrition and arthritis, who refuse to look at the literature and refuse to look at the studies."

TREATMENT

Dr. Rich Ribner from the Friar Center suggests we try to listen to the body and realize it has an intelligence. In other words, if you are following a certain lifestyle and your problems are the result of this lifestyle, then possibly a change in lifestyle will change the illness.

People say that as the body gets older, the most natural thing in the world is for it to get decrepit. But give the body credit for the intelligence it has. When the body tells you something, if you will listen and follow what it says, you will improve.

What is arthritis? It's pain. Why is it painful? Well, what have you been eating? Maybe you say, "I have a very good diet. I have pancakes in the morning with sausages. Then orange juice. I use saccharine"—precisely a diet loaded with substances that will bring complaints from the body. So we must think of detoxification. Our air is noxious, our oceans are polluted and so is the body. So we have to help the body heal itself by first cleansing.

Eating Right

Peter Agho, M.D. of The Tri-State Healing Center, says, "I do diet. Not just for arthritis. The thing about the whole diet is this. Change the diet, and the arthritis—along with obesity, high blood pressure, and other problems—will get better. The diet should include fresh fruit, including fresh fruit juice, and vegetables. You should eliminate animal fats and cut high fat foods."

Dr. Ribner adds, "Eat natural foods as close to their original states as possible."

Dr. Howard Robbins, of the New York Healing Center, outlines his treatment: "We use a complete vegetarian diet, including a lot of green leafy vegetables. These are important because of all the phytochemicals and phytoestrogens that help in all the chemical processes that are necessary to being well again. We give them juices, six to eight fresh green juices a day—the best way to take in these chemicals."

Dr. Luke Bucci, author of *Pain Free: The Definitive Guide to Healing Arthritis*, notes that part of the reason people get arthritis is because of the lack of essential nutrients in a highly processed, refined diet. Sure you get plenty of calories, protein, and fat—usually the wrong kind of fat. What you do not get is just as important—the minerals: magnesium, zinc, copper, manganese, boron. Many people are not aware of boron as a nutrient, but boron might turn out to be essential to our joints' health. These are what you do not get with our current, typical American diet. We lack the substances that prevent the joints from repairing themselves from the damage they get. That is why you want to start eating a whole food diet, rich in organic vegetables, fruits, and nuts.

Dr. Ribner tells this story: "Recently, a woman came to the clinic with a terrible case of arthritis. She was in terrible pain and had been taking anti-inflammatory medication and tranquilizers. She was miserable. She said she thought about killing herself. I said, 'Stop this nonsense. I'm going to ask you to do something. You may not even want to do it.' She said, 'Anything.' So, I said, 'Between now and next week, I want you to drink six to eight glasses of water a day, but it has to be distilled or spring water. And eat nothing but brown rice, just brown rice.' 'But, but...' she began. 'Wait,' I said, 'You were talking about killing yourself. So, listen, I'll add a few green vegetables to that.'

"You have to make sure there is a cleansing. Make sure they drink the water. Have a bowel movement daily.

"Well, this woman was so desperate that she stayed on the diet one week. When she came back there was marked improvement. She still had a long way to go, but there was a change."

Supplements

Dr. Bucci believes that special nutrients can help and prevent rheumatoid arthritis, and the most important substance for healing arthritis is glucosamine. There are several types of this. For glucosamine sulfate, you should take 1,500 mg a day in divided doses; glucosamine hydrochlorides work quite well also.

They "convince" your joint tissues to repair the damage. If the situation is not too far gone and you still have cartilage, you can rebuild it to normal which means being pain free or greatly improved status.

Another very important nutrient is chondroitin sulfate. Chondroitin is one of the things glucosamine gets synthesized to in your joints. Chondroitin is one of the molecular "cements" or "glues" that holds together cartilage and lets the collagen protein be laid down forming the actual tissue.

Another interesting finding has been the value of our friend vitamin C. This should be taken as 4,000 mg/day in 2 or 3 doses with meals. We have thought about using C for many other problems but is it also a very important nutrient for the joints. Along with glucosamine, it is the only other substance that can stimulate the cartilage to repair itself. The drugs have not been able to do this.

Another substance of value is vitamin E. Take 400 IU/day in one pill. It helps reduce pain as has been shown in human clinical trials. Also useful is vitamin B_3 (niacinamide). This should be taken in 150-200 mg dose 3 to 4 times a day. It will not kill pain right away—it takes time, maybe up to one or two years. But you'll see a gradual improvement, as range and function of the joint are bettered.

Magnesium and the obscure mineral boron are valuable. Areas of the world where they have low soil levels of boron show more osteo arthritis. Several human studies have been done that show that a very minor dose of boron, some 3 to 6 mg a day, can reverse the symptoms of osteo arthritis. This is very promising and exciting. I think boron is related to another mineral, magnesium, which has not had as much clinical trial. But we know it is extremely important for every healing process in the body. So there is a very definite link between boron and magnesium.

Interestingly, if you do not eat your fruits and vegetables, it is almost impossible to get a dietary intake of boron, since it comes almost exclusively from vegetables and fruits.

"One of the questions I get as I go around the country," Dr. Bucci continues, "trying to spread this message of the connection of nutrition and arthritis is: 'Where is the evidence? No one's heard of glucosamine.'

"Well, I'm not the one who thought this up, though I may have rediscovered it. There is valid, strong scientific research and human clinical trials on this substance, millions of man hours of use of glucosamine sulfate by doctors, mostly in Europe. Others in Europe are using substances they extracted from the cartilage itself, such as the chondroitin sulfate.

"There is a very large body of literature on the topic, with dozens of human studies and even more with animals. We know how and why these substances work because this is how the body heals itself. So I answer their question about where are the studies with my own question: 'Where's everybody been?' Why have people not read the prodigious literature available? Why don't people just open up their eyes and read?"

Allergies

Dr. Levin makes the point that another important aspect to look at is allergies to foods and chemicals. Removing the offending substance from the patient's environment—whether internally with food externally with chemicals—we see dramatic changes over and above what we see with just vitamins and minerals.

Dr. I-Tsu Chuo says the apparent cause of arthritis is common foods, what the patient eats all the time.

Dr. Teich elaborates that the food the patient wants the most is the problem, like milk, for example. He cites a study by Richard Pettish (*Arthritis and Rheumatism*, February 1986, "Food induced arthritis. Inflammatory arthritis exacerbated by milk") that shows milk can cause severe allergy and arthritis.

Many studies indicate that food definitely causes problems; the nightshades, for instance—the family including potatoes, tomatoes, tobacco, coffee—bring on allergies. They also crossreact with ragweed.

He warns, also, of the glyco proteins in milk, wheat, corn, and cinnamon, as well as inhalants such as dust, mold, or pollen. Chemicals are also vitally important in causing allergies as are additives in foods.

CHIROPRACTIC

Many arthritis sufferers we interviewed for this chapter said of all the things they tried to eliminate the pain, going to a chiropractor helped the most .

Dr. Mitchell Proffman, a chiropractor at the Tri-State Healing Center, showed me two x-rays. The first showed bones nice and clean and square in shape; the second showed degeneration of the bones.

He showed what arthritis looks like in the human body; thinned disks and a little lip or spur, the body's defense mechanism to heal or shore up the area so it does not totally disintegrate. He said to think a person has a pinched nerve somewhere in his or her body, in the neck, for example meaning it is out of alignment. He administers a gentle push with his hand, which is not painful, to move the bone back into position. The nerve energy comes through and the joint can start to heal.

RECONSTRUCTIVE THERAPY

Noted physician Dr. Arnold Blank has used reconstructive therapy as an important means of treating arthritis. He mentions that thousands of patients complain to doctors each year of chronic pain and of joint, muscle, tendon, and ligament dysfunction. Frequently, the doctors aim to relieve the symptoms but do not deal with the cause of the illness. People take pills, anti-inflammatory drugs, steroids, even use surgical procedures. Many times, they're worse off after the treatment than they were when it started.

Reconstructive therapy, created in the 1920s by osteopathic physicians Gedney and Schumann, is a healing approach that works by stimulating the body's ability to heal itself. Their design was to help stimulate the body's ability to heal ligaments, tendons, and cartilage. The doctors found that by injecting substances that caused a slight irritation to these tissues, they would help the blood vessels grow into the region, thus bringing more oxygen, vitamins, and minerals as well as the fiboblast growth factor, into the cartilage, promoting tissue growth.

Dr. Blank introduced me to one of his patients. "George has had an injury to his shoulder due to chronic overuse. I have been injecting into the ligaments in and around his shoulder joint.

"This therapy works best when the patients are in an optimal nutritional state. Vitamin and mineral levels are important in our healing response and ability.

"The injection consists of a variety of different liquids. Primary liquids I use are calcium, lydicaine, and saline. They take a moment and really aren't painful.

"The majority of patients feel improvement after the first three or four treatments, developing some strength and feeling less pain, even increasing the range of movement.

"The nutrients we may use, natural ones, include ones that have an anti-inflammatory effect, such as vitamin C, shark cartilage, sea cucumber, glutathione, and glucosamine sulfate.

"All of these substances are used once reconstructive therapy has begun because the new blood vessels going to the tissues will enhance healing. These nutrients may not work well when there are no blood vessels going into the area, so they should be administered after the therapy has begun its work."

Another male patient recounts his experience:

"I injured my back and didn't realize it until I started getting aches in the back of my leg. I had heard about reconstructive therapy so I started on my back, had so many treatments, then I went to the hip, knee, and shoulder. They all feel great at present."

HERBOLOGY

Letha Hadady, an herbalist, asks what role herbs, used each day by millions of individuals, can play in helping with arthritis.

She relates an important thing to remember about arthritis is that it is essential to eliminate the underlying problems that make it possible. Killing the pain is not enough, you need to eliminate the toxins that result from poor digestion and poor circulation.

She shares some of her herbal secrets for total health—using produce and herbal remedies, substances you can find in the grocery store, the health food store, or through mail order.

In dealing with arthritis, one thing you must have everyday is alfalfa. You could chew ten tablets a day with a little water to eliminate much of the uric acid that could build up to create joint pain. Rhubarb also eliminates acid. It is a laxative but it also breaks apart the crystals that form around your joints to give you pain.

Another wonderful food, full of vitamins and minerals, is dandelion greens. Anything green will be a rich source of calcium. Dandelions break down pain-giving acid too.

Star fruit is a sweet delicious fruit you can find in your grocery store or vegetable stand. Juice it. Add a cup and a half of cold water. Drunk three times a day, it will eliminate inflammatory joint pain, bleeding hemorrhoids, and burning urine—it is cooling and cleansing.

It is important to realize that not everyone's arthritic pain is the same. Do you wake up in the morning with your joints feeling stiff and sore? Do they feel better after you move them around and after you exercise? If so, you need to take warming, tonic herbs that build vitality, increase circulation and warm joints Adding a pinch of turmeric to your stews will do this. Turmeric and cinnamon are a good combination for achy shoulders. If you have rheumatism that gets worse in cold weather, add a quarter of a tea-spoon of turmeric and cinnamon to a little water and drink it as a tea.

Asafoetida is a spice available in Indian stores. A little added to cooking beans or other hard-to-digest foods will help cleanse the body and warm the joints.

One other thing you can use is the resin myrrh; a few drops added to your tea makes your joints feel warm and your blood move, bettering cir-culation.

Hadady says Asian medicine uses many herbs that can be added to cook-ing. For example, Tang Kuei increases circulation and warms joints. Another very safe and classic Chinese remedy is Du Huo Jisheng Wan, one that Chinese doctors have used for generations, which makes arthritis in all parts of your body feel better.

Her favorite, Guan Jie Yan Wan, translated as "walk as smoothly as a tiger." This remedy brings blood circulation exactly where you need it—your hips, legs, and joints.

The wonder of Asian remedies is that a combination of herbs take the painkiller where it needs to go. There are so many, including Raw Tienchi ginseng, Efficacious Corydalis, Tien ma, Three Snakes Formula, Mobility 3, Clematis 19, Eucommia 18, Leigong Ten Pian, Rinchen Dragjor-Rilnag Chenmo.

ACUPUNCTURE

Acupuncture has been used by countless people throughout the world to help alleviate the pain and suffering of arthritis. Dr. Yuan Yang of the Tri-State Healing Center reminds us arthritis around the joints causes much pain. "We put the needle around the joint to create circulation, taking the pain away. There may be cold, blocked blood and low energy, so I apply the needle for smooth blood. Moving blocked energy takes the pain out."

I asked her, "Are you saying that putting acupuncture needles around the joints where they are swollen will stimulate better blood flow and help relieve the symptoms?"

"Yes," she responded, "then we have to do energy points. We must find the whole body energy points. Maybe we will work with the spleen point, the meridian and kidney points. These points will help circulation any-where in the body and will make for better circulation and digestion."

PHYSICAL THERAPY

Shmuel Tatz works at Medical Arts at Carnegie Hall with an exercise physiologist doing mostly hands on treatment, going directly to the problem, to the arthritis. He works with people who have arthritic problems from overuse syndromes or accidents.

They go directly to the joints. For example, working with a pianist who has problems with the hands they will try to move the bones, separating the joints to make more space.

"Today in physical therapy we use many modalities. One of these is magnetic pulse therapy. We know of the positive effects of magnetism on the body. Scientists have developed a machine with different programs so that we can make adjustment for every different situation.

"We put electrodes on the body. For example, on the hip joint. Here it stays for 15 to 20 minutes. Usually, patients report a very mild relaxing sensation and the pain decreases.

"Many people with pain from osteo arthritis are afraid to be touched. People with a swollen knee, for instance, can do reflexo therapy. For the knee we touch an acupuncture point on the ear which gives relief."

Once this manipulation has had an effect, they start to exercise the knee by putting the legs in slings, relieving the pressure on the joint, making it easier for the patient to move the body. By trying to open the joint and make more space around the bones, it allows better circulation.

The same can be done for every part of the body—for the shoulder, neck, and so on—movement is very important for people suffering with arthritis.

Lori speaks about her improvement:

"Here at Medical Arts, I was able to receive physical therapy, which has enabled me to avoid surgery and has greatly improved the quality of my life. I'm still dancing."

YOGA

Molly McBride, a yoga instructor, believes you do not have to stop working on your health simply because you may have some physical limitations. You will see how easy it is, even working with something as simple as a chair, to stay fit and help yourself with the problems of arthritis.

The basis of yoga is breath and breathing practices, she says, which helps circulation and also helps flush the body out by collecting toxins to exhale them. Breath is the foundation of all the yoga stretches.

We start with just taking a simple breath; the basic beginning exercise is a three-part breath. Let the air fill the abdomen, then the ribcage, then the upper chest. Exhale, letting the breath exit the upper chest, then ribcage and then abdomen. Inhale, exhale.

It is important to take time everyday to do these breathing exercises. A really good time to do them is first thing in the morning when your stomach is empty or, if you have eaten, wait a few hours before you start the practices. These breathing exercises can be combined with some simple joint lubrication exercises. To regenerate the body and increase the flow of oxygen through the whole system, to help relieve all of the toxins that get built up in the muscles and the protective cartilage around the joints, try simple yoga exercises.

CONCLUSIONS

To understand the nature of the treatment, you have to understand the first rule to health is good hygiene, personal and internal.

What does that mean? Well, a lot of Americans are eating fairly good diets some of the time, but not all of the time. Whenever you eat something bad for yourself, you undo whatever a good diet was accomplishing.

Not all diets are the same. I say get a good diet. But what does that mean? Does it mean eat hamburgers and cheeseburgers? No! It means eat a diet that is rich in live food. Does live food mean raw food? Not necessarily. It means nutrient-rich food loaded with life-supporting live enzymes. Give up meat, yes. Caffeine, absolutely. Sugar, yes. And give up chicken. Eat fish, the ones that are rich in the Omega fatty acids that help lubricate joints and will help your heart. Mackerel, cod, salmon and sardines. These are the fish that are the most important for a good diet that helps prevent arthritis.

Take six g1lasses—and I'm talking about 12 to 14 ounce glasses—of fresh, organic juice. These juices should be aloe vera, cabbage, cucumber, celery, apple, and carrot. These are the mainstays, the primary beverages. (The aloe vera should be taken from the bottle, not as a plant which has diarrrheal properties.) Concentrate on these unless you are hyperglycemic or diabetic, in which case you will have to stay away from carrot and apple because they make your blood sugar level too high. Add such things as dandelions and a small amount of mint. Almost all the other vegetables can be juiced, and these are outrageously good, particularly for arthritis.

Make sure you are getting the right nutrients—to find out, you can check your blood. Make sure you get folic acid, niacinamide, pantothenic acid, vitamin D, and vitamin E (400 units/day). You can take from 2,000 to 20,000 mg/day of vitamin C, adjusting what you need each day, depending, for example, on how much stress you are under. Under stress, increase your dose. If you have a disease like cancer or chronic fatigue syndrome, increase your dose even more. The necessary nutrients are vitamin B_{12} (1,000 mcg), vitamin B_6 (50 mg/day), vitamin B_2 (50 mg/day), vitamin B_1 (25-50 mg/day), vitamin A, a lot of which you'll get from the juices and fish oils (25,000 units/day), and MaxEPA (1,000 mg/day).

The minerals we need are calcium-magnesium (1,200 mg per day), iodine, and sea vegetables, which are wakame, kombu, nori, and hijiki. One four-ounce serving of these vegetables a day is good for the trace minerals. Also take phosphorous (700 mg), potassium (500 mg), sulfur, which can be found in garlic (2000 mg), onions—an onion a day keeps the heart and blood circulation in good order—and manganese (25 mg). There are also the more esoteric minerals such as evening primrose oil (200 mg/day), superoxide dismutase, Co-enzyme Q 10 (100-200 mg/day), silicon extract, boron (5 mg), copper lysinate (2 mg), methionine, and selenium.

Selenium, by the way, is not in our soils. And if it is not in the soil, it is not in the plant and so it will not get in our bodies.

Methionine is an amino acid found in soy. Take enzymes. People with arthritis often have deficiencies in liver enzymes. Rebuild the intestine, the liver, the pancreas. Take the plant-based enzymes which are the primary nutrients.

Here is what it comes down to. You must eliminate milk, red meat, sugar products, green peppers, eggplant, tomato, tobacco, alcohol, salt, deep fried foods, preservatives. Then you have made a major step in re-balancing the body chemistry.

You are doing two things: detoxifying so you do not have those triggers going off and damaging your body, and fortifying your body with those green vegetables, supplements, minerals, phytochemicals. You are exercising and doing other good things; in total, something has to work.

I know it sounds complex, but look at the benefits.

The average person with arthritis does none of the above. He will try simply to take a drug and hope for a miracle. But the miracle does not come. Who are you going to blame. The doctor? No. The pharmaceutical company? No. It is our expectation that something outside of ourself is more important for helping us than our innate healing capacity.

I hope you have been enlightened about many of the different treatment possibilities for arthritis. We did not give you a prescription for cure, but the idea that there are more options and choices and being able to see and make those choices is vital for healing.

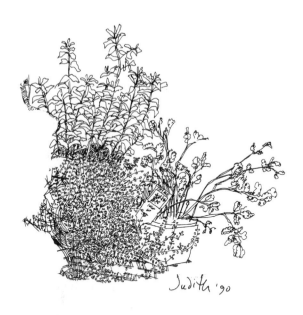

Judith '90

24 · CHRONIC FATIGUE SYNDROME

"Why is it that for ten years Americans with a debilitating illness were not recognized as having a disease? They were simply told that chronic fatigue syndrome does not exist. Dean Black says, 'You have to go back to the last century and you will read about women suffering from nervous disorders—so many of them that clinics had to be set up to care for them. There was always the search for a cause, but one couldn't be found and so, without a cause, doctors wouldn't say it was a disease. It had to be in the patient's mind. This is not a new way of sweeping things under the carpet.'"

CHRONIC FATIGUE SYNDROME poses a major problem for traditional medicine, which has fumbled in its treatment to the point of sometimes claiming the illness does not exist.

But chronic fatigue is a major problem in the United States. Millions do not have the energy they once had. This goes from those having just a little bit of energy to those with a maximum depletion, who are in bed, unable to function. This chapter will look at different courses and natural therapies, nutritional and psychological, to help people, especially as many traditional healers have abandoned the field. We ask: What is the natural approach?

DEFINING CHRONIC FATIGUE SYNDROME

Our readers may recall Charlotte Perkins Gilman's classic short story, "The Yellow Wallpaper," written at the turn of the century. It focuses on a woman who feels lethargic and constantly worn out. However, since her husband, a doctor, cannot find any organic cause, he refuses to believe she is really sick. He keeps telling her to lie down, although this "rest cure" is not working and even making her sicker. As we will see in a minute, when we hear the opinion of Dean Black, this common female complaint in the nineteenth century provides a striking parallel to the reception of chronic fatigue syndrome, which many practitioners, not finding its cause, have tried to ignore.

Neenyah Ostrom, author of *America's Biggest Cover-Up*, underlines that chronic fatigue syndrome is very difficult for the average doctor to diagnose especially because the government agency charged with creating a definition of the illness has come up with one so misleading that nobody can figure out what the illness is supposed to be. In late November 1995, there was a meeting at the Centers for Disease Control in order to discuss changing the definition of the disease. It turned out researchers wanted to define it out of existence, so that anyone who is tired can be said to have chronic fatigue syndrome. Ostrom argues, "If you speak to any clinicians who see people with this condition, they will tell you it is very easy to diagnose. They can tell within moments of talking to a patient whether the patient has it, since the symptom complex is so unique."

Why is it that for ten years Americans with a debilitating illness were not recognized as having a disease? They were simply told that chronic fatigue syndrome does not exist. Dean Black says, "You have to go back to the last century and you will read about women suffering from nervous disorders— so many of them that clinics had to be set up to care for them. There was always the search for a cause, but one couldn't be found and so, without a cause, doctors wouldn't say it was a disease. It had to be in the patient's mind. This is not a new way of sweeping things under the carpet."

Ostrom mentions, "Since there are debates in the government on whether chronic fatigue syndrome exists or not, very few therapies have been tested for chronic fatigue patients."

Dean Black brings up another historical example to explain the current difficulties traditional medicine has in coming to grips with chronic fatigue syndrome. He says that we need to go back to the origin of the current paradigm, in the 17th century, when Rene Descartes promulgated his doctrine of universal doubt, which held that one could know nothing without scientific method. "People would say things to Descartes, but he would explain them away, saying, 'I can see this, this, or this equally plausible alternative.' He felt we could only know things for certain if we have a scientific method whereby we can define truth in a rational, cause and effect manner. Now that method had a certain amount of rules, one of which was there had to be a straight line between a single cause and a single effect. Deviate from that and you introduce so much complexity that the idea of certainty is lost.

"Medicine's power base is the idea of its basis in certainty, which hinges upon the concept of a single, linear, cause-effect relationship. That's why medicine is always looking for a single causal factor. This is called the theory of specific etiology."

In reference to chronic fatigue syndrome, Black alludes to the situation of Epstein Barr, which was initially thought to cause chronic fatigue syndrome, although later this theory was debunked. "That is why they were so happy to discover this EB virus," Black explains. "It seemed marvelous to them because it served to justify the single cause idea. Yet, as has been frequently pointed out, everyone may have Epstein Barr [it is so widely distributed]. Chronic fatigue syndrome is caused by many factors operating together. But this idea has been excluded by traditional medicine, which refuses to come to grips with multi-factorially generated disease. So medicine's reluctance to accept this multi-factorial explanation is because it holds to this idea of absolute truth, which requires simplicity and must have one cause and one effect."

Andrew Gentile, Ph.D., stresses that we need to be able to differentiate between chronic fatigue syndrome and other health problems. Since chronic fatigue syndrome has no known cause, we need to rule out other disorders that we know the cause of. The working definition provided by the government for this disease says there is no other illness at the root of it. Distinguishing it calls for great care, since feeling fatigue is ubiquitous as a symptom of many diseases, such as anemia, low thyroid, hypoglycemia and a variety of other illnesses. These other illnesses must be clearly ruled out.

Gentile calls chronic fatigue syndrome a degenerative disorder that causes fatigue and has flu-like symptoms. The fatigue is not a simple tiredness, it is an exhaustion accompanied by feelings of unwellness. Often patients are bed-ridden for months. The chronic fatigue syndrome—a syndrome is a disorder that contains a collection of symptoms, but is not necessarily a disease entity—includes sleep disturbance as one of its manifestations. The patient is not able to fall asleep or stay asleep and does not feel refreshed or restored after much sleep. The other symptoms have to do with cognitive and intellectual functioning. As Gentile describes, "Patients will go from one room to another and when they get to the new space, they can't remember why they are there. They can't remember the name of a colleague they worked with for years. There are difficulties in concentration and an inability to read complex texts. So there are cognitive symptoms, sleep disorder, flu-like symptoms, frequent sore throats, tender lymph nodes and often fevers and chills."

DIAGNOSIS

Dr. Martin Feldman says the first step in the analysis of any patient who comes to him with fatigue, whether mild, moderate, or severe, is to profile the patient to see how he fits with the five major categories or possibilities of the syndrome. It is not, by any means, that every patient with the syndrome has these problems, but they are a good place to begin tests in case of weaknesses in the areas. These five indicators, with Feldman's comments, are 1) An immune viral breakdown, leading to low adrenal function. "You'll find that almost all chronic fatigue syndrome people have low adrenal function once you test the adrenals properly"; 2) Thyroid imbalance. "A large proportion, though a little less than half, have these issues"; 3) Vitamin B deficiency; 4) Hypoglycemia; and 5) Cerebral allergies. Within those five are found almost all people with chronic fatigue syndrome.

For Feldman, after these tests, the next phase is testing thymus, spleen, and the lymphatic system. He states, "It's very easy yet very hard to test the thymus because you have to use electrical energy. You could test the T and B cell counts. That's easy to do but it's very expensive; so, in daily practice, it's easier to test thymus electrical energy. You can also do this for the spleen. When we have a circuit, like a weak thymus circuit, we can try any aspect of therapy within the weakened circuit to obtain a resonance in a way that will help that circuit be strengthened and come up."

Dr. Gentile is more concerned with self diagnosis. "If you feel you have chronic fatigue syndrome, ask yourself these questions: 1) Am I not just tired but have had debilitating fatigue for six months? 2) Do I have flu-like symptoms? 3) Can I not find any physiological cause? 4) Do I have pronounced sleeplessness? 5) Do I have low stress tolerance so that if I take a short walk or try any sport, I feel vaguely ill and tired? If you answer yes, you may want to consider a fuller assessment of yourself by a physician."

Majid Ali, M.D., states that most physicians have a tendency to focus narrowly on one or two aspects of a problem But, he says, "I don't think trying to find a diagnosis for one or two symptoms is terribly important. What is important is how the patient describes his suffering. We need to think of what things we can do at a molecular and energetic level to relieve his suffering and restore his health.

"I've seen patients whose lives have been devastated by chronic fatigue syndrome. They've gone through all these drugs, anti-virals, steroids. With each drug, they get better initially and then nose-dive. What do we do?

"Think of chess. In chess, the queen is the most powerful and the pawn is the weakest piece. But as a good chess player knows, there are many games in which the lowliest piece, the pawn, can take that all-powerful queen. This can be done by a player who is able to 'read the board.' And I think what a good holistic physician has to be able to do is read the board. What I mean is look at the patient's whole situation and then, as a doctor, ask yourself: 'Should I first work on the kitchen, what the patient eats, or should I first work on self regulation, control of breathing and so on, or must I first create some hope, make them talk to other recovering patients and take a workshop?'" Making the correct choice of initial therapies should take precedence over minutely analyzing the symptoms.

CAUSES OF CHRONIC FATIGUE SYNDROME

Viral Possibilities

Although many resist the multicausal explanation for chronic fatigue, as Dr. Gentile notes, some healers have been able to develop such an explanation. "There is now the feeling that a single cause is not sufficient, and, moreover, in the world of treatment, it is now much more productive to work on caring for the symptoms than on continuing on a quixotic search for a single cause. Healing is really the charge of medical research."

Feldman tells us that chronic fatigue syndrome is an entity of severe fatigue with a 50% reduction in capacity. There is a continuum of fatigue problems, and chronic fatigue is on the low end. "One will find two factors involved," he states, "first, a flu-like infection, either a new or renewed one, and often, though not necessarily, a history of such infections, whereby the viral mix—for there may well be more than one virus involved—weakens the immune system. The second point is that this immune system difficulty somehow pulls down hormonal function. Almost all patients with this syndrome have low adrenal function and many have low thyroid function. So we have a hormonal mix-up causing fatigue, but behind this is the viral disease pulling down the immune system."

According to Ostrom, "What is probably behind the chronic fatigue disorder is a virus that was first found in AIDS patients. It is called Human Herpes Virus 6 (HHV-6). What is interesting is that there are two types of this virus, one form is found very widely in the general population and the other is found in people with cancer, AIDS, chronic fatigue syndrome, and other immunological problems. That virus can attack the immune system very effectively and I believe it will eventually be found as instrumental in causing chronic fatigue syndrome, AIDS, and some forms of cancer."

Gentile adds that a plethora of studies look at viruses in connection with this syndrome. One theory has it that there is a single viral agent. In fact, he states, "I have heard chronic fatigue syndrome being called a number of things: from Epstein Barr to mononucleosis.

"Epstein Barr was brought into the discussion by way of a lab in Philadelphia, which exclusively studies this virus. One of the lab assistants was negative for current and acute Epstein Barr virus, but during the course of the study the assistant developed the symptoms of chronic fatigue syndrome. He was treated and found to be positive for Epstein Barr virus. So we had the first studied case in which a person went from Epstein Barr negative to Epstein Barr positive at the same time as he had all the symptomatology for chronic fatigue syndrome. That began a flurry of studies investigating the Epstein Barr connection. We now know there is not a high degree of correlation between the symptoms of chronic fatigue syndrome and Epstein Barr serological tiders. So Epstein Barr is probably not the cause of chronic fatigue syndrome."

Gentile goes on to note that the EB virus is widely distributed in the populace. Most people have it by age eight. So there is not a clear discrimination between those who have it and those who do not. We would expect many more people to be ill with chronic fatigue if it was indeed Epstein Barr that was causing it. As a result, this candidate for being the cause of chronic fatigue syndrome has fallen into disfavor.

"However," he persists, "several other candidates have presented themselves, including HHV-6 (formerly called HBLT), which is a B lymphocyte virus and was being studied by the National Institutes of Health. But again, studies showed that this virus is very widely distributed and thus could not be the distinguishing agent that was responsible for the syndrome. There are other studies proceeding. Wistar, a renowned laboratory in Philadelphia, is looking at a retro virus, HTLV-2, as a possible cause."

Neil Block, M.D., reminds us that quite a list of viruses have been implicated in some forms of fatigue syndrome. These viruses include, along with Epstein Barr, Herpes, Coxsacki, Adeno, and Entero viruses as well as a number of lesser known ones. He echoes Gentile in saying, "The one that has received the most attention, Epstein Barr, has not panned out as an answer and, indeed, in some sufferers, it plays either a very minor role or no role at all. But it can't be dismissed. And most cases deserve to be tested with an Epstein Barr viral tider to determine the antibody status, whether there is or has been current or past infection with the Epstein Barr virus."

Other viruses that have been implicated are the long-lasting sequalae or aftermath from the hepatitis virus, the mononucleosis virus or influenza virus, all of which have been known to cause a fatigue two or three months after the original virus has disappeared.

Dr. Ali says, "It's very enlightening to look at Epstein Barr. I come from Pakistan and for us Epstein Barr was not a kissing disease. Because of poor sanitation, all of us were exposed to the virus as children. But we came through the exposure with intact immune systems. Our immune systems fought off the Epstein Barr and we acquired a certain resistance. In this country, people will get infectious mono or Epstein Barr (those are the same thing) later. They get it in college or high school. It's the so-called kissing disease. They will be sick for four or five weeks and lose some weight. They'll be tired for some months and then snap back."

However, he states, there is a different possible scenario. Think of people in their 30s and 40s, with good jobs. They are not fit and are under tremendous stress. Their nutrition is awful, and now comes Epstein Barr and it floors them. "The problem," Ali states, "is not that Epstein Barr is more virulent; the problem is their molecular defenses are shattered. Their bodily ecosystems are destroyed and so they have no ability to fight back. So whether Epstein Barr is a devastating terminal attack on their immune system or a garden variety illness they can easily get over depends on the state of their previous health. You give Epstein Barr to little children and they generally survive very well. In fact, they generally don't even know they have this disease. So the issue is not the power of the virus but of our defenses."

Gentile states, "The consensus among practitioners is that a single virus probably does not cause this illness. We have to carefully distinguish between cause and trigger. Clearly, a virus may trigger a cascading set of events in various body systems: neural, endocrinal, cognitive, hormonal. A variety of abnormalities may be found in these systems, but if viruses do trigger these imbalances, then they quickly hide within the normal cells—

which does usually happen with viral behavior—while their effects wreak havoc in the body system."

It is as if the virus triggers something in the immune system wherein the system cannot find its way back to homeostasis, failing to self regulate. There is a breakdown each time the immune system is stressed by toxic load from the environment or food allergies or when infections are reactivated. The flare-ups and relapses occur and reoccur frequently, reproducing all the symptoms. These relapses then compound themselves. If a patient is not sleeping every night, then symptoms like exhaustion and a deranged immune system crop up.

"We know, by the way," Gentile adds, "that the rhythms of this illness dovetail nicely with 90 minute circadians. In sleep, we have a REM cycle that occurs every 90 minutes, and this is the cycle by which our immune system is synthesizing proteins. The immune system works lock and key with this cycle. But if one has a sleep disturbance caused by a virus or a set of viruses from this disorder, one's sleep will be off and so the immune system will be off."

Environmental Factors and Allergies

Dr. Ali looks to the surrounding environment and lifestyle as playing causal roles. He relates that the immune system gets injured by environmental pollutants, such as mold, formaldehyde, and pesticides, as well as by allergic foods or by nutritional aspects, by stress and by lack of physical fitness. He gives equal emphasis to all four areas.

Dr. Michele Galante also sees the importance of allergies. "The patients I have seen have been very allergic, not only to pollens and airborne agents (as from grasses and trees) but especially to foods and to chemical sensitivities. These are people that are so sensitive that they cannot be exposed to perfume, nail polish, gas fumes, carbon monoxide, or even just paint, as from a freshly painted room. They are so debilitated that a short exposure will give them headaches, a weakened condition, even emotional states. Chronic fatigue syndrome is closely connected to allergy."

Dr. Ostrom seconds this notion. People, he says, who have chronic fatigue syndrome will often develop allergies they have never had before. For instance, they will exhibit violent allergic reactions to medicines and show new food sensitivities. In patients with chronic fatigue syndrome as well as AIDS, a portion of the immune system shuts down, another portion, which causes immune reactions, is revved up, almost 100%. These people respond immunologically to things that, before they got sick, their immune system would not have recognized.

Some of these allergy causing substances are unavoidable. Chemicals in our environment, aside from those in our foods (the coloring, preservatives and so on), are everywhere. There is chlorine in our water, the air is filled with pollutants; things that were not in our ecological system 50 or 60 years ago. Recent phenomena that accompany technological advances, such as the mercury in silver amalgam dental work, is weakening our systems. These chemicals in and of themselves do not necessarily have so strong an impact, but all together, day after day, for many years, overloads the liver and immune system. Electromagnetic influences, previously ignored, are now under discussion. Many believe the cathode rays from computers influence the electromagnetic fields of the body, for instance, as well as the electromagnetism of cellular phones, radio waves, TV waves, things relatively new to our environment." (For a fuller discussion of this topic see the magnet therapy section of our chapter on Pain Management.)

Foods and Yeast Infections

Dr. Ali says we should take children as our models since they learn quickly and change eating patterns to ensure health. He sees children with fatigue and attention deficit disorders. After tests you find the child is allergic to wheat, dairy, peanuts, sugar. You tell the mom she has to change everything she feeds him and she is ready to collapse. But talk to her six or nine months later, once she knows all the other wonderful food options she has, and she is happy. The child resisted at first, but then his problems began to clear up. Halloween came, he nose-dived. He began to clear up again. Thanksgiving, he nose-dived. Christmas, he nose-dived. Children learn more quickly than stubborn adults. Knowledge allows us to change in accordance with what we learn.

Dr. Galante also turns his attention to food, pointing to processed foods, white sugar, white flour, hydrogenated products, and chemicalized foods, all lacking vitality. People are eating these foods in far too great a quantity. Through food therapies which remove these foods, at least in the less severe cases, he has seen relief from hypoglycemic reactionssuch as mood swings and manic depressive symptoms.

Another problem in chronic fatigue syndrome is candida, both external and internal.

Ali reminds us, however, not to go looking for a doctor to cure us of yeast since it is in our bodies. "You do not want to get rid of it, but rather achieve 'gut balance,' and restore the gut ecosystem." Candida is just one possible problem; he tests for the nine different kinds of yeast. Of the yeasts, candida is not number one in terms of the body making antibodies against it, though candida is number one in terms of total population.

Metabolic Regulation, Vitamin and Hormonal Deficiency

What about the relation of chronic fatigue to metabolic regulation? Pavel Yutsis, M.D., believes we can understand metabolic immune depression in relation to chronic fatigue syndrome. When glucose production is up it brings on a level of hypoglycemia, with a high degree of glucose in the blood causing an increased level of insulin in the blood. Because of poor utilization of glucose, fatty acids come to the surface, increasing in the blood in order to provide a sufficient level of energy. A high level of triglycerides will occur and the immune system will be depressed because it needs a new army of T lymphocytes, which are not being produced because of derangement in lipid metabolism.

Dr. Block relates these problems to lifestyle. Those who do not have the best lifestyle, such as the smokers, drinkers, and those who do not breathe the best air, often lack B nutrients, which affects the immune system. Even if you are taking a number of vitamin B pills, make sure you are on a multi B regimen, so none of the B vitamins begin to get scarce in the body.

Lack of C, E, and beta carotene can also affect your immune system, as well as a lack of minerals, particularly, calcium, vanadium, copper, magnesium, potassium, molybdenum, boron, iodine, selenium, and chromium. The trace minerals are especially important for organ function.

Block also points to hormonal imbalances, particularly thyroid imbalance (especially hypothyroidism) found in females in a prevalence of six to one over males. It tends to come spontaneously between the ages of 20 and 50, although it can come at any time, often from unknown causes. The rare causes, which are the ones known for this disease, are because of a superabundance of iodine in the body or a deficiency of iodine, the latter being unlikely in our society, where we have iodized salt and other sources. Another rare cause is that of a person consuming too many of certain vegetables, such as cauliflower, broccoli, or Brussels sprouts, which tend to bind the active ingredient and inhibit thyroxin production.

Other hormones frequently out of the normal range are the adrenals. "There are a number of tests we can run for this, none of which is perfect," Block continues, "for, we have to remember, the adrenal gland is really two organs in one. On the inside, the adrenal medulla is making adrenaline and its brother noradrenaline. And then there's the outer coating, the adrenal cortex, making cortisone-like substances, related to our immune system and blood sugar control, and corticoid steroids. The last thing the adrenal cortex is important for is modulating the male and female hormones that are in conversation with the pituitary gland and primary sexual organs.

"And, lastly, some chronic fatigue syndrome patients have imbalances in gender hormones. It is not unusual to have imbalances in the estrogen that governs the ovary function or to have imbalances in other governors such as LH from the pituitary gland or in progesterone."

People will come to him with complaints, such as lack of menstruation or milky discharge from the breast, breast tenderness or more menstrual cramps than usual. Meanwhile, every month he has one or two men come who are low on testosterone blood scores, though with this one must test the degree of free testosterone to validly interpret the blood test. This last group makes great strides when given carefully measured dosages of male androgens.

Galante remarks, "The allopathic drugs, conventional drugs, antibiotics, and steroid usage are major influences. The use and abuse of these drugs, in childhood, for example, sets up chronically weakened conditions that will extend into adulthood and contribute to a predisposition for chronic fatigue. These drugs are suppressive in nature, not curative. They themselves impose an illness upon the system. This may be one of the largest of the causal factors."

Ali heard of a young person suffering from chronic fatigue syndrome who went to a medical clinic and was given a prescription for steroids. We know steroids suppress the immune system, so why would anyone give someone with this disorder these drugs? Steroids can create a sense of euphoria for a couple of days, of well being which is false. An unenlightened patient will take the steroids; an enlightened one will reject them.

Psychological Factors

Dr. Gentile tells us that the disorder seems to reduce stress tolerance. Sufferers cannot exert themselves or will relapse into a fatigue, whether they try to walk or swim. He has had patients who had been marathoners before contracting the illness. They report the same onset. They had been working hard then got sick with fever and chills. The illness waxed and waned. They would feel better at times and go back into running but then quickly relapse. For these patients, stress cannot be tolerated, either in physical or psychological form, and will exacerbate the illness again and again.

Dr. Block adds that the stresses that affect and elevate the chronic fatigue syndrome patient are the same ones that affect us in everyday life. These cause faltering in many bodily systems, such as in the neurotransmitters, which are missed in examinations by many doctors who are not aware of GABA, dopamine, serotonin, and other neurotransmitter chemical levels.

Dr. Paul G. Epstein says a key tenet of naturopathic medicine is to do no harm and treat the underlying cause. If a person has chronic fatigue syndrome, that is a diagnosis—they have a suppressed immune system (another diagnosis) documented by blood tests and other measures. What caused this? It may be improper diet, then the patient will need to eat properly. But we need to ask why he adopted that diet in the first place. It may be stress, but we can ask what caused the person to follow certain patterns of reaction to stress. As we treat the patient, going through all the different problems layered one on top of the other, we eventually get in contact with the person's core self.

One way to get into this is through the inner child. A lot people have been influenced by John Bradshaw's work on recovering and healing the inner child and on seeing the connection between the wounds and scars of childhood which may have led us to create lifestyles that are addictive. So, even as I help the person medically, by advising on diet, stress reduction and so on, I remember this. If we do not touch deeper problems, healing may not occur.

OUTLINES OF A HOLISTIC APPROACH TO CHRONIC FATIGUE SYNDROME

Difficulties of the Current Paradigm

Dr. Dean Black states that we were born to interact with the environment in a particular way. So we ask what is right for the body as it exists in the natural world. If we interact out of line with the body, we become sick. If we act properly, we become better. It is as simple as that. Natural health does nothing more than sustain the body's operations as they ought to be sustained.

"If you look at the body from an overall point of view," according to Dr. Galante, "from an environmental point of view, focusing on the bug is not going to be productive. As sophisticated as modern medicine is (so advanced we can tell all the amino acids and proteins in the body and get pictures of them), we cannot help the person who's got the difficulty. That seems to be a problem."

Dr. Ali thinks this is because so many doctors proceed from a flawed paradigm, the prevailing model of disease medicine. "A physician read one of my monographs and said, 'Ali, I know what you're talking about. We are disease doctors, while you are a health physician. I have difficulty relating to you because unless you give me the name of a disease, I don't know how to behave.' That's a paradox. I believe there'll come a time when people will not even go to doctors. They'll be coming to me, not so they can get drugs, but so they can get off drugs."

Dr. Galante summarizes his ideas in this way: "Why is medicine having so much trouble today? Because it doesn't have the answers. That's why we're in a crisis. That's why people are turning to natural therapies as they see the conventional approach is not curative but suppressive. That's why I exist."

FINDING THE RIGHT TREATMENT

Dr. Gentile brings forward some related ideas. "Several key points about finding treatment for chronic fatigue syndrome involve the choice of an empathetic expert who believes the disease exists. It has reached the level of scientific respectability and most practitioners and medical examiners believe it exists. It is important to have someone up to date on in the literature and who has seen, minimum, 50-100 patients—someone who understands the ups and downs of the disease and is aware of the number of different treatments that have developed."

He points out a number of ways to locate a credible expert. For one, there are chronic fatigue syndrome support groups in every major town in our country and now worldwide that have lists of physicians who have tended to specialize in the disorder. There are national groups such as the Chronic Fatigue Syndrome Association with offices in Charlotte, North Carolina; Kansas City, Kansas; and Portland, Oregon. They maintain a list of doctors who understand the disease and have treated it and are sympathetic and believing.

"This last trait is so important," Galante explains, "because many sufferers have gone through scores of doctors. We're treating a woman now who has already seen 75 physicians all over the world. She was ready to give up because she feels people do not believe her. So, a critical part of treating this illness is belief. A second thing to bear in mind is, this being a chronic illness with a wide range of symptoms, it will tend to fall between the cracks of all the medical sub-specializations. With this disease, it will not be adequate to go to a single physician. It would be worth considering putting together a team, which would include a GP/internist, one who works both with traditional and alternative therapies; an allergist/infectious disease specialist; and a psychologist/psychiatrist. This team could coordinate so as to work out a treatment plan. They could collaborate and work so the client understands what is coming next. And if these treatments don't work, they could determine why that might be, and what would be worth trying next."

THE SPIRITUAL ELEMENT

Dr. Ali tells us that when dealing with a chronic, devastating illness like this, hope and the spiritual element are two elements essential for long-term success. She has had case histories that truly stretch the bounds of credulity. "Creating hope is a very easy thing to do; sustaining hope is difficult but it is central to healing. Before I see a patient, he or she has seen at least seven specialists. They've had biopsies, CAT scans. When they come to me, it's not that easy to simply reassure them that they'll get better, after they've seen the previous failures. But, fortunately, by the time they get to me, they've listened to some of our tapes, read our books, and, most importantly, have talked to some of the other patients who have gotten better. So when they come in, and they've seen our nursing staff, our ancillary staff, they see we are all serious. If they ask how my program differs, we say this: they do not have the option to remain sick."

TREATMENTS

Vitamin Therapies

A nurse is making up an IV chronic fatigue syndrome protocol with vitamin C, magnesium sulfate, pantethene, calcium, pyridoxine, and a multi-vitamin formula. She says patients who come in are very tired, have joint pains, headaches, and memory loss. These IVs help repair cell membranes and boost the immune system, which will then hopefully function better. About 90% of her patients have responded well. Dr. Ali will usually order a set of five to begin with, she says, and after that he can measure their response, see how deep their problem is and whether they require further drugs.

"I see these drips as jump-starting the cellular enzymes," Ali says. "The enzymes, which are detoxification enzymes, are dependent on minerals and vitamins. If I feel there is enough time, when the patient is not acutely ill or has been chronically ill for a number of years, I will try to use a more conservative approach. But when I see people with severe, incapacitating fatigue, I use the IV. In fact, in one of our studies where we compared one group who had the IV and one group who didn't, we saw the IV speeds up the recovery process."

Ali continues, "We have 14 different formulations or protocols to manage different clinical problems in our IV drips. For chronic fatigue syndrome, we use C, magnesium, calcium, pyridoxine, pantethene, zinc, B vitamins, molybdenum, potassium, copper, and selenium. Most of our protocols have 15 to 18 items, and we change their quantities depending on the individual's state."

Dr. Ostrom notes that the anti-oxidants, with C, E and A, will be efficacious in treating chronic fatigue syndrome, as they are with AIDS, since in both cases they are entering the same immunological battle. In these cases, the systems are under fierce attack from free radicals, viruses, and, in some cases, bacteria. The supplements help to re-equilibrate and repair damage done by the molecules and help boost the immune system.

"First, we have to get the vitamins really right," Dr. Feldman urges, "since they are the building blocks of the immune system. People suffering from chronic fatigue syndrome are deficient in such things as A, B_5, B_{12}, E, bioflavonoids, the essential fatty acids, zinc, selenium, and GLA (gamma linoleic acid). All those must be put into order before we can proceed further."

For immune strength or immune power the following supplements are recommended.

A (as pure A)	10,000 to 20,000 IU
Beta carotene	15,000-25,000 IU
B_6	100-200 mg (be tested for reaction first)

C (buffered) to bowel tolerance (try a sago palm not a corn source. Buffering neutralizes acid)

E	300-600 IU
Quercetin	250-1,000 mg
Pyncnogenol	50-150 mg
Essential fatty acids	100-350 mg (obtainable from sunflower, sesame,

safflower, evening primrose or soybean oils, and black currant, a tablespoon a day)

Zinc picolinate	20-50 mg
Selenium	100-300 micrograms (oceanic)

Dr. Neil Block discusses his treatment: "If proteins or amino acids come out low, we can try to individually supplement the amino acids. If minerals are lacking, they can be given individually or in tandem, trying to operate by an economy of scale, so a patient doesn't have to take from more than 10 to 15 bottles at a time. As for hormonal imbalance, I have 20-25% of my chronic fatigue syndrome patients on thyroid. I prefer to use the more natural brands of thyroid. Again, I believe in giving both the male and female hormones. We also have to try to adjust the pancreas and adrenals. For the pancreas use chromium or chromium picolinate. For adrenals, the glandulars or homeopathics and sometimes things like licorice tend to help multiple hormones. If we are working on the pituitary, use glandulars, the homeopathics, and on rare occasions, I use a lot of the amino acids to try and build neurotransmitter activity. The amino acids to be used are arginine, tryosine, and phenylalanine. Tryptophan was also once useful to me until they took it off the market. I'm also not afraid to use, correctly and in small doses, items obtained from the pharmacy. What I tend to shy away from are the tranquilizers, such as Valium or Librium. I do make use of anti-depressants on occasion."

Often his patients have seen other physicians and holistic healers and they may need only one or two things to turn the body around on multiple levels. With neurotransmitters being easily adjusted nowadays, with items like the less toxic anti-depressants such as neuro-trytamine, neuroiptamine, and the newer Paxil and Zoloff, which lack drastic side effects and have a response beginning in two to four weeks, they're worthwhile. It's nice for a patient who has suffered two, four, six years, to take these new agents and, within two to four weeks, get at least some indication of the direction in which they are going."

Dr. Ostrom mentions another new drug which may yet be helpful: Amplygin, currently in FDA trials, appears to fix a very important immune system anti-viral pathway. Found to work on AIDS, it has yet to be proved against chronic fatigue syndrome.

Dr. Galante opines antibiotics can certainly be called for when all else fails, where the system has been debilitated, perhaps by too much drug use before. However, the state we are aiming for is where the energy in the body will overcome all problems.

Herbal Therapies

Herbologist Letha Hadady says that the tradition of herbology is very rich in China with many herbs to choose from for healing the immune system. One is a form of ginseng called Dang Shen. Another is astragalus. In her view, when used together, the first lifts our energy up and the second sends our defenses to the surface.

After using these herbs, we should act to kill germs and viral infection with such herbs as honeysuckle flower, andrographis, and dandelion. When we have built strength and killed germs, we must build blood using Chinese blood tonics, such as Han Yin Sow, called eclipta alba in Latin and growing wild in the American Southwest. It builds blood without any side effects, such as inflammation. You can take this every day in powdered form. Other immune strengthening agents are Chinese ginseng, dandelion, false ginseng, astragalus, andrographis, eclipta alba and honeysuckle.

She also mentions, Fo Ti, which builds blood while it keeps us cool.

When you fight viral infection with herbs, she reminds us, you have to do a number of things. One part of herbal treatments is taking antibiotic and anti-inflammatory herbs., like dandelion, a cleansing agent that keeps us cool. It can be put in salads, soups and found in the health food stores as capsules.

Honeysuckle flower grows outside in the garden. Boiled as tea, it will eliminate a sore throat and fever as well as kill pneumonia, stapf and strep germs.

There are three types of ginseng: American, Chinese, and false. The American type provides more moisture, more saliva and is good after a fever. Chinese ginseng, called Ren Shen, gives us enery. Dang Shen, or false ginseng, makes us feel stronger, without feeling hotter. All can be used in soups.

Cayenne pepper plays a role in health, increasing circulation and making us feel stronger. It can be used by those who do not find it irritating.

There are also herbs for relaxing the nervous system. One is Siberian ginseng, which can be taken as an extract or in capsule form. Valerian, taken in capsules, can quiet the nervous system. "For people who are depressed," Hadady says, "we need to bring them to their center as a way to be grounded and to feel more whole. Use ginger and mint. Mint helps to bring the worries out of the head and ginger helps to burn them away, because it is digestive and heating so it brings us warmly to our centers. They make a good combination."

High Energy preparation is the name of an herb mixture that uses Western and Oriental ingredients. It has guttacola, American ginseng, demi-anna, red clover, peppermint and cloves, which strengthens the adrenals and lungs.

Hadady adds that cloves and hot water will pick up your energy, and make you breath deeper.

Dietary Changes

Dr. Ali sees eating right as a measure to prevent or combat chronic fatigue syndrome. Carbohydrates, like corn and wheat, are big culprits. One should eat healthy substances, such as wild and brown rice or unusual grains such as fatigue and spelt. Soy products are also very good, as is teff. The other good sources of carbohydrates are lentils and different types of beans. Tomatoes, potatoes, and yams are okay, but in moderation. Foods which have white flour are a no-no, as is white rice. The best sources among the grains are brown rice, amaranth, quinoa, soy, teff, and spelt.

Lentils, beans, eggs, and protein drinks are good sources of protein. Egg is excellent, but many people are allergic to it. Dr. Ali also recommends protein drinks in the morning—their amino acids give sustained energy. Sugar and carbohydrates, by contrast, provide a roller coaster effect—they are useful only when doing an endurance type of physical activity, in which case you need carbohydrates. But most people do much better without sugar and carbohydrates.

Dr. Ali does not insist his patients follow a vegetarian diet, but recommends little beef. Unusual meats, like venison or pheasant are better, he states. "We provide a list to patients of places where they can order such meat. Cornish hen and turkey are fine. Hunted fish (deep sea fish) are good. Cultured fish are not recommended. They're beginning to put fungicides into fish raised in fisheries. If you are going for fish, do the deep seas ones. (Unless you have serious mercury sensitivity, then you should avoid fish.)"

He feels eating certain fats is essential, but one should avoid oxidized, processed, denatured fats or animal shortening, corn oil, palm oil, and coconut oil. If you do not have milk sensitivity, butter is possible. You can make ghee by taking butter, warming it and taking the white part off. It is delicious and those who cannot tolerate butter can still tolerate ghee. Use virgin olive oil, the type you find in Italian stores. Avocado oil is an excellent source of monounsaturates, but if it is processed stay away. For supplemental oils, flaxseed is excellent. People should make a habit of using flaxseed on their salad dressing.

Dr. Galante prescribes using a lot of live foods, that can be taken right from nature without cooking like raw fruits, vegetables, and sprouts. They can provide tremendous energy, with a lot of enzymes and nutrition. They take little energy to digest and give much energy back.

Think of all the varieties of vegetables: red leaf and green leaf lettuce, mustard greens, red and green chard, arugula, broccoli, beets, carrots. Turnips and parsnips, both root vegetables, are very high in calcium. Green leafy vegetables give needed chlorophyll and oxygenate your blood. Radishes, red and green peppers, eggplants are excellent and ginger can be used to flavor any juice. Celery is a good diuretic and cabbage is high in beta carotene, as are all the green leafy vegetables. Sprouts are the best source of protein, put into a salad it will add to anything you are eating. An ounce of wheat grass, which is high in chlorophyll, is equal to 22 ounces of the choicest vegetable you can imagine.

Homeopathy

Homeopathy is Dr. Galante's specialty; it has been very effective against chronic fatigue syndrome, and is probably quite different from what people are experiencing with other treatments. Homeopathic remedies are given in micro-dosages, all made from natural substances, effective in treating and curing many conditions.

To talk about one particular therapy, though, is not appropriate, Galante explains, since the essence of homeopathy is that each individual will have selected for him or her a remedy based on his or her unique physical constitution and manifestation of symptoms. He points out that the homeopathic healer will select a remedy that is uniquely fitted, mentally and physically, for a particular sufferer's makeup.

Acupuncture

Abigail Rist-Pidrecca, R.N., O.M.D., points out that the *chi*, or bioelectrical energy, flows through pathways in the body. When there is a disease process occurring, she says there is a blockage. Acupuncture needles—there are actually 365 points that can be used—open the blockages and let the energy flow smoothly through meridians. The other thing that occurs is that the needles dilate the blood vessels, so you get more blood flowing through the area, more oxygen and more nutrients into the area, and this aids all forms of health.

Needles are pre-sterilized in ethylene gas. After they are used, they are thrown away in an infectious waste container so there is no cross contamination question in the process. "If you do go to an acupuncturist," Rist-Pidrecca cautions, "one of the first things I would ask as a patient-consumer, is whether they are using presterilized needles."

Tai Chi

One of the benefits of *tai chi* is that it increases one's awareness both internally and environmentally. "Then you can choose which to work on, whether there is something physically wrong or something in the environment that needs to be corrected," says Eric Schneider of the Northeastern Tai Chi Chuan Association.

He tells us the practitioners can use the energy in their bodies to go toward the conflict and resolve it rather than spend time worrying. We are born with a certain amount of energy, called pre-birth *chi*. You may know a person who can go out and party all night and wake up the next morning at 6 a.m. fine. Another person will do the same partying but the next morning be unable to get out of bed. This is due to differences in the natural reservoir. The practice of *tai chi* can increase the natural storehouse.

According to Schneider, the environment has energy, brought into the bodily system through the simple breathing apparatus. You have to cultivate a part of your body that can observe phenomena dispassionately, without having to grab onto every experience and run with it, to get yourself in stressful situations and say quietly, 'Oh, so this is what is happening now. What can I do about it? What are my options and how am I feeling?' In this way, you can soberly assess your experience.

Tai chi is a ten year practice. Practitioners say, 'ten years great gain, three years small gain.' It takes ten years to get what is called the *gung chi*, the task framework so the body has a certain way to contain energy. Gradually, as the mind starts to cultivate and stay with the body, the whole system starts to grow. This is not a quick fix. "In fact," says Schneider, "in my opinion, any practice that is to have profound value cannot be done quickly. Everything that has lasting effect takes time."

IMAGERY AND HEALING

Dr. Paul Epstein uses a type of visualization in his practice. He says imagery is a therapeutic technique that assists people to explore through words and symbols so they can understand the language of the subconscious.

"In exploring this," according to Epstein, "usually what comes up is the issue that is at the core of what will be the healing. When we are dealing with people, they may get in touch with childhood wounds or abuse from the past that needs healing. Perhaps they'll get in touch with the fact that the work which they are doing is not real work.

"In one such case, with a person suffering from chronic fatigue syndrome, we found the illness was a case of a person trying to get love. She had not let go of trying to get love from mom and dad. She was still stuck at that place. And the pain and the grief of not having that love were not only weakening her immune system, but keeping her stuck in the unhealthy way she was living her life."

Dr. Ali reiterates some of Epstein's message: "What I demonstrate to my patients is that the way you look at the world around you determines the biology under your skin. If you can be in a self-regulatory, healing mode, your brain activity, heart activity, muscle energy, skin energy, will all be functioning positively. Or you can be trying to figure things out, think everything through in an overly intellectual way, and your biology will be as up and down as the New York skyline. This is the stress mode and it causes disease. Another mode is an even, steady state mode and that is a resting mode.

"Our goal is to perceive this energy in these modes and understand how the energy profoundly affects the electro-physiological profile. Can we allow this energy to guide us into the healing mode? We want a transition from an ordinary, thinking, nervous stressful mode that causes disease to a non-thinking, meditative, deep respiring mode that makes us well. That is our goal."

A HOLISTIC HEALTH MODEL

Dr. Michele Galante ties it all together: "A homeopath will tell you that a person cannot be well if he or she is feeling ill at ease in mind or heart. Just having a physically healthy body is not enough. People want more. We are not saying the doctor and homeopath has the key to make people happy, but we can say that homeopaths do work to make people feel emotionally better. There is a realignment of what's called the vital force, which causes the person to get well. We all have this capacity. The body is a living, tremendously powerful organism and it can heal itself. It healed itself before there were antibiotics and it will heal itself long after antibiotics fall out of favor."

Epstein elaborates his earlier position: "What's needed in treating chronic fatigue syndrome or AIDS or such problems is a new approach. Not looking for the quick fix or what will work for everybody, but for an approach that is individualized, holistic and one that empowers the patient to get involved in the cure and gives that patient belief and hope that healing is possible.

"There are two points in my treatment that I've been told by patients have helped them most. That I have given them hope and belief that healing is possible, and I have shown them that there are things they could do to help themselves. I don't heal anybody. Doctors don't heal anybody. They support people as they heal themselves."

A physician's work, in his opinion, is to support the self healing of each individual and to help them through the process.

Dr. Epstein wants to help patients listen, explore and understand the message of their disease, which is the key to unlock the door to recovery. After the diagnosis, medications, natural or other, there still has to be an exploration healing for this person. We might have conditioned immune-suppressant responses built into our attitudes, beliefs, the way we live our life, the way we think and the way we eat. An illness cannot be fixed from the outside; there is no magic bullet for chronic fatigue syndrome. People heal themselves by engaging in a self-healing process, by looking at their life and its meaning.

It may seem rather complicated, but it is not. It is based on the knowledge that we do not get sick over night. The condition may manifest suddenly in certain symptoms, but it took years and years to arrive. And it was not from one virus; not just Epstein Barr or herpes or parasites, low blood sugar or electromagnetic pulsations. It was a combination of all of them.

In order to detoxify, it takes time. It might take you a year to really cleanse. You need a rational diet so you can get rid of the food polluting your system. Bring in the healthy foods, exercise, meditation, acupuncture.

If you are what you eat, eat what you appreciate becoming. Remember, the mind is a powerful healer and also a powerful slayer. Surround yourself with positive thoughts and people who will support your endeavor to live a natural lifestyle. Chronic fatigue syndrome can be cured. Everyday you can be processing health and overcoming disease.

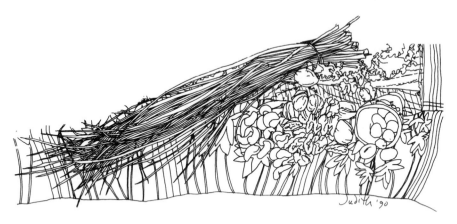

25 · HOLISTIC DENTISTRY

"The mouth is indicative of the body's general state of health. If you have a cavity, it is the end result of general physical problems of the whole body not just the isolated tooth.....Teeth are not like rocks embedded in there with no relation to other parts of your body. They are like a coral system, a crystalline structure and minerals go in and out all the time."

TURN-OF-THE-CENTURY AUTHOR and editor Frank Harris wrote, "Doctors tell us that men commonly dig their graves with their teeth." Not only is this done by improper diet, but by not taking care of one's teeth or even by putting poisons in one's mouth. In this chapter, we want to look at how eat-

323

ing right can add to the health and capability of your teeth, while eating the wrong substances, such as sugar or chocolate, can damage your teeth by reversing the natural fluid flow in the mouth.

We will also evaluate the way people treat their teeth when they are diseased. We will find that typical treatments for repairing damage, such as silver amalgam fillings and root canals, are much more hazardous than claimed. More shockingly, we will find that many say the fluoridation of water, a public health practice established in most major cities, is not only dangerous to our bodies but has no positive benefits for teeth at all.

NUTRITION

The first thing to think about when it comes to healthy teeth is whether we are following an appropriate diet. which will be reflected in the condition of the gums and teeth.

Think of the general practitioner of yesteryear. One imagines this doctor making a house call on an ailing patient. His first request on seeing this patient was "Stick out your tongue." He wanted to see the tongue's color.

Victor Zeines, D.D.S., the author of *The Natural Dentist*, reminds us that this practice, far from being quaint and outdated, can still be used to make a good, first diagnosis of medical problems. In fact, Chinese doctors, who also ask to see the patient's tongue, have a book that discusses 280 diseases that can be detected from the state of the tongue. Today, such problems as the following can be diagnosed by inspecting the tongue:

- a white tongue—toxins are coming out of the body. This will be observed in people with a cold or the flu.
- cracks in the tongue—vitamin deficiency
- yellowish gray or yellowish green tongue—gall bladder or liver trouble.
- brownish or grayish green tongue—intestinal or stomach problems

The mouth is indicative of the body's general state of health. If you have a cavity, it is the end result of general physical problems of the whole body not just the isolated tooth.

What is decisive for the health of the teeth? It is simply eating a proper diet. Let us look at the research in this area.

Famed dental researcher Weston Price wrote a book, which he worked on in the 1920s and 1930s, based on studies of the teeth in people in native cultures. People that followed traditional ways, eating simply prepared food, indigenous to the region where they lived had teeth in good condition with no malformation, or crowded placement. As soon as they adopted a

Western diet of canned processed food with white sugar and white flour, their dental health deteriorated. Children born to parents on a Western diet had occlusion and malformed teeth. Price even saw that children born before the introduction of Western foods had healthy teeth, while children in the same family born after the new diet was instituted had poor teeth.

He concluded reasonably that the nutrition in Western cultures is the main cause of dental problems.

When a person is not eating properly the body becomes acidic, so minerals are pulled out of the mouth to travel into other parts of the organism. The teeth weaken in an acid environment while acid-based bacteria begin booming. A cavity arises from a mineral deficiency followed by an invasion of bacteria.

Sugar is a main culprit in this process, though not in the way popularly understood. Many believe sugar gets in the mouth and sits on the tooth, wearing it down. The real problem with sugar is that it reverses the fluid flow. This flow normally goes from the tooth's pulp chamber into the mouth. Sugar alters this, sending materials in the mouth into the tooth's internal environment, irritating the inside of the tooth, creating cavities. Caffeine, found in coffee, tea, chocolate, soft drinks, and pain medication also creates this inversion, based on a change in the hormonal balance; it also encourages diseases such as MS and arthritis.

We know what you should not eat, but we still have to ask what foods are best suited for our mouths. The way the human jaw is set up and the chewing motions made are geared toward a fruit diet. Such a diet of fruit, along with nuts, seeds, and root vegetables will create an alkaline state in the body as opposed to the acidic state current American diets support. This is another reason to adopt the vegetarian diet we talked of earlier.

In Chapter 4, we saw supplemental vitamins are necessary for good health; the same is true with respect to healthy teeth.

Grayshu Pearlstein, author of *Wild by Nature*, points out why supplements are so needed in our environment. In the United States we have a high level of stress, a polluted environment and deficient diet. Food often comes to us shipped over long distances, losing many of its nutritious qualities in the trip. We need to make up for those lost qualities with vitamins and minerals.

The average person should first take a calcium and magnesium vitamin, from 800 to 1,500 mg/day. Men need about 800 mg while women need higher dosages, with the largest dose needed by pregnant women. A calcium supplement is necessary for strong teeth, while a B complex will help people keep up their energy levels.

Folic acid can help the body utilize nutrients, aids the functioning of the nervous system, and is particularly useful for pregnant women since it prevents neural tube damage.

CoQ 10 will oxidate cells, while vitamin C taken in dosages of 6,000 mg/day will keep the gums healthy and strong. Mineral supplements are also helpful.

Drinking juices is a good way to obtain the recommended five vegetables a day in your diet. Carrot juice is an excellent beverage, high in calcium. A 12 oz. serving of carrot juice can have as much as 600 mg of calcium.

Green leafy vegetables are also high in calcium. Traditional culture held that chewing on kale was the fastest way to get white teeth. This idea probably is based on recognition of kale's high calcium content. Kale can be juiced and mixed with carrot or apple juice, perhaps with a drop of lemon.

MERCURY FILLINGS

Even a person eating a healthy vegetarian diet can have problems with their teeth and go to a dentist for help. Yet the shocking fact is, a patient can go to a dentist to solve one problem and leave, apparently cured, but actually in a more imperiled state.

The common treatment for dental caries are fillings. But what are we putting in our mouths? A large percentage of the commonly used filling is mercury. The current silver filling is typically composed of 14% silver, 1% zinc, 12% tin, 26% copper, and 52% mercury. This amalgam has a higher proportion of mercury than fillings had 20 years ago. Eighty-five percent of the American population has these fillings

For over 150 years we have been told these fillings are safe, the most durable available. This is not true, argues Lydia Bronte, a health researcher. The amalgam in the filling constantly leaks mercury into the mouth and saliva, where we swallow and inhale the mercury, which then gets into the tissues.

Her claim has been substantiated by a 1996 Toxicological Profile released by the Department of Health and Human Services. In discussing the dangers of mercury it states, "One of the most likely forms of exposure is by absorbing mercury vapor released from dental fillings. Most silver-colored dental fillings are about 50% metallic mercury and slowly release small amounts of mercury vapor."

In the early 1970s, Hal A. Huggins, D.D.S., the director of the Huggins Diagnostic Center, found that mercury could leak from the fillings and damage the body. As he puts it, people with these fillings have "little time bombs in their mouths." Huggins says mercury is coming out in measurable amounts. This opinion is backed up by Dr. Warren Levin, director of Physicians for Complementary Medicine, who remarks that studies have shown if you chew gum, then put a probe in your mouth to test the air, the level of mercury vapor registered is enough to exceed what OSHA (the Occupational Safety and Health Agency) classifies as a safe level for industry.

Up until 1985, the American Dental Association (ADA) repeatedly declared that mercury never escapes from fillings. Then they had to acknowledge that it did leak. Still, even with the leakage, ADA Online, the ADA's Website, declares the fillings safe.

What effect does mercury have once it gets in the body? Mercury will act to deactivate enzymes that utilize zinc and other agents. Dr. Alfred V. Zamm points out that this inactivation will affect every cell making them slowly dysfunctional. The enzymes are shut down when mercury substitutes for the minerals necessary for enzyme operation.

Other diseases or health problems will be exacerbated by the presence of mercury, including such illnesses as Multiple Schlerosis, Lou Gehrig's disease, leukemia, tremors, Chronic Fatigue Syndrome, Parkinson's disease, and Alzheimer's disease. Moreover, memory is affected adversely and depression and anxiety can occur.

The most common symptoms of mercury toxicity are fatigue, depression, inability to concentrate, memory deficit, gastro-intestinal tract problems, kidney problems and frequent infections.

Further symptoms include brittle nails, lack of energy, sensitivity to cold and heat, dry skin, dry hair, irritability, and mood swings. The neurological symptoms include nervousness, headaches, and hypo-thyroidism. Everyone who has the fillings is bound to have some problems with the thyroid since mercury interferes with its operation and with the absorption of the thyroid hormone into the body. A person who has a hypo-thyroid condition due to the presence of mercury will test normal on thyroid blood tests but will have all the symptoms.

Mercury will also effect the presence and functioning of the T-cells, which control the human immune system. An important study on this subject is "Effect of dental amalgam and nickel alloys on T-lymphocytes" by Eggleston, D. (1984) *Journal of Prosthetic Dentistry*, Vol. 31, No. 5. The study took patients' T-cells counts. The subjects were then given mercury fillings and the count was taken a second time. and the amount of T-cells went down 35%. The fillings were then removed, and lo and behold the T-cell count climbed back to its previous level. The article's conclusion was that mercury and nickel in these fillings adversely affect the quality and quantity of T-cells.

Other important studies drawing attention to the danger of mercury are Palkiewicz, P., Zwiers, H., Lorscheider, F. (1994) *Journal of Neurochemistry*, Vol. 62, pp. 2049-2052, and Duhr, E., Pendergrass, C., Kasarskis, E., Slevin, J., and Haley B., (1991) *FASEB Journal*.

When patients have mercury fillings removed from their mouths, they often see improvement, although it may be held back by the mercury already in the body. Dr. Michael Schacter, medical director of the Complementary Medical Center, has seen patients both whose blood tests have gone from abnormal to normal once silver fillings were removed and victims of MS and Chronic Fatigue Syndrome whose conditions have markedly improved once fillings were taken out.

Dr. Zeines has seen improved memory, better sleep and less nervousness. He notes patients suffering from arthritis, cirrhosis, MS, auto-immune diseases, Chronic Fatigue Syndrome, and heart disease have registered marked improvement.

Removing these fillings is not an easy task and the process is potentially dangerous since taking out the amalgam could accidentally release mercury.

Howard Hinton, D.D.S., a holistic dentist, stresses that the removal must be done under the care of both a physician and a dentist. The patient must be on a good diet and should undergo laboratory tests to determine how he or she is eliminating the mercury. Ideally, the removal should be carried out in a sterile, bubble chamber—a round room with a laminar air flow circulating through the space; negative ion generators, to charge particulates in the air; and processed water and air. A rubber dam is used in the mouth to reduce exposure and the filling is removed with extreme care. (The highest absorption in the body is in the mouth.) During the operation, high suction and lots of water is used to reduce the presence of mercury vapor.

Once the fillings are removed, one still has to detoxify the body. A lack of health improvement may be due to the fact that mercury is still in the body.

Elmira Gadol, D.M.D., another practitioner of holistic dentistry, speaks of a treatment to aid the body after the fillings are out that detoxifies the brain. When a cell is toxic with heavy metal, it can not easily eliminate it since the cell wall has a changed ionic balance, but an anesthetized cell will release the metal.

Garlic supplements will help the body eliminate the existing mercury toxins and selenium can be taken to neutralize the metal. Mercury found in fish from polluted waters is less toxic than that from fillings, since the fish's body will have produced selenium to neutralize the poison. (Note that caffeine will act to retain mercury in the body.)

Once the fillings are removed, hair analysis should be done to see what other heavy metals are in the body. These metals interfere with cell processes, such as the oxygen going in and the carbon dioxide going out. These metals also have to be drawn out or problems will remain.

Some patients can be helped by taking intravenous vitamin C. Also, various chelating agents can be prescribed. These agents will attach to the mercury and take it out of the body in urine or feces.

Hot baths with Epsom salts and baking soda are also recommended as a way to bring out the mercury. In working on detoxification, various methods should be tried alone and in combination. Whichever is doing the best job should be used.

ROOT CANALS

A second common dental procedure, root canal, poses another problem; it may leave hidden bacterial pockets that prove a breeding ground for disease.

In theory, root canal procedures are worthwhile. A root canal is undertaken when the tooth's pulp cavity has been entered by decay and the nerve is infected and dies. The tooth too may die, its insides, cleaned out by decay, may fill with pus. A root canal treatment cleans out the ruined area and, as Dr. Warren Levin, director of Physicians for Complementary Medicine, explains, fills it with gutta percha (a substance derived from tree resins).

Remember that the tooth is filled with dentin tubules, running from the inside of the structure to the outside in which bacteria could sit, producing toxins which transfer into the system. A study some years ago took teeth that had root canals and ground them up. Some of the powder was placed under the skins of rabbits. They found that if a patient had arthritis, the rabbit got it. If the patient from whom the original tooth came had heart disease, the rabbit contracted it, and so on. Clearly, bacteria was still carried in the teeth after the root canal had been performed and it could carry disease into the body.

This research was never publicized until the book *The Root Canal Cover-Up* by George E. Meinig, D.D.S., recently appeared.

Huggins, explaining the process of bacterial transfer in detail, says that whenever you put anything in the tooth for the root canal, bacteria will get into the dentin tubules and flow from the pulp chamber to the outside of the tooth. Though in a root canal procedure bacteria is cleaned from inside the tooth, it cannot be cleaned from the tubules. Sometimes on the surface of the tooth dentists are finding toxins extruded from the denal tubules that are similar to those produced by botulism.

A second problem may arise. The teeth sit in a kind of hammock, called the periodontal ligature. When a root canal is performed, the dentist must take a round drill, or burr, and cut out about 1 mm of the bone of this hammock to clear out the toxin deposited in the layer. When this is finished, there still may be a hollow space, called a cavitation, with a layer of bone on top. This space could fill with toxins. Serious illnesses may arise if this cavitation exists, especially in the wisdom tooth area. Of course, in proceeding with a root canal, this area should be cleaned out, but it can be and is often, missed.

Although more systematic study has to be made of the possible hazards of this technique, clearly it should not be engaged in as thoughtlessly as it has been.

FLUORIDES

Dentists have been using root canals and mercury in fillings blithely, ignoring the hazards and accepting traditional methods as necessarily reliable. Before the evidence began to accumulate, especially on the dangers posed by mercury, there was no reason for them to doubt the efficacy of what they were doing, since the fillings had proved themselves.

This is not the case for the last topic we wish to take up. As we look into the shady history of fluoridation, we learn that this procedure was tainted from the beginning, pressed on the gullible common people, not by medicine but by public relations men and their industrial paymasters.

David Kennedy, D.D.S., from the International Academy of Oral Medicine and Toxicology, puts it quite well when he states fluoride is a poison. It kills rats and insects; so, certainly, it will kill bacteria if it is scrubbed on the teeth.

Fifty percent of the people in the United States drink fluoridated water, and 42 of 50 major cities in the U.S. have fluoridated water. When water is fluoridated there is 1 part to a million in the water. In toothpaste, there is 1,000 parts to a million and in the dental rinses used by dentists, there is 10,000 parts per million.

All this, when the largest study ever conducted in this country on the effects of fluoridation, which looked at 39,000 school children, saw no significant differences in incidence of tooth decay between cities that had fluoridated water and cities that did not. It was found in this study that Butler, Kansas, which had the lowest evidence of dental caries and did not use fluoridation in its water supply.

It has no positive effects, but what about its down side? Fluoride is carcinogenic, and an immune suppressant that causes dental fluorosis (white or brown spots on the teeth). It increases the tendency to hip fracture by poisoning the bones.

Why did this dangerous substance, with no real protective qualities, become so widely adopted? In the 1940s there was a crisis in the aluminum industry, with big companies such as Alcoa being sued for polluting and killing cattle and other livestock. Edward Bernays, one of the fathers of public relations, and a nephew of Sigmund Freud, came up with the idea of selling the public on the beneficial uses of fluoride, one of the dangerous byproducts of aluminum production. It was said it could prevent dental caries and the publicity campaign would help the public forget the recent aluminum scandals.

The economic motivation behind this sales effort, which was triumphantly successful, was not the millions of dollars that could be made by marketing fluoride products, but the billions that would be saved by industry if it did not have to clean up the fluoride it was putting into the environment.

In a nutshell, companies have fluoride to dispose of so they are using people's bodies as hazardous waste dumps.

The health hazards of the substance have been discussed in a number of places. In 1977, an executive of the National Cancer Society documented that there is a 5% increase in cancer in communities that began fluoridating their water.

An even more notorious study and an attempt to suppress it involved Dr. William Marcus, a senior science advisor at the Environmental Protection Agency's Office of Drinking Water. He read a study that was done to test the dangers of fluoridation concluding there was an increase of bone cancers in animals that took fluorides. In April 1990, he went to a meeting at Research Triangle Park where the National Toxicology Program was to review the study and found that the program's staff had downgraded every cancer reported in the study.

Marcus states that in 25 years in the field, he had never seen such a downgrading. Occasionally one or two cancers would be downgraded, usually for terminological reasons, but nothing like this. He returned to his office and asked an investigator to look into it and the investigator found that scientists at the program had been coerced into making these downgrades.

He wrote what is now called the May Day memo, calling the public's attention to this chicanery and was subsequently dismissed from his job. He won a whistle blower's lawsuit brought because of his unlawful firing and was reinstated.

Fluoride is a poisonous substance brazenly passed off as health enhancing.

Thus we see proper care of teeth depends on eating sensibly and on being aware of the lurking dangers of accepted practices in dentistry. You should think carefully and consider alternative medical strategies before filling your mouth with silver fillings and having root canals. And you almost should be careful before you turn on the tap; your water may be poisoned with fluoride.

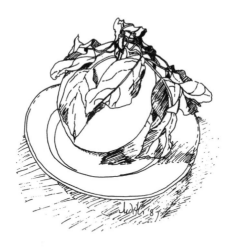

26 · HAIR CARE AND HAIR GROWTH: A NATURAL APPROACH

"I asked a beautician who has treated hundreds of people's hair whether she saw any connection between the things a person ate and their lifestyle, on the one side, and hair health, on the other.

"She told me, 'Definitely, I see that when people eat well the hair is healthy looking. It's a reflection of what they eat and the habits they have. Everything is shown in the hair.'"

BEFORE WORLD WAR II, Karl Popper came out with a book revolutionizing ways of thinking about science. Where previous philosophers thought there was a way to prove a theory correct, he said this was impossible; the best one could hope for was that it would not be proven wrong. In fact the strongest theory, in his definition, was the one for which it could be said: There were many failed attempts to prove it erroneous.

Nowadays in science you start with a theory and then see whether you can substantiate the theory or see if it has no merit. In good science, you try to disprove more than prove yourself. If you cannot disprove yourself, then pretty much you have made your point.

Is it possible that the reason we lose our hair, and that our skin gets droopy, our nails brittle and fungusy, and our gums bleed more easily as we age is because we have done so little to feed the immune system and our overall body chemistry?

Throughout history, men and women have been concerned about their hair, for religious reasons, social reasons, interpersonal reasons and for grooming. Sometimes the hair is long, sometimes a person is nearly bald. One thing is for sure, no one looks forward to getting bald. No one is happy about it. People don't like looking down at their feet in the shower and seeing a clump of hair. So I simply kept asking a basic question. Is it possible, using major changes in our diet, lifestyle, amount of exercise and stress management, to reverse, slow down, or in some way limit the process?

Traditional science says no; if it is in the genes, then it is inevitable. Yes, there has been some small change for those taking the medications, but that is incidental. You might get a little peach fuzz on the site of some former hair, but you pay a price since there are side effects to the medication.

A person had tried the drugs and told me, "My hair was falling out at a pretty fast rate. I was in the Rogaine treatment for five years, and the reason I had to stop it was my blood pressure went up excessively. I was very frustrated. This seemed to be the last stop."

Another man told me, "I wanted to look into this problem of falling or shedding hair, a scaly scalp, and some irritations at the temple and crown. The first thing I did was I went to a dermatologist just to get some consultation. She said I had eczema, dermatitis of a sort. She gave me one direction. She said there was a hot product on the market, monoxodil, that I should try and there should be some results. I tried it for several months and there were no results. Not that it was a waste of money. It was an attempt."

I wanted to see if you could do it without medication, by rebuilding the body chemistry without a magic bullet, salve, potions, or shampoo.

REASONS FOR HAIR LOSS

I asked a beautician who has treated hundreds of people's hair whether she saw any connection between the things a person ate and their lifestyle, on the one side, and hair health, on the other.

She told me, "Definitely, I see that when people eat well the hair is healthy looking. It's a reflection of what they eat and the habits they have. Everything is shown in the hair."

Dr. Danise Lehrer, a licensed acupuncturist and a doctor of homeopathy, noted that in traditional Chinese medicine, hair is viewed as a sign of the health of the kidneys, liver, and blood. So if you have healthy hair, then you have healthy blood and healthy energy.

Dr. Martin Feldman, a physician who practices complementary medicine, believes that an overabundance of junk food, processed food, sugar, caffeine, dairy, caffeine, wheat, chicken, additives, salt, yeast, chocolate, alcohol, meat, refined food, preservatives, antacids, and smoking as well as the use of aluminum cookware contribute to hair loss. "Eliminate these and not only will you grow more hair but you will be totally better and will gain longevity and a healthier life span."

Colette Heimowitz, a clinical nutritionist, notes that as alternative physicians and clinicians we have to look at the whole picture and not just at the single symptom of hair loss. We have to constantly replenish our bodies and let the biochemistry and cells function optimally at all times. She adds that the need for replenishment can be seen in light of the danger of free radical molecules in the body. In a free radical pathology, a molecule loses a hydrogen electron and attacks other healthy cells, trying to regain its lost balance. An anti-oxidant lends a free radical a hydrogen molecule without destroying itself, stopping free radical pathology in its tracks. However, once pathology begins, the radicals duplicate themselves by the billions within a minute, so the anti-oxidants have to be constantly replenished throughout the day.

A hairstylist put it like this, "Your hair is fed by the blood stream so if there are any difficulties in that area it will be carried through into the hair and the skin. You could be losing your hair, it could be brittle or dull. Nutrition does have an effect on everything in your body and so your hair is an appendage of what is going on. It is a reflection of who you are."

Hair and skin are last on the list of priorities. Your heart, your liver, your kidneys, your brain are all more important to the body's functioning. Your body has innate knowledge of itself, about what infections or what cancer cells or what viruses are present. It says to itself "I will selectively have to take care of what I can and fight those more important battles first. Whatever is left over I will give to the hair." Well, the average American never has anything left over. They're always drawing more out of the body. There's always a greater assault against the body going on than benefits flowing in.

DRINK GREEN JUICES

Graysha Pearlstein, a clinical nutritionist, tells us for hair and overall body health, we should consume six freshly-prepared green juices a day with organically grown vegetables because, they are free of pesticides, fertilizer and other artificial residues. Also, the soil used in organic farming is very vital and alive and mineral and nutrient rich, far more vital and health-promoting then commercially grown vegetables.

Increased circulation to the scalp is important so exercise should be part of any program, along with juicing, to support the body nutritionally.

I recommend the following 4 stage program to provide increased vitality to your hair and scalp.

STAGE 1
DAILY PROTOCOL FOR THE FIRST THREE MONTHS

B complex (50 mg)
B_{12} (100 mcg)
garlic (500 mg twice)
aloe (1 oz three times)
protein (9/10th g per kg of body weight)
[1 kg = 2.2 pounds]
6 glasses of dark green vegetable juice or 6 scoops of chlorophyll rich powder

STAGE 2
DAILY PROTOCOL FOR THE SECOND THREE MONTHS

sea vegetables (one serving)
flaxseed oil (1 tablespoon)
evening primrose oil (500 mg)
choline and inositol (500 mg twice)
PABA (100 mg)
folic acid (400 mcg)
biotin (500 mcg)

STAGE 3
DAILY PROTOCOL FOR THE THIRD THREE MONTHS

sea vegetables (1 serving)
zinc (50 mg)
l cysteine (500 mg twice)
evening primrose oil (300 mg twice)

pantothenic acid (100 mg twice)
vitamin E (400 IU)
co-enzyme Q 10 (100 mg twice)
biotin (500 mcg)
choline and inositol (500 mcg)
B complex (50 mg of each)
B$_{12}$ (100 mcg)
silica (150 mg)
PABA (250 mg)
folic acid (800 mcg)
6 glasses of dark green vegetable juice or 3 glasses dark green
   vegetable juice and three of green plant extract of 6 scoops of chlorophyll
   rich powder

STAGE 4
DAILY PROTOCOL FOR THE FOURTH THREE MONTHS

PABA (500 mg)
pantothenic acid (500 mg)
garlic (1,000 mg)
onion (1,000 mg)
sea vegetables (6 oz.)
biotin (500 mcg)
choline (1,000 mg)
inositol (1,000 mg)
niacin (250 mg)
borage oil (500 mg)
omega 3 oil (1,000 mg)
cayenne (5 mg)
protein (9/10th g per kg of body weight [1 kg = 2.2 pounds])
6 glasses of dark green vegetable juice or 3 glasses dark green vegetable juice
   and three of green plant extract of 6 scoops of chlorophyll rich powder

Phytochemicals

What is it in these vegetables and fruits that is making a difference in
health?

Dr. Feldman informs us that drugs have potential in genetic-overcoming,
like Rogaine, which has been somewhat effective. There are better ways to
deal with the problem, however, like extracting phytochemicals in fruits
and vegetables via a very low temerature process.

"In a study I did I gave participants as many as 15 to 20 separate fruits and vegetables that were extracted via the low temperature method, giving a total of approximately 300 different phytochemicals per day.

"My study in reversing hair loss did not rely on phytochemicals alone, but was holistic in scope. The program overcomes the genetic threshold through a multiple assault on the problem, by removing stress and doing exercise, becoming vegetarian, and detoxing by removing bad food.

"I should stress that though this approach is multi-factorial, phytochemicals are still crucial. We can do it without medication, with phytochemicals, which are probably the medicine of the future."

EXCURSUS ON PHYTOCHEMICALS

Phytochemicals are substances found in edible plants that exhibit potential benefits in the prevention and treatment of disease. There are thousands of phytochemicals in the foods we eat and scientists are just beginning to discover their healing properties. According to the Journal of the American Dietetic Association (April 1995): "It is the position of the American Dietetic Association (ADA) that specific substances in foods (e.g. phytochemicals as naturally occurring components and functional food components) may have a beneficial role in health as part of a varied diet. The Association supports research regarding the health benefits and risks of these substances. Dietetics professionals will continue to work with the food industry and government to ensure that the public has accurate scientific information in this emerging field."

The report goes on to say phytochemicals are present in many frequently consumed foods, especially fruits, vegetables, grains, legumes, and seeds, as well as in such less common foods as licorice, soy, and green tea. In addition to naturally occurring phytochemicals, scientists are developing what they call functional foods, which consist of any food or food ingredient providing health benefits beyond the traditional nutrients it contains.

Phytochemicals and functional food components have been associated with the prevention and/or treatment of at least four of the leading causes of death in the country—cancer, diabetes, cardiovascular disease, and hypertension—and with the prevention and/or treatment of other medical ailments including neural tube defects, osteoporosis, abnormal bowel function, and arthritis.

Dr. Potter, professor of epidemiology and director of the University of Minnesota Cancer Prevention Research unit, has been studying the relationship between diet and cancer for more than 15 years. He found that people with diets heavy in fruits and vegetables have lower rates of most cancers. Limonene in citrus fruits, for example, is known to increase the production of enzymes that help the body dispose of potentially carcinogenic substances. Even the National Cancer Institute estimates that one in three cancer deaths are diet related and that 8 of 10 cancers have a nutrition/diet component.

Phytochemicals have been used by pharmaceutical companies in making many of their products. According to a report in Business Week (February 15, 1993), 25% of modern pharmaceuticals are derived in some way from plants. The heart medicine digitalis and the cancer drugs vinicistine and taxol are just some examples. Pharmaceutical companies may soon be motivated to isolate components in foods into pills or supplement form to market the individual elements for their health benefits. However, due to regulatory problems, such companies will have to market naturally occurring components as drugs.

What makes phytochemicals new in the public ranks is their potential health benefits before people get sick, and the saving of both lives and health-care dollars. Unfortunately, according to Dr. Stephen L. DeFelic, head of the Foundation for Innovation in Medicine, the field is still in its infancy because of too few large-scale clinical trials focusing on the health benefits of foods. Since phytochemicals are not patentable, companies are reluctant to finance long-term studies that could cost as much as $200 million.

Nevertheless, epidemiological evidence and small human trials point to benefits which may well be sleeping giants in the nutrition arena. Such is the case with licorice root. In one USDA study, licorice root, an extract, proved to be 50 times sweeter than sugar without promoting tooth decay. It contains prostaglandin inhibitors that may guard against cancer and ulcers, and it is being pursued by many companies as a food additive.

In another study, Michael Gould, professor of human oncology at the University of Wisconsin Medical School, found that d-limonene, the major component of orange peel oil, protects rats against breast cancer. In addition to findings such as these, the ADA report notes that well-designed clinical trials indicate the beneficial effects associated with high fruit and vegetable diets cannot be duplicated by nutritional supplementation alone. Clearly, there are more benefits in the healthy foods we eat than are obtained from the most common nutrients often associated with them such as vitamins C, E, A, beta carotene, and so on.

For more information on phytochemicals, see the extensive electronic database assembled by Stephen M. Beckstrom and James A. Duke at the National Germplasm Resources Laboratory, Agriculture Research Service, United States Department of Agriculture, accessible on the World Wide Web (http://www.ars-grin.gov/~ngrlsb/).

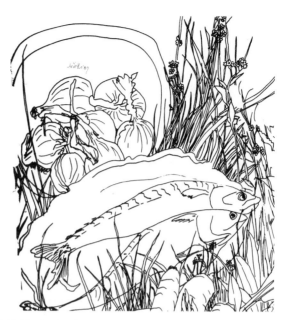

27 · HEART DISEASE

"My clients often have conditions that are not related to heart disease, according to them; but with my special training as an herbalist, I see a connection to the heart. Mind, body, spirit, all are interconnected and our heart is affected by all of these things. Depression, for example, is a problem we see connected to a weak heart and poor concentration is another. Insomnia, poor concentration and palpitations are all signs that poor circulation could be touching the heart. As herbalists, we strengthen what is weak so the heart will not falter."

—Letha Hadady

W.B. YEATS' POEM, "The Circus Animals' Desertion," concludes, "I must lie down where all the ladders start / In the foul rag-and-bone shop of the heart." His metaphor is meant to suggest a mature person's heart that has been lacerated by romantic and political betrayals. However, given the lifestyles of many Americans, who fill their arteries around the heart with plaque and debris, we might take the poem literally. With heart disease being the number one killer, we are certainly driven to ask if there is any way to clean up our foul hearts.

If we ask the opinions of some of the leading doctors and nurses in the field of alternative heart disease therapies, we find reason both for hope and despair. The hope comes from the stories of dramatic reversals of coronary problems, while despair comes from pondering the persistently hard-line doctors who refuse to consider alternative approaches fly in the face of much evidence that newer therapies work. Hidebound doctors are encouraging to patients who do not want to alter their diets, exercise or do anything else to change their lives, though they are veering toward disaster.

Dr. Robert Roberti, a cardiologist at Dean Ornish's Program for Reversing Heart Disease at Beth Israel Hospital in New York City, gives us hope. We have understood for the past 10 to 12 years, he relates, that coronary heart disease is not an irrevocable process. Changing diet, reducing stress, stopping smoking, getting exercise can reverse the blockage of arteries in coronary disease.

Dr. Stephen Atkins points out that we can remove plaque from the veins. He recounts stories of patients who had problems walking who now jog and run. They were told they must have bypass surgery because of total reduction in blood flow, but the hardening of the arteries was reversed and so too was the need for the bypass.

Dr. Ronald Hoffman of the Hoffman Center uses chelation, oxidation, lifestyle modification and other techniques to reverse heart problems. Delores Perri, M.S., R.E.D., argues that doctors should be taught about nutrition and if they do not know, should be open enough to tell their patients to consult someone else.

Heart disease is an illness that kills more Americans than any other, 1 in 5. In every year for which we have records, except 1918, heart disease has been the number one killer in the United States. The heart attack is the largest killer. Every 33 seconds an American dies of heart disease. There are 945,000 deaths annually. Heart disease accounts for 42% of deaths each year. On average, we have a stroke a minute and someone dies from a stroke every 3.5 minutes. Stroke is also one of the leading causes of long-term disability. We spent $151.3 billion in 1996 for cardiovascular medical costs. Sixty million people (more than 1 in 4) have some form of cardiovascular disease.

Many people are confused about heart disease and the question arises: Whom do you believe? Do you believe the physician who says there is not a shred of evidence that nutrition, diet, homeopathy, and other alternative routes to dealing with the problem are valid? The physician who says this in the face of dozens of articles in peer-reviewed, respected medical journals that say these therapies work and that deficiencies in such areas of proper diet and exercise lead to heart disease while proper use of these regimens reduce the risk?

Do you believe your doctor who says you do not have to change your diet, lose weight, exercise, reduce cholesterol, even though much literature says you do have to make these changes?

Perhaps after you read this chapter, which looks at new therapies that can help with this condition, you will be in a better position to know whom to believe.

WHAT IS HEART DISEASE?

What is the biology of heart disease? The arteries supply blood to the heart's muscles for the pumping action. These arteries are designated coronary because they surround the heart like a crown. If part of an artery is obstructed, the muscle which serves the heart is deprived of blood and nutrients it needs for the pumping action, resulting in a heart attack.

Obstruction does not occur suddenly; it is a slow, usually painless process that takes years to form through a process called arteriosclerosis, or hardening of the arteries. The cholesterols that build up in the arteries are carried by the blood in complex molecules called lipoproteins. These are combinations of fat and protein that are much larger than a normal blood cell. The LDL (low density lipoprotein) is a molecule that has a large amount of fat and a small quantity of protein. Having large amounts of LDL in the blood is a major risk factor for coronary heart disease. Another lipoprotein, HDL (high density lipoprotein), has large quantities of protein and small quantities of fat. It is thought that these help reduce the amount of cholesterol in the bloodstream.

The beginning of heart disease is thought to be in childhood. By the third decade of life, lesions (plaque) develop in the artery walls, characterized by an over-accumulation of cholesterol, other body fats, and debris which can completely shut off the blood flow in the artery. Usually the final stoppage is due to a blood clot that forms in the damaged artery, shuting off blood flow and resulting in the death of the muscle that the blood was supplying. Commonly, this is called a heart attack.

WHY ARE ALTERNATIVE REMEDIES NOT GIVEN A FAIR HEARING?

Before beginning to discuss alternative heart treatments, it might be eye-opening to note the reasons so many doctors prefer to ignore them; traditional doctors are often enthralled by the dazzle of high technology and the promise of large financial rewards.

I asked Dr. Hoffman about this situation. Why, with so many indications that traditional therapies are not working, physicians, cardiologists, and other healers do not take a step back and see if other modalities might be in order?

Dr. Hoffman's opinion is that we have become the victims of a "medical-industrial complex" run amok. The cardiovascular unit where heart operations are performed is the crown jewel of many hospitals, a major profit center, and the source of hundreds of referrals to physicians who derive their livelihoods from hospitals. The heart unit is a high-tech wonder, very easy to develop and expand and very hard to cut back.

According to Hoffman, many respected cardiologists, professors at major universities, are decrying the current trend by saying we should get away from high-tech, expensive procedures. Hoffman thinks we should simply use medicines when necessary but handle the majority of heart cases by natural dietary modifications, sending the few remaining cases to centers of excellence scattered around the country. Unfortunately, instead, the high-tech centers are spreading like wildfire.

NATURAL REMEDIES

Diet

There is not a lot of controversy over what is wrong with the American diet, with its high amount of animal proteins, saturated animal fats, dairy, deep-fried foods, and refined carbohydrates. The average American diet is 43% fats, 14% proteins, and the rest mainly carbohydrates. The average daily intake of cholesterol is 450-500 mg.

The American Heart Association recommends we cut fat intake to 30% and only 10% of this should be saturated fats (fats found particularly in land animals, palm and coconut oils, hydrogenated vegetable oils.).

(Note: We have been told that margarine, made from "polyunsaturated fats," is good for our hearts and will lower cholesterol. That is simply not true; it is loaded with the fatty acids that contribute to heart disease. Instead of margarine, use olive oil, canola oil, or other oils such as flaxseed, almond, safflower, sunflower, or soy. Of these, olive oil would be on the top of my list. But don't have margarine.)

No more than 10% of the oils you eat should be polyunsaturated fats, like those found in vegetable oils (such as corn and cottonseed oils). According to the American Heart Association, we should get the rest from monounsaturated fats, such as olive, and be taking in less than 300 mg of cholesterol each day.

Maybe former President Bush did not like broccoli, but perhaps if he knew some of the things that were in this marvelous vegetable, he would have changed his mind. Broccoli and other produce is the first thing to turn to for heart-benefiting foods.

We eat broccoli and all kinds of produce, seeds, legumes, and grains to get our beta carotenes and maybe the vitamin C, but they also contain important phytochemicals. This includes beta carotene, but also alpha-carotene, ascorbic acid, ash, boron, caffeic-acid, calcium, chlorophyll, chromium, citric acid, copper, glycine, iron, linoleic acid, lysine, magnesium, niacin, oleic acid, phosphorus, potassium, riboflavin, selenium, thiamin, tryptophan, and zinc, among others—there are a 1,000 different phytochemicals, so important in protecting us from cancer. Among them are also the phyto estrogens, which guard against prostate, breast and lung cancer. These chemicals have all kinds of healing properties. Chlorophyll, for instance, helps purify the blood and acts as a detoxifier.

If you want to lower your blood pressure, you can do this with vegetables such as garlic, broccoli, or asparagus. Do not forget, you should have at least five servings of vegetables and three of fruits each day, raw, steamed, or juiced. Once you start, you will notice a world of difference in overall vitality.

Other invaluable heart foods are rice and beans, complete proteins rich in fiber and B complex vitamins.

We grow up with the pernicious myth that if it is not an animal protein, it is not a complete protein and so not really nutritious. I did studies at the Institute of Applied Biology that proved conclusively that beans, legumes, and all grains contain complete proteins just like animal proteins, without the saturated fats. They do not have the high calories, and are rich in vitamins, minerals, and essential oils.

Hence, cultures that have rice and beans as a dietary staple have been so healthy. There are thousands of ways to prepare them, too. Go into a health food store and look at the different preparations along with all the other foods sold. When you see the variety, you will not feel deprived by not having steak and potatoes.

It is worth mentioning the division over the proper foods for those with heart disease. There are over 60,000 dietitians in the United States and they have been a primary source of information on what a sick person should be eating. After all, the physician has little training in nutrition, graduating medical school with only an hour or two of learning about the subject. The dietitian is well trained, yet even within the field of dietetics there is a split. A very small percentage believe the standard American diet has played a large part in causing diseases we are beset with, including heart disease.

Dolores Perri, M.S.R.D., discusses proper diet for the heart. Blood pressure medications are natural diuretics and deplete the system of magnesium, needed for heart function. Moreover, she notes, many Americans do not eat many vegetables, and it is in vegetables where you get lots of magnesium. We need to increase the magnesium content of our diets, she says, with vegetables, seeds, nuts, and beans.

Luanne Pennesi, R.N., B.S.N., a holistic nurse, also emphasizes diet as a means to deal with heart problems. She will sit down with a patient and assess his or her eating habits and lifestyle, getting patients to recognize the different facets in their lives and how they connect to their health.

The holistic nurse, she tells us, will discuss the problems with dairy in a diet and the options, such as rice milk. The nurse will tell them about the effects of raw vegetables in the diet, how many types of vegetables exist, and what the difference is between organic versus processed food. She'll mention the effect of pesticides in the soil and how they affect fruits and vegetables, having them taste the difference between organically grown and non-organically grown produce. When we take away the stigma of organic food, the idea that it is bland and tasteless, and let patients taste it for themselves, they find it is easy to shift to organics.

GARY NULL'S TOP TEN LIST OF SUPPLEMENTS OF A HEALTHY HEART

1) Coenzyme Q-10. I have seen over 100 studies, minimum, that show how important this substance can be in helping oxygenate the tissue as well as giving a great boost to the heart.

2) Vitamin E. I would not imagine there is a doctor in America who is not aware of the literature on this vitamin. It keeps the red blood cells in the body from clumping together. It is estimated that between 400 and 800 units are useful in preventing stroke. You may go higher, to 1,200 or 1,600 units, unless other medical conditions preclude this usage. I believe we would cut the incidence of stroke by 20%, saving 50,000 to 100,000 people a year, just by having everyone take this little, inexpensive supplement.

(Let me mention at this point that I remember interviewing Dr. Wilfred Shute, a man who, with his brother, had worked for 35 years on over 30,000 patients whom he treated with vitamin E. I went to see his clinic and while I was there I interviewed 50 people who were his patients, including a woman who kept photos of her toes, that had been covered with giant gan-grenous sores. They were going to be amputated and it was vitamin E that saved them. It all seemed too good to be true.

This was at the very beginning of my career when no one believed vita-min E had such potency. People wouldn't take it. You couldn't even find it in most vitamin pills. Today every other medical publication is extolling the anti-oxidants in vitamin E. Do you ever wonder about all the people that died in the interim, who did not have to die and would not have if doctors had been more progressive and flexible?

Dolores Perri points out, "The knowledge of vitamins' value was there for 25 years. I remember talking to a doctor when I was working in a nurs-ing home and telling him about vitamin E. He said, 'There's no definitive study on that.' The doctors just wouldn't look. Many of the elderly who could have been helped, were not.")

3) Chromium Picolinate. A lot of people have heard about this. It has been shown to be beneficial both for the heart and blood sugar.

4) CSA (chondroitin sulfate A), also very good.

5) L-carnitine. This is one of my favorites. If every American took 500-1,000 mg/day, we could really make a dent in heart disease. When I race—and I am an American Class racewalker, holding American records in indoors, outdoors, and all distances from the 1 mile to the 40 k—and I take the L-carnitine, I find I have a greater capacity for breathing. I am not as fatigued, and my recovery is much quicker. Now you should take L-carni-tine along with vitamin E, because they work synergistically together and they work terrifically.

6) Vitamin C. If there is one vitamin everyone needs to take everyday, it is this one. If a person has a cold or flu, he or she may require 50,000 mg of C for quick recovery; we should realize for heart disease we may require substantially more. So get over that old-fashioned idea that all you need is one glass of OJ and you have got the necessary vitamin C. That idea went out with the horse and buggy. Now we have thousands of studies in the lit-erature of the valuable properties of C, which can help with everything from cancer to heart disease and diabetes. I would take 500 to 1,000 mg/5 times a day, because vitamin C washes out of your system, so we need to take it throughout the day. By the way, two physicians, specialists in coronary heart disease, recommend their patients take vitamin C before going to bed at night because they find it helps prevent heart attacks during sleep and in the morning. This is when the majority of heart attacks occur.

7) Lecithin. Lecithin is made from soy. Not only does it keep our arteries strong and healthy, but it helps with the emulsification of fats, helps the brain and is good for memory as well as the heart.

8) EPO (Evening Primrose Oil), 1,500 mg daily.

9) Vitamin B_1. Of all the Bs, this is the most important for the heart: 25-50 mg daily.

10) MaxEPA (EPA and DHA). This is better know as fish oil. They are part of the Omega 3 and Omega 6 fatty acids that you find in salmon, sardines and mackerel. But many people do not eat these fish so they should be getting them in MaxEPA. They should take 500 to 1,000 mg of this supplement. It is worth noting that clinical and epidemiological experience as well as scientific studies have found that people who have a lot of fish in their diet have less heart disease than people without such a diet.

Those are the ten natural nutrients to take to prevent or treat heart disease. Taking them is not a panacea but must be done as part of an overall program.

Stress Management

Virtually all the authorities agree that if you are going to get a handle on heart disease, and that includes the hypertension, the high triglycerides, high cholesterol (particularly the elevated low density lipoproteins, the bad part of the cholesterol), the overweight body, and all the other conditions that frequently contribute to coronary heart problems, then you are going to have to deal with stress. Stress or distress is a major problem for the American psyche.

For a long while we have known that stress is a contributor to heart disease, but only recently have we begun to understand the physiological basis of the connection. We will look at how this occurs before turning to stress management techniques that help dissipate this problem.

Richard Friedman, Ph.D., Harvard Medical School, remarks that most of us, when we are confronted with stressful situations, try to over-solve the problem. In our society, we constantly try to fit square pegs into round holes, and when we find that is not going to work, we turn inward, brood, and look for ways to dissipate stress, frequently by acting inappropriately, such as by overeating, drinking or taking inappropriate drugs or medications, contributing to the disease process.

Friedman tells us there is a link between stress and cardiovascular disease. Very recent research supports that when we are stressed, due to a fear of physical or psychological danger, the body exhibits a fight or flight response, as it prepares to fight an enemy. One of the important things happening internally, as triggered by the response, is your body readying itself not to bleed if you get cut or injured, which makes a lot of sense from a biological and evolutionary perspective. However, if the threats are psychological and you have a bad diet, you may be going through stressful incidents 20 or 30 times a day, triggering the fight or flight response. Each time this happens, the body prepares not to bleed by making your blood platelets stickier. This internal clotting takes place every time you get angry whether on a supermarket line or in a traffic jam. As this goes on for weeks and months, this continual clotting can contribute to the plaque in the arteries. A heart attack that may occur when you are 50 years old, would not have occurred until you are 80 years old if you had undergone less of the buildup induced by platelet stickiness.

When you are exposed to a biochemical or psychological stress, a host of changes are taking place in addition to platelet stickiness. The body's ability to fight off viral and bacterial infection will be lessened by the weaknesses induced by stress. Stress compromises the immune system's ability to fight off opportunistic diseases.

There is some good news, though, about our ability to fight off the debilitating conditions leading to heart attack. Friedman notes that just as continued stress leads to a weakening of the system, there is an opposite effect, labeled by his colleague at Harvard, Dr. Herbert Benson, as the relaxation response. Eliciting this calming response on a daily basis makes it less likely you will have high blood pressure or the arteriosclerotic plaque buildup or a heart attack down the road.

The relaxation response should be combined with other behavior modifications to create a healthier response to stress and all should be combined with the best medical care. That is the way to optimize your health.

Dr. Friedman tells us how the relaxation response is engendered: Use whatever strategy you have available to let go of any muscle tension you may be experiencing. Make sure your muscles are loose and your jaw lets go. After you are feeling a bit more comfortable, focus your attention on your breathing. If you find yourself having any distracting thoughts, do not let them bother or take you away from the process. As soon as you have a distracting thought, simply say to yourself "Oh well" and return to a concentration on your breathing and to a thought or image that allows you to stay calm, peaceful, and relaxed. Become aware of the cool air coming in and the warm air going out. Keep this up till you are deeply relaxed.

Chelation Therapy

Chelation therapy is a process of cleaning the arteries, that costs about $95 per treatment. Dr. Atkins says, "We recommend about 20 treatments with the patient taking a treatment once or twice a week. Then a maintenance regimen can be kept up by having the patient come every four to six weeks." Bill, a patient of his, says it definitely works.

But what about the cynics who say the so-called benefits from chelation are all in the patients' deluded minds? Bill explains his medical history.

"I was beginning to feel very tired, very lethargic. and the doctors said they could do nothing for me. There was nothing wrong, they said. After about 20 chelation treatments, I began to feel a tremendous difference in the way I felt . People have told me I look younger and I feel more energetic.

You have to be motivated, willing to stick to a diet, take vitamins. People who have had serious heart problems have taken this course and improved. I've seen people who've had two angioplasties and those failed, then they've taken this course and they've had better results than with the two previous angioplasties. A friend of mine wasn't able to walk one block, had shortness of breath and angina. Now she walks twenty blocks a day and swims for an hour, with no problems."

One thing Bill mentions is that none of these therapies can work alone. Although chelation has brought an improved, more vigorous life to Bill, he has done chelation in combination with exercise, eating right and making other modifications of his life. He has done this as opposed to looking for medications or other more conventional solutions.

Dr. Ronald Hoffman has estimated that upwards of 50 million Americans take medication for hypertension. He states, "It's been shown that one third of the patients on high blood pressure medications are being given them incorrectly and that simply withdrawing the medications would be the right solution for them. But with our type of proactive program, we could reduce to a 10-20% core of patients who could really benefit from these medications. For them, lifestyle modification with exercise and dietary supplements is too little, too late. But for the vast majority, who work at it, meditate and use biofeedback, this is the right solution."

Dr. Hoffman thinks patients like Bill deserve a lot of credit. Many have been influenced by mainstream medicine. They have been told alternatives do not work, that if they use them their life will be hanging by a thread. Many have been berated into complying, but some patients have the gumption to say, "Look, the angioplasty you gave me doesn't work. The medicine is making me sick and I want something else."

What is gratifying for Hoffman is that skepticism and rebellion are being rewarded, because, as many studies are now showing, the medical therapies of the past are being discarded as unsafe and outmoded. Skepticism in approaching conventional treatments is a good idea. Studies are showing the wisdom of therapies like chelation and taking anti-oxidants, whose value is being borne out by positive results. Exercise and stress reduction are being shown to be beneficial, while conventional treatments turn out to be too expensive, ineffective, and downright harmful in some cases. The scientific current has been turning around in recent years.

Homeopathy

Ken Korins, M.D., explains how his specialty, homeopathy, offers another alternative practice that seems to get results with heart disease: "Homeopathy works by giving very small doses that are extremely individualized to the person's symptoms and physical state. These doses work on a type of vibration or energy that stimulates the body much in the way that acupuncture works."

Many traditional practitioners dismiss the benefits of this technique due to a colossal ignorance of the evidence. These physicians say this therapy has never been proven by randomized, double-blind studies in the way more scientific procedures have been. Korins argues that is absolutely incorrect. He tells us that in 1993, in a British medical journal there was an article by Kleinsman, which reviewed 107 clinical studies of homeopathy. About 80% of them found that homeopathy had positive effects. And many of these were extremely rigorous studies. In the *Journal of Pediatrics*, a very rigorous double-blind study showed extraordinary results from homeopathy.

What are the kinds of heart problems that improve with homeopathy? Hypertension is a big one. It will help people recovering from congestive heart failure, cervo-vascular accidents, arterosclerotic heart disease and a very wide range of conditions.

In classical homeopathy, the specialist selects a single remedy. Korins elaborates, "For our work, we don't rely on a lot of tests and the high technology that goes with them. We prefer to look at what symptoms a person has and how they present themselves. For example, if a person is having angina, tightness, a squeezing sensation, a remedy like songea or cactus, which is extremely effective in treating angina, would be called for. Sometimes there is a congestion in the head, a hot feeling when the blood pressure goes up. The prescription there might be a remedy like gloline.

"What you are looking for is an idea of what physical state the patient is in. A particular heart patient may not have any manifestations of heart disease per se, but you are looking for the particular homeopathic remedy that will stimulate the body's healing properties. In that case, it will really be the body itself that is doing the curing and not the homeopathic remedy." (See the chapter on Chronic Fatigue Syndrome for details on homeopathic methods.)

Qi (Chi) *Energy*

An Oriental treatment that has some success with heart patients is the manipulation of *qi* (*chi*) energy. Dr. Jeie Atacama, D.D.M., LAC., uses *qi* energy to accomplish healing. With this practice, one does not use needles as in acupuncture, though it does share with acupuncture the concentration on meridians of the body. In a technique he learned from his father, Atacama uses his fingers directly on the skin of patients. As Bill Moyers showed on his television reports on Oriental philosophy, such healing practices as *tai chi* and *qi gong*, depend on channeling internal *qi* energies to rebalance the body.

Atacama has not counted the numbers of patients he has helped, but it has been, he estimates, between 3,000 and 5,000 in 20 years of practice. Rebalancing *qi* energy can help greatly with heart disease by rebuilding the body's health and restoring its self healing powers.

This practice works exactly like acupuncture. U points are found on either side near the base of the spine. One point is connected to the large intestine, which is part of the bodily system particularly in touch with the qi energy, which involves all the non-liquid, biological energy that circulates through the body. The treatment should be done three times a week, lasting for as many weeks as is called for by the condition. If the problem is cramps in the leg due to poor circulation, ten sessions would get rid of the problem.

Herbs

More Americans will be buying and using herbs now than they have been in the last 100 years. Dr. James A. Dukes at the USDA has written a major textbook and has become a major authority on the use of herbs for health. But not many doctors have caught up with Dr. Dukes. One person who has is Letha Hadady, one of the leading herbalists in the United States.

She says most Americans do not go to the doctor when they are a little sick; they wait until they are really suffering. They might have chest pains, difficulty breathing, but they generally are not going to the doctor and, of course, not to their herbalist. They say, "I'm tired; I'm under stress," and ignore it. But that is a terrible approach because some of the underlying problems of heart disease are the ones they are complaining of: fatigue, stress, and poor digestion. Poor digestion and fatigue lead to cholesterol buildup, which leads to pain and heart congestion. People try to breathe more deeply and reduce stress when they experience these early symptoms, but it does not help. But changing your diet, taking herbs and foods that reduce cholesterol, that will definitely help.

Her clients often have conditions that are unrelated to heart disease, according to them; but with her special training as a herbalist, she sees a connection to the heart. Mind, body, spirit, all are interconnected and our heart is affected by all of these things. Depression, for example, is a problem connected to a weak heart. Insomnia, poor concentration and palpitations are all signs that poor circulation could be touching the heart.

Many Western doctors will say herbs, especially Oriental ones, are not tested. This is a prejudiced answer because when you go to a public library or consult a computer indexing service like Med Line, which is available to all medical students and any interested person, you will find 3,500 studies on Chinese herbs alone. The majority of the research is done in Asia and for Americans to say this research does not count is racist.

There are quite a number of these remedies available in health food stores, by mail order, or in your local Chinatown.

She points out that one of the major underlying problems associated with heart disease is fatigue. Now Chinese doctors link the heart's health to the strength of the adrenal glands, not an obvious connection. "If I had a patient complaining of fatigue and being overweight, I would suspect heart problems if not then, somewhere down the line, so I would work on the adrenals. To strengthen the adrenals, you can get the herbal preparation from Chinatown called Goldenbook. It adds to immune energy and will help with kidney and heart problems. We strengthen what is weak so the heart will not falter."

She goes on to mention that clove, a spice we have at home, is a strong stimulant. A pinch in the late afternoon will act as coffee. Coffee is a major problem because it increases stuck, painful circulation in the gastro-intestinal tract which will affect the whole circulation, meaning the heart will not run smoothly. A pinch of clove will replace coffee better than anything else.

Siberian ginseng, a mix of various ginsengs, is good. The ginsengs are adaptogens, that is, they will help us maintain energy as well as aid us in living under a high level of stress. They support the nervous system. Raw Tienchi ginseng, one Americans are less familiar with, comes in powdered form. When you take a little bit (1/2 teaspoon) in cool water every day, it will reduce cholesterol and pain around the heart.

Two Chinese remedies that are especially valuable in relation to heart pain and congestion of the blood vessels are Dan Shen Wan, which combines salvia and camphor. The camphor dilates the blood vessels while the salvia increases the heart's action. The other is Guan Xin Su He Wan, which contains frankincense. This is mentioned in the Bible, you may recall, along with myrrh; both increase circulation. Frankincense for stuck circulation increases blood flow around the heart. You can take it once a day to prevent heart attack. It can be chewed and swallowed. Hadady recommends it even if you have no heart problem symptoms. It has healthy ingredients such as liquid amber, and sandalwood, which keeps the esophagus and chest cool.

Yan Shen Jia Jiao Wan is a combination of ginseng and other herbs that work on brain circulation, freeing the circulation of the blood in the brain, so it is not just for heart difficulties, but for victims of heart attack, stroke and hemoplegia (which paralyzes and cramps on the whole side of the body). It is taken as a preventive measure when you have high cholesterol and are at high risk of heart trouble. One a day prevents problems.

Baoxin Wan is a remedy for heart attacks. If you feel faint and experience pain and weakness, you sniff it like a smelling salt. If the pain is great and you feel the onset of an attack, then take it orally. It includes ginseng and liquid amber. The ingredients are always in English or Latin on the back. It treats the congestion of the blood vessels around the heart and frees the blood vessel.

Some of the underlying problems leading to a heart attack are well countered by herbal remedies, like excess weight and cholesterol. The best way to lose weight is not to get rid of your appetite or jazz up your energy level with a stimulant, but to take a sensible diet that reduces fat as well as take some herbs that are valuable additives. One preparation with a self explanatory name is "Keep Fit, Reduce Fat" capsules. The ingredients are ginseng, hawthorn, and other herbs that are good for the heart. Hawthorn is a slightly bitter, slightly sour berry and works as a digestive. You can take a capsule of Keep Fit after meals. Cholesterol is reduced and the muscle of the heart is made stronger.

Evening primrose oil is another useful way to reduce cholesterol. Chinatown is an excellent place to purchase this remedy since the prices are apt to be considerably lower than those given for comparable items in health food stores.

Another popular remedy in Asia is green tea, which has been reported all over, including in the *New York Times*, as a very good remedy for reducing cholesterol. "This," Hadady mentions, "is a good alternative to other caffeine teas, because the caffeine in it is very low. It gives the satisfaction of a bitter tea while reducing cholesterol."

Bojemni slimming tea is protective of the heart. It has hawthorn in it. Also beneficial is Xiao Yo Wan, a digestive remedy that boosts circulation and combats depression. It contains ginger, mint, and other herbs, eases the flow of bile, eases the digestive process, and reduces chest congestion.

Digestive Harmony is an American-made product that uses Chinese herbs, one of many such products now on the market, sold door to door or through mail order. "This is part of a trend now," Hadady explains, "a very important trend in herbalism, of using Asian herbs manufactured with American standards. Digestive Harmony can be ordered from Oakland, California. It will ease the underlying troubles related to heart disease.

Remember depression is in part a heart problem, Hadady says. The heart is not just a digestive center, but is for our emotions. Depression is rightly associated with heart disease since it affects the heartbeat. When we are not happy and our emotions are not smooth, then we feel it in the heart.

Some remedies that combat depression come to us from China. Co-schisandra strengthens the energy levels and keeps us from losing the energy we have. It is good for both the adrenals and the heart. It fights against poor memory, poor concentration and depression. Also try Anshen Bu Nao Pien, available in all the Chinatowns in the United States. It is for depression, blood deficiencies and heart-related problems such as panic and anxiety.

Also useful is Mao Dong Qing, which is the chinese name for holly, and it comes in capsule form. It is for chest pain and prevention of heart trouble. You can take several of these capsules each day as a preventive. If you already have heart problems, it reduces cholesterol, congestion and pains.

"In general," she concludes, "Chinese remedies for the heart also treat emotional problems, not just pain, but sadness, anxieties and other mental suffering."

FULL ALTERNATIVE MEDICAL PROGRAMS

Dean Ornish's Program for Reversing Heart Disease

Deborah Matra, R.N., works at the Ornish Program at Beth Israel. It opened in 1993 and has enrolled 200 patients over the past two years. Dr. Roberti, also at the program, explains that it has four components:

1) Moderate, supervised exercise.

2) Stress management, involving stretching exercises and some yoga poses as well as the teaching of relaxation and meditation techniques.

3) Low fat, vegetarian diet, with no animal products and no added fats.

4) Group support sessions where patients meet to learn more about their problems and act to express themselves.

Dr. Roberti explains that everything they try to do is to modify risk factors known to increase the dangers of coronary disease. It is not that different from a general medical program. The goal is to reduce weight, lower cholesterol and blood pressure, control diabetes, stop smoking, and control stress.

He talks of a study in the 1989 British medical journal *Lancet*, where two groups of heart patients were studied. One group followed the Ornish guidelines, the other took the regular medical treatment for coronary disease. One year after starting this Ornish program, there was a reversal (improvement) of the coronary artery measured through an angiogram. This same group has done a follow up, five years into the program, and when they evaluated the blood flow to the heart with a PET scan (a state-of-the-art procedure), there was a significant improvement in flow even after five years of doing the program. In September 1995, the study came out in the *Journal of the AMA*.

"One thing we remind patients who enter this program," Matra says, "is that they need to regard what is required as a prescription from their doctor. They need to stick with the diet and exercise, do the stress management routine daily, stay with it as they would honor their doctor's prescription."

The Tri-State Healing Center: IV Vitamin and Ozone Therapy

We have been led to believe that genetics has a primary role in all diseases, and it probably does in many. We must see, however, the connected symptoms. We must see that diet and lifestyle play an enormous role and far more of a role than genetics, though genetics is a contributing factor. The Tri-State Healing Center, a place that is unique in the United States, takes a holistic approach to healing. They use state-of-the-art, even avant-garde, techniques, vitamin C drips, dietary counseling, acupuncture, massage therapies, chelation, body therapy, all things done by qualified individuals and they have had some magnificent results. Let's talk to some patients who've been helped at the center. John talks about his experience:

"I'd say that I'm 95% responsible for my ill condition, out of sheer laziness and neglect. I weigh about 600 pounds and I realize I am apt to get various diseases because of my weight. I have already suffered some: high blood pressure, fatigue, severe viral and bacterial problems, edema of the right leg that causes cramps. I have trouble flexing the joints."

In the African-American community to which John belongs, there is, unfortunately, a high incidence of death from coronary heart disease and far too many cases of high blood pressure.

The patient mentions that much of his disease arose from faulty lifestyle habits, growing up eating too much fat, a lot of meat, drinking alcoholic beverages, all of which undermine health.

Howard Robins, M.D., from the Healing Center, says he is trying to motivate people to take a holistic view by cleansing, detoxifying, and rebuilding the body's immune system. "We try," he says, "to let the body heal itself from all its injuries and weaknesses. We do not focus on one illness, but on the body as a whole. This is how holistic medicine was originally formulated.

"In our program, we have a medical doctor who assumes charge of the patient's medical condition, a homeopathic practitioner, a nutritionist, who does extensive nutritional counseling with each patient on vitamins, herbs, and minerals, an acupuncturist who uses this technique as well as prescribes Chinese herbal remedies to strengthen a weak organ system; and a dentist who removes mercury amalgam fillings, which cause fatigue and weaken the immune system. We also have a chiropractor who will rebalance the back structure so there will be better nerve innervations so the system won't misfire and damage the organ system. Since all the body's systems are interconnected, we need to put everything back in order."

Dr. Robins' particular specialty is to work with intravenous vitamin C and ozone therapy. He tells us that in vitamin C therapy a person is built up very rapidly to large doses, up to the 100,000 mg range and eventually to the 200,000 range. High levels of vitamin C cleanses the artery walls of calcified fatty plaques. They also use EDTA in the drip which functions by melting the calcium bonds to the walls so the plaque is freed and the EDTA and C can wash it out of the body's system. Then the solution goes on and cleanses and heals the scars left by the low density lipoproteins, healing the walls so that plaque will no longer adhere to them.

They also use ozone therapy—called major auto hemotherapy. They take out a certain amount of blood, about 300 ccs or 10 ounces, and mix in an oxygen/ozone combination. They then put the blood right back in, taking about 30 minutes. The ozone helps oxidize fatty plaques, sort of liquefying them and removing them from the walls while making the red blood cells more flexible, so they can slip through these clogged arteries. This last measure is very important in preventing the need for bypass surgery and getting rid of angina pain.

You might wonder how ozone therapy originated. Robins traces it back to World War I. It was found that men who had been burned by mustard gas or injured or shot and were kept in the back of the hospital tent, where the electric generators for the field lights were kept, were getting well. Eventually, they realized the cause of the improvement was the ozone gas created by leakage from these generators. That began the work on ozone as a means to heal and prevent the amputation of limbs with gangrene. "We've seen some miraculous results of ozone therapy at the Healing Center, for it's one thing that really does work."

CONCLUSIONS

Five years ago I suggested to a leading cardiologist that use of vitamin E, stress management, exercise, dietary changes, power walking, and proper supplementation would make a vast difference in the prevention and treatment of heart disease. He looked at me and responded, "No way. It's not scientific. It won't work."

Today if you were to read JAMA (*Journal of the American Medical Association*), the *New England Journal of Medicine*, the *Medical Tribune, Lancet*, or any other major medical journal, they recommend the same treatments disparaged five years ago. Thanks to the pioneering work of Dr. Dean Ornish and others, the concept of alternative treatment is less controversial and people are not willing to accept these treatment if they seem to offer the best possibility of health. Hopefully, in the future we will not have to reject one or the other, but accept the best features from each as they lead to better health.

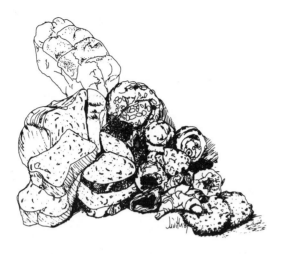

28 · REVERSING THE AGING PROCESS NATURALLY

"With the proper diet, we found we could lower cholesterol, lower the triglycerides, lower the percentage of body fat, aid digestion, shorten the transit times of food almost by half, remove constipation and create better sleep habits, so we could shorten a person's needed sleep (often cutting this by two hours a night). That's reversing the aging process."

IN THE LARGELY UNREAD, fourth book of *Guilliver's Travels*, the hero comes to an island, near Japan, where a race has realized mankind's dream of living forever. The irony is that these immortals all wish they were dead, because, though they have lived hundreds of years, these have been miserable years, since they have all the infirmities of the aged, such as blindness, deafness, arthritis, and senility. Jonathan Swift's satirical thrust can be applied today, when we consider the following facts. Americans are living longer than ever before, but most are unable to enjoy longevity because its potential pleasures are canceled out by the early, prematurely early, encroachments of aging.

This is why, when we start to get older, especially when we have not been living the healthiest of lifestyles, we begin asking: Can I detoxify? Can I reverse premature aging? Can I get back more energy, energy I didn't have since I was young? As we will see, if one is willing to take the steps to live in a healthy and natural way, the answer is Yes.

In this chapter, we will look first at what causes premature aging, both physiologically and in our deficient lifestyles, and then look at a program to reverse this aging. The program is all-sided and includes proper eating habits, exercise, the use of muscle and mental relaxation techniques and the adoption of a mental attitude that faces life bravely and honors it in all its forms: human, animal and vegetable.

CAUSES OF PREMATURE AGING

Why do so many of us look older than our years? What are the forces, inside and out, that seem to pushing so many people to an early grave, or if they don't literally kill them, weaken them so their vitality, strength and *joie de vivre* are far below what they could be?

In our society, we have accepted the idea of being overweight, of having high blood pressure, high trigylcerides, high cholesterol and arthritis, as inevitable accompaniments of getting older. Since so many people have these problems, we think of them as normal. Even the doctor will say, when you get to be a certain age, these situations are to be expected and, since they are irreversible, accepted.

Ross Pelton, Ph.D., disagrees. "We can live to be 100 to 120 years old, staying healthy until the end of the maximum life span," rectangularizing the aging curve.

Martin Feldman, M.D., supports this stand. "We need to have optimum energy as we grow old, not accept the diminishment many find encroaching as they grow older."

Joint disease, Feldman points out, is an area where medicine has accepted a reversible condition as inescapable. There is now an epidemic of joint disease in the United States. The majority of people over 60 have either early, moderate or late osteoarthritis. Conventional doctors call it a wear-and-tear disease of the joints that appears naturally, which sounds nice, as if the joints wear out like the parts of a car, but it is nonsense. The disease is the product of deficiencies and occurs when the joint is not being nourished. A nourished joint will remain healthy.

Feldman has seen marathon runners in their 70s and 80s who use their joints tenfold or even fifty fold more than a normal person and yet their joints remain robust.

Dr. Richard Ash says the body may age before its time because it is carrying too much toxic load due to things the body is exposed to environmentally and biochemically, coming especially from the dust and chemicals we ingest daily. This assault weakens the repair mechanisms and leads to a vitamin and nutriment deficit.

According to Dr. Pelton, the primary cause of premature aging is free radicals. Dr. Denum Harman of the University of Nebraska first developed the theory of how these radicals act to accelerate aging. The radicals are electrically imbalance molecules that do tremendous damage at the cellular level. If we look down into the body, into the cells, we find their individual powerhouses, the mitochondria. In the mitochondrias' folds are super coiled strands of DNA. An invading oxygen free radical can zoom into the mitochondria and hit one of the DNA's paired bases, distorting the whole segment. A repair enzyme will quickly move to the site and return the DNA to its original shape. But this is a process that gradually wears the body down.

Dr. Eric Braverman of New York has mapped brain aging and how nutrients influence this process. Using a test called the Brain Electronic Activity Map (or BEAM), a technique developed at Harvard Medical School and refined, strengthened, and expanded by Dr. Braverman, the brain's level of electric activity is studied. This is a crucial area of concern because such things as substance abuse, hormonal imbalance, chronic fatigue, anxiety, hypertension, and even lyme disease, may affect the brain and cause premature aging. Often an EEG or MRI will show nothing wrong, while the BEAM test reveals the brain has been suffering from stress. It gives a window on the brain and how it is aging. So, as Braverman says, he is using "the BEAM that lights the path to wellness."

He relates that one thing this test registers is the speed of brain cycles, since slowing is a key marker of aging. The normal healthy rhythm of the brain is 10 cycles per second of Alpha waves. Compare this to the heart's normal rate of 1 cycle per second. Since the brain is intense and complex, it functions more quickly than the heart. As people age, though, their brain rhythm will decrease to nine, eight or seven beats per second. There will be a drop out of Alpha rhythms and an increase of Theta waves.

This can occur prematurely for many reasons including head trauma, Alzheimer's and abuse of such substances as cocaine, marijuana, and alcohol. When these causes operate, the frontal and temporal lobes will be found to be aging in an accelerated manner. Aging will also be increased by whiplash, metabolic disorders, loss of circulation and the "toxic home syndrome," which refers to the damage that can be done to the body by things such as cleansers that vaporize, pesticides and herbicides that are found around the house or garden. Add to that possible harm from fluorescent lights and electromagnetic pollution. The latter is caused by the electromagnetic grid we all live in, surrounded by digital clocks, VCRs, CD players, computers, sleeping blankets, cellular phones and beepers, and microwave ovens. These appliances transmit negative electrical resonance—the opposite of what our bodies need, causing damage to our chromosomes and tissues. These stresses hurt us slowly, in small ways, causing cumulative degeneration, creating subtle discrepancies in how the body functions.

Braverman notes that a computerized spectral analysis will pick up how these factors have affected the brain. A PET scan, which tells about the metabolism of the brain, can be correlated with a BEAM test, which may be recording not only weaker brain electrical activity but a loss of metabolism of the neurotransmitters.

Finally, Hal Huggins, D.D.S., highlights another cause of premature aging, the mercury in silver amalgam fillings. Mercury does not just sit there—you inhale it and it goes into your lungs. You eat and chew, wearing it away, so it goes into your stomach and digestive system. There it undergoes metastasization, forming methal mercury, a highly toxic substance. (In our Holistic Dentistry chapter, we have a section devoted to this hazard.)

ANTI-AGING NUTRIENTS

Supplements

In the next ten years, 50% of the United States population will be over 40, but unlike their parents these baby boomers are not accepting diabetes, high blood pressure, arthritis, overweight conditions, and high cholesterol as the necessary companions of aging. They are looking for ways to stop premature aging.

The first thing to look at as a means of reversing aging is supplements. Most people do not know how to properly take vitamins and minerals. You must follow the law of compensation. If you smoked, used sugar or caffeine, if you have been an angry person who held in your anger, if you have not honored the life force, not exercised, not been fulfilled, you must work to compensate for these deficiencies.

One-a-day supplements are the easy way out. I have met people who say, "I eat meat. I eat sugar. But it's all right because I take my one-a-day vitamin."

My friend, that does not work. The body cannot be lied to. After 30 or 40 years of the body's debilitation by an unhealthy lifestyle and environment, a little pill will not do the trick. You need to detoxify and cleanse the body.

Another illusion is the idea of the recommended daily dose, given by drug companies and conventional physicians. This is not the best way to think about health. These recommendations are like the minimum wage. Is that what we are interested in, minimal health. Or do we want optimal health? These dosages of supplements, which are now called recommended daily values, are very substandard if one wants a long-term healthy lifestyle.

You have to know what your bodily state is and plan accordingly. I would suggest one level of usage for healthy people who know they are healthy, while, for those processing diseases, there is a quite different level of use. The person becoming conscious of his or her health will need to consult a nutritionist who can design a personalized supplement program to meet an individual's needs.

Dr. Ash has talked to his large New York City radio audience about the revivifying power of DHEA, called the mother of all hormones, which is a key underlying ingredient for the productions of the adrenal gland. He tells us when the body is under stress, the adrenal gland requires cortisone and adrenaline, more highly in demand during such times. If these hormones are overused, they will become depleted as will DHEA, the precursor of these substances.

A lack of DHEA, he explains, will cause all sorts of negative consequences for the immune system. Often at age 80, a person will have 1/20th of the DHEA he or she had at age 20. Once the capacity and reserves of DHEA have been eaten up, chronic diseases will be harder to combat due to a weakened immune system. One of the earliest signs of DHEA depletion is an inability to get REM sleep, which will cause insomnia. An uninformed doctor may prescribe sleeping pills, which will not get at the root of the problem. This deficiency will also cause poor sugar regulation, a hyperglycemic symptom, since with low DHEA, a person will not be able to tolerate sugar in the diet, so will have to eat more frequently. Other common symptoms are palpitations, sweating, confusion, poor concentration, and not being able to cope with everyday stress.

Braverman has found that counteracting the aging process has to be undertaken on an individual basis. His treatments look at each patient's individual hormone imbalance, brain mapping, attention span, memory problems and cardiac and exercise capacities. Once this is examined, the patient needs to be nutritionally correct. He recommends natural yam extract which contains PET (progesterone, estrogen and testosterone), all the hormones that are essential. Progesterone has anti-cancer properties and helps with the calming of the brain. Estrogen strengthens the bones, has anti-cancer effects, especially in the colon, aids memory and gives cardio-vascular protection. Testosterone reduces the side effects of other hormones, and helps keep the sex drive vigorous through a person's 50s, 60s and beyond. For a woman, the ovary produces all three of these substances, but as Braverman puts it, "If the ovary dies, you must resurrect it. If you permit an organ to die, you allow yourself to die. We must stop this if we want abundant life. We replace depleted hormones with PET, and missing adrenal with DHEA."

Dr. Ash points out that with a low amount of DHEA, there will be less salivary IGA, which is a substance found in the gastro-intestinal (GI) tract. When IGA is depleted or absent, there will be more antigen penetration in this area as well as food and chemical sensitivity reactions. There may be inflammation of the tract, a condition called "leaky gut," whereby certain unwanted foods and chemicals get into the body system. Then auto immune disease may rises when the body attempts to defend itself against these unexpected intruders. Ash notes, that by administering DHEA and building back up salivary IGA, we can diminish food sensitivity, lower toxic load and restore the GI tract, getting back an intact immune system, treating the cause not the symptoms.

Dr. Pelton has studied drugs that enhance learning and intellectual capabilities while slowing down brain aging and senility. They help you get smarter and keep you from getting dumber—so you don't lose what you've already got. One of these substances is hydergein, which is available by prescription in the United States in a 1 mg tablet, while it can be obtained in the rest of the world in a 4 1/2 to 5 mg tablet. It will enhance cognition in the elderly. Moreover, studies show it increases learning, memory and recall abilities in young adults. It increases neural pathways and electrical energy flow in the brain tissue.

The reason such supplements are crucial is that, as a person ages, certain fatty acids, amino acids, and members of the four main groups of nutrients are lost. Scientists are looking into this issue and already know that choline, tyrosine, glutathione, cyctine, vitamin E, zinc and chromium are poorly absorbed and deficient in older people. Meanwhile, as these substances grow scarce, there is a buildup of heavy metals, such as aluminum and lead. These can be removed from the cells with chelation. Vitamin C and zinc are also useful in flushing them out. Most importantly, as the body loses necessary nutrients they have to be put back in for optimum physical and mental functioning

At the same time, free radicals, growing more common in the body as we age, have to be fought. Remember, when you eat meat, drink alcohol, and are around pollutants, then the body creates free radicals. They cause skin to wrinkle in the sun, they foster cancer, arthritis and heart disease. However, nutrients, called anti-oxidants, such as beta carotene and vitamin A, are able to neutralize the effect of the radicals, slowing down the aging process.

Another invaluable supplement is the citrus bioflavonoid complex, which can be obtained from lemons, plums, and oranges among other fruits. With an orange, one can cut open the skin and right below is the nutrient, the bioflavonoid. Another bioflavonoid that is good is rutin, which comes from buckwheat. If one is going to take the bioflavonoid in pill form, I would recommend 300 mg per day for a healthy person, while a person in poor health should take 500 mg. As for the rutin, the proper dosage for a healthy person is 25 mg per day, while the ill person may take up to 50 mg.

Blueberry extract is good for the eyes. During World War II, the RAF gave this to its pilots to improve night vision and strengthen the immune system. Red cabbage extract is also important. There are cultures that lack a variety of foodstuffs, but they eat cabbage and obtain its anti-bacterial, anti-ulcer properties. Cabbage, eaten juiced or steamed, will prove very healthful.

Red wine concentrate also has life-enhancing effects. A few years ago a study was made of the people living in a certain area in France. This was a group who had a high cholesterol diet, who ate creams, cheese and meats to such a degree that one would expect them to show a high level of cholesterol and heart disease, seeing that coronary trouble and high cholesterol go hand in hand. Yet, they did not have many heart problems, and the only thing that seemed to be counteracting the effect of this diet, distinguishing them from other groups with similar diets, was red wine. This is what the study showed.

I looked into it. It could not just be the wine, because alcohol in general is not beneficial, in fact, it destroys nutrients. It had to be something in the wine. It had to be the bioflavonoids, anti-oxidants, in the red wine. If this is so, you don't need the wine. Why not take just the grape, for from the skin and seeds comes an anti-oxidant, which can be obtained as a pill. Recommended daily dosage for the healthy is 50 mg, and for those not in good health, up to 200 mg.

If you lived in China, you would probably be drinking green tea and taking green tea extract. We know it has anti-cancer properties. It is an immune system stimulator. Decaffeinated green tea is very beneficial.

Beta carotenes are helpful and can be obtained in all the green, red and orange fruits and vegetables. As I've said previously, six to nine servings a day of fruits and vegetables are ideal.

Glutathione is good for the immune system but it is not easily assimilated by the body so it should be taken with something that produces it in the body, such as intacytelsistine. Recommended dosage is 200 mg a day for the healthy and up to 400 mg for those not in the best of health.

I might also mention L-cyctine, which is useful in detoxifying the liver and for problems with the liver.

Of all the nutrients, though, the single most important is vitamin C. Its benefits are multiple. This vitamin is important for the skin, giving it that youthful elasticity. This is because it produces collagen, the connective cell tissue, which holds the muscles and skin together. It helps the body produce interferon and increases leukocyte activity. It aids the thymus gland, the liver and the brain, while acting to prevent arthritis, cataracts and heart disease. It seems it helps with everything. A healthy person should take 2,000 mg a day, spread out over the course of the day. For the unhealthy person, I have seen them take, under medical supervision, up to 150,000 mg in IV drips. (We discuss this further in our chapter on the heart.)

Another life-giving supplement is vitamin E. People with Herpes IV, chronic fatigue syndrome, hepatitis and even AIDS have miraculously improved by taking large doses of the vitamin. Dr. Wilfred Shute, up in Canada, working with his brother, has treated over 30,000 patients in his decades of medical practice. He has helped with intermittent collodication, diabetes, gangrene and so many other conditions. (More details of his treatments appear in our discussion of heart disease.) Recommended dosage of this vitamin may be 800 units, sometimes 1,000 or up to 1,600 units.

A recent book, *Anti-Oxidants and Coronary Heart Disease*, written by a doctor from Dallas with a conventional background, confirms the thesis we are advancing—that taking anti-oxidants can prevent heart disease. His book shows the medical literature is full of studies supporting this assertion.

When we consider that millions of Americans are dying of heart disease every year and that many of these deaths can be prevented by taking the anti-oxidants, then it might be asked: Why aren't more people taking them? If you wait for your average physician to prescribe them, a physician who probably has no training in their use, and probably is in bad health himself, then you could be waiting until the ambulance comes. Whereas, if you want to wait until society as a whole catches onto their use, you will be waiting at least for another five years.

Nutritionists and physicians point out that giving a supplement orally is good, but even better is taking it intravenously. In this way, you can take large doses and absorb it all at once.

At the Tri-State Healing Center of New York City, they use IV drips of vitamin C and other nutrients to counteract the aging process.

Howard Robins, D.P.M., points out toxins and free radicals are stressful to both the body and mind. When the body is in pain, fatigued and under attack from heavy metal and other pollutants, which we come in contact with on a daily basis, this weakens us as well as affecting our minds adversely. With the IV vitamin C, we cleanse the body. The Tri-State Healing

Center also uses drips with other nutrients, such as EDTA, as a way to cleanse the heavy metals from the body and keep viral problems under control, by destroying viruses and keeping them from replicating. These drips will also help boost the energy level.

DIET AND NUTRITION

America's SAD Diet

We are living in an unhealthy world, eating empty calories, so as a result we cannot get the nutrition we need. We end up with GI manifestations and an inability to uptake all the nourishment from the foods we eat, so eventually we get to the point where we can not take in the proper minerals and nutrients even if we ate all the right foods. To combat this, we need to take supplements as well as change our eating styles.

I like to go out west, to Albuquerque, Santa Fe, and other cities. When I travel, I observe the eating and health habits of people, comparing people in the city with those in the country or suburbs. Not surprisingly, people in the country live longer. Why is this?

Dr. Pelton reminds us that for hundreds of years, people have been eating fresh fruit and vegetables, allowing the immune system of the vegetable kingdom to add to our immune protection. It is only in the last one hundred years that we have gotten into factory farming and processed food. With such foods, we are not getting the vital phytochemicals. One important yardstick of the healthiness of your life, is how many of these plant-based phido chemicals you get into your system, which translates into how many fruits or vegetables you regularly eat.

We have been eating four food groups for nutrition. Everyone, from our home economics teacher to our parents, told us to eat meat for our muscles, drink milk for bones, and, maybe, eat some spinach and fruits when in season. Back in the 1950s, the economy was booming, and families thought they were prosperous if they ate meat; meat showed you had arrived. We also began to eat convenience foods. We did not want to waste time in the kitchen. We wanted to be in front of the TV, so we could be encouraged to buy things we did not need. The lessons learned in the '30s about conserving resources and living frugally were lost.

Many of us are living with the old mindset. We eat meat three times a day. For breakfast, we eat sausage or bacon; then lunch calls for pizza or a cheeseburger or hot dog, maybe fish or a ham sandwich; then for dinner, pork or a two-inch cut of beef. With dinner, we may have a potato, but probably French fries, for the fry is the most commonly consumed form of potato in the United States. We finish that meal with coffee with sugar and, of course, a dessert. Then we wonder why we are sick.

Most countries cannot imitate this diet, and, so, they do not imitate our disease patterns. Look at Africa. In the African diet there is no dairy, and the people have no osteoporosis. They have no animal protein to speak of and no rectal or colon cancer. There is no coronary heart disease and no arthritis in any significant numbers, no spastic colon or appendicitis or any of the gastric distress we have. Daily, they eat 50 grams of fiber and we eat 15 grams.

Our diet is an abomination. We are not only eating the wrong things, but those things are being made worse by the way they are processed in industrialized food.

Humans and animals are hit by many bacteria that are resistant to antibiotics. To combat them, we feed our animals even stronger antibiotics along with the tranquilizers, growth stimulating hormones and other chemicals they get. We do not preserve, we embalm our meat. If you ever cut your finger, you will see as the blood oozes out, it is red at first, but very shortly, as it hits the air, it turns brown. The same thing should happen to beef or other meats. Fresh cut it would be bright red, but, in a couple of hours, it would grow brown and then begin to stink. So, the butchers shoot it up with a color fixative, sodium nitrate, since they know people would not buy it otherwise. We know this fixative is a cancer-causing agent. This is not in dispute.

Another problem with meats is amines. You can get these from meats as well as other foods and beverages. Then add them to nitrates, which are also found in much food and drink. Eat a ham sandwich or corned beef with beer and you are getting amines and nitrates. Together they create nitrosamines, one of the most powerful, cancer-causing agents. Dr. Lijinsky at Oak Ridge showed nitrosamines can cause cancer even at low dosages. We are not talking about high amounts for this substance. So why are Americans surprised that they have a high incidence of colon-rectal cancer, one of the worst cancers?

According to Dr. Virginia Livingstone, we should not only avoid red meat but chicken. Chicken can get leukosis, a precursor of leukemia, which anyone who eats diseased chicken could contract.

We did not have such incidence of any of these diseases, but then, we did not eat so much animal protein and what we did eat was not preserved in the way we preserve it today.

Set aside the purely physical effects of eating meat for a minute and think of the ethical issues. Have you ever been on a farm? Seen a lamb? They are cute. Each one has its own unique, individual personality. If you have a flock of them, each one is different. They respond to love and they are fearful of people who do not love them. Where does that love come from? The soul. They are not just projecting love to get fed. You can't go around and say the lamb has no soul, but your dog or cat does. Does your dog or cat have feelings and understand you? Does it bond to you? Do you think a dog is just a dumb animal? It has sense. It has a spirit. It is alive.

I will tell you something from my heart. If we want to honor life, we cannot take a life just because it tastes good. That would be a denial of the spiritual value of life. What if we did not take any energy in except that which has been given us by nature: the grains, the nuts, the seeds, the legumes, herbs, tubers, and spices—all we need to be healthy? And if we are taking in something we do not need, we are not honoring life. Part of being healthy is honoring life.

The health of the body begins with the intestine. We used to believe it starts in the artery, but now we know the artery is secondary to the intestine. If it is bad going into the intestine, it is all the worse when it reaches the artery. You do not see the digested elements from fruits clogging the arteries and laying down plaque. You do not see legumes, vegetables, beans, nuts and seeds laying this down. No, you see meats and fat clogging them and creating congestion.

I mentioned other cultures do not eat all the animal fats we do, or consume so many saturated fats. They may consume even more fats than we do, but not the unhealthy fats we use. The Italians, for instance, use the monofats: olive oil, linseed oil, almond oil, walnut oil, which are rich in the essential fatty acids, the Omega 3 and Omega 6 acids which keep our arteries clean, our heart strong and our joints flexible.

Deleterious animal proteins are also found in dairy. Did you ever notice how much mucus dairy creates. You wake up in the morning, your eyes are puffy, you're clearing your throat, you've got flatulence, distention, congestion in the lungs. I've seen brain fatigue from dairy.

Dr. Feldman notes, "Part of the problem is people trying to get their calcium through milk. Milk is not a good source of anything. Milk is a commonly allergic food. Many people cannot assimilate the calcium in milk well. It is a myth of the dairy industry that this is a worthwhile place to get your calcium." Calcium, we should note, is manifestly deficient in those with osteoporosis.

Another thing to eliminate is sugar. I remember reading in a British medical journal from the beginning of the century an article where the doctor was complaining about the diseases he was seeing in people who were consuming excess amounts of sugar. He worried about what would happen if people consumed more than what he considered an already gargantuan amount. People were consuming six pounds a year. Now, it is estimated that every American eats an average of 150 pounds a year. No wonder diabetes is one of the leading killers and people are grossly overweight.

Get rid of the caffeine. I think I know a lot about that substance, since my doctoral dissertation was written on it and my laboratory work was done on the subject. (I have Ph.D. in human nutrition and public health science.) If you knew what I know about caffeine, you would not have it in teas, medication, chocolates, colas, and coffee. It is a poison. If it were invented today, it would be banned as being too toxic. The fact that billions consume it every day does not make it any safer. For one thing, cola, with the phosphorus, sugar, and caffeine, chelates out the body's calcium.

Beyond thinking about what we eat, we should consider how much we eat. There are 90 million American chronically overweight. Cultures in which people have long lives eat less food than other groups.

Dr. Roy Warford did a study in which he give different amounts of calories to groups of rats with one group getting substantially less than the other. The group with fewer calories was semi-fasted and lived longer.

Dr. Mark Lane at a gerontology research center in Baltimore, Maryland, has been doing studies of caloric restriction on rhesus and squirrel monkeys. We have known for years that if you feed a lab rat or a mouse about 30% less of the normal caloric intake than they would eat if allowed free rein, they will live significantly longer than their counterparts, allowed to eat as much as desired.

Dairy, meat, saturated fats—all seem to wear down the body prematurely. We have a choice. We can believe these scientists, the ones hired by special interest groups that make 100 billion dollars from selling dairy and sugars, processed food and meat. The ones we know are out to protect their $100 billion investment. We believe them or we believe what our body tells us. We believe in our body's cause and effect. We know that when we eat right and eat vegetarian, we feel better, eliminate better, our skin is better, even our hair is growing thicker.

Dr. Pelton puts it aphoristically, "There are a lot of things wrong with the American diet. I call it the standard American diet or SAD. It's sad because it's low in nutrition. With the farming process that has developed in this country and the tremendous processing of food undertaken, people do not get the nutrients they need."

EATING RIGHT FOR LONG LIFE

I was pleased, both by what I saw and what it signified, when I went to the Dallas market, one of the largest in the United States. In it, there are hundreds of fruit and vegetable stands. Most cities in the U.S. have a farmers' market, open at least one or two days a week, but the Dallas one is open 365 days a year. It has six large hangers, each the size of a football field. Six are for fruits and vegetables and it has an additional six for selling flowers. The success and popularity of this market signifies that people in the area are into buying fresh, healthy, and inexpensive foods. Many Americans who want to get back to what is important are going back to organic. Looking at the vastness of this market, one realizes how much variety one has to choose from. This is where your good nutrition comes from. This is where we should be shopping for our meals if we want to reverse the aging process.

Take the papaya. It enhances digestion, is rich in beta carotenes, rich in calcium and magnesium.

You can buy an organically grown head of broccoli at the Dallas market and it may have 90% more nutrients than a commercially grown head, taken from land where the soil has been denatured. If you do not have the nutrients in the soil, you are not going to get them in the produce grown in that soil. Buying these organic foods and paying a few cents more, is certainly an improvement over the $1,000 or $100,000 you will pay fighting the diseases acquired from a lifetime of bad eating habits.

A number of doctors testify to the benefits of a healthy vegetarian diet. Dr. Feldman, talking about patients in his nutritional program, says his group is doing better on lowering cholesterol than any comparable group. He states, "We did not select people to come in to work on cholesterol problems. We are using a total assault on the lifestyle without focusing on cholesterol. The level of reduction is superior to that found in any prior drug study [where drugs were used to cut down on cholesterol]. It is extremely important that we can achieve this reduction without drugs. Drugs are expensive and have side effects. Also, we do not know what long-term problems may arise with them."

A doctor in Connecticut was able to eliminate arthritis—chronic intermittent arthritis—in 88% of his patients through the use of a simple elimination diet, having them cut out various foods to see which ones were adversely affecting them.

Dean Ornish has shown a vegetarian diet can help clear the arteries. The findings of my study group supports this claim. We found we could lower cholesterol, lower the triglycerides, lower the percentage of body fat, aid digestion, shorten the transit times of food almost by half, remove constipation and create better sleep habits, so we could shorten a person's needed sleep (often by two hours a night). That is reversing the aging process.

Nina Anderson, author of *Over 50, Looking 30*, notes that organic foods are also valuable because they contain enzymes. Our present diet depletes our body's enzymes. Anderson says the problem is we eat too many cooked foods, which are overly processed, causing the pancreas to work overtime. Americans have some of the largest pancreases of any human being.

What happens after you eat a Thanksgiving dinner? Anderson asks. Ninety percent of the food at the dinner is cooked. After we eat, everyone wants to go to sleep. That happens because the pancreas is going crazy trying to put out enough enzymes to digest the meal. (Enzymes are what allow nutrients to be used. For example, you have enzymes in the heart that allow magnesium to be used. Without that enzyme, magnesium will not get to the heart.) It has to call for reinforcements from another source of enzymes, the metabolic enzymes. They are in the organs, killing the viruses and fighting disease. All of a sudden they are called out to help digest food. But what do you think happens when they have left the front lines?

"If you want to avoid degenerative disease, those debilitating diseases," says Anderson, "then you should take enzymes. They'll fight the battle for you. You'll stay young and you'll look young."

Your skin is a reflection of your internal health. With proper diet and the use of enzymes, she tells us, your age spots will disappear, moles will shrink, and the lines on your face will thin. Those are some things you will notice. They are external changes and not as important as internal regeneration. Still, they have value since people are concerned with not looking old. If you keep taking enzymes, your internal organs will stay young and healthy and you will feel good.

Now where do we get these enzymes? Enzymes are the catalysts of life. Raw foods are loaded with enzymes. Fruit and vegetable juices are filled with enzymes. When food is processed, the first things taken out are enzymes. Why? Because the enzymes are what allow the food to ripen, though, if it ripens far enough, it rots. So to stop it from ripening and rotting, so that it can be sold longer, these enzymes must be destroyed. But if you destroy the enzymes, you destroy the food's life force. It will have carbohydrates, vitamins, fats, and minerals, but not its life force.

All in all, our diet is crucial to our outward and inward appearance and health. Think of Italy and the Mediterranean. You see people with magnificent skin, lovely and supple, and this is because of the oils and other healthy foods in the diet. The Mediterranean diet includes a lot of oils and beans, a lot of white beans, garlic, onions, herbs, fresh food, a lot of organic. They have wines, but ones rich in bioflavinoids and the essential nutrients. They eat food that helps the heart, and deoccludes the arteries.

Diet is crucial. Eat less. Eliminate saturated fats and the excess protein that we take in which creates toxicity in our body, in our liver, while making us feel sluggish. These fats and protein creates edema and dehydration. Go vegetarian and organic. That is a major part of the recipe for maintaining vitality and health.

KINESIOLOGY

Now that we have seen what eating habits and supplementation are conducive to reversing the aging process, we can look to a number of exercises and therapies that can help us to grow older gracefully.

John Etcheson, expert in kinesiology, says this discipline is an acupuncture related science developed by the Chinese. It focuses on learning what foods and herbs are best used and assimilated by an individual. With this knowledge, a proper supplementation and diet can be devised that is finely calibrated to an individual's biology.

Etcheson, also a herbalist, states, in kinesiology, "First we need to test a patient's polarity to find out if it's balanced."

He demonstrates with a female client. She extends her left arm, shoulder level, away from the body. The patient has placed her other hand flat on the top of her head. That's a positive energy position. Etcheson pushes down on her extended limb, asking her to resist the pressure. She can hold her own against his pressure. Now she turns the hand on her head over. That is negative. This time when the hand on the head is reversed, the extended arm can be pushed down more easily. Etcheson explains this is a normal reaction based on the differences in polarity. If the patient were strong either way she placed her atop-head hand, she would probably be dehydrated or need to work with his thymus to balance her body.

Next, again with the left arm extended at shoulder level, the patient holds a nearly empty canister against her solar plexus with her other hand. The extended arm is weak and can be forced down easily. Next the right hand holds a canister filled with honey or another organic substance against the solar plexus. Now the arm is stronger and cannot be forced down. This is because the body knows the honey's nutritional value. In the nearly empty canister was a little table sugar, which is without value to the body. This same experiment might have been done, by the way, by placing alternating substances under the tongue. This is one way we can see the body's reaction to different herbs and foods.

In kinesiology, these food reactions are studied more precisely to determine proper individual diet.

EXERCISE

What kind of exercise can slow aging?

One valuable type is power walking or racewalking. Franco Pantoni, a U.S. National Champion racewalker and the racewalking coach for the

Natural Living Running and Walking Club, discusses this exercise. He compares racewalking to running. "The difference from running is the speed at which we travel. This exercise was established in 1908. It's great for both the body and mind. Most people don't know that Harry Truman and Albert Einstein were walkers. I have a picture of Einstein walking—he was a very fast walker—and a journalist is trying to keep up with him."

This exercise will increase the amount of oxygen in the blood. One reason the body ages is free radicals cause cellular damage. Free radicals are generated by a lack or low level of oxygen in the tissues. A slight decrease in oxygen in the tissues will be accompanied by an increase in the pesky free radicals. Vigorous exercise will combat this problem.

Pantoni describes the exercise by saying that the posture for free walking is to keep oneself very straight and light on the feet as if an invisible wire pulled one up from the top of the head. The hips are kept very loose. The inclination forward is 4 or 5 degrees, bending forward from the ankles, not waist. He tells us to lean forward as if you were about to fall forward. Stride forward, planting the heel first, keeping the leg straight, toes up. The arms is are bent at a 90 degree angle at the elbow and held in front of the chest. The hands are closed but not clenched tightly. The arms are held about six inches in front of the chest. As you move, swing them between the chest and waist, with a pumping motion, an easy, natural motion, working all the muscles in the upper body. The faster you go, the faster you pump, bringing your heart rate above 120.

"But as you go, think about relaxation," Pantoni coaches. "You have to think relaxed. Sometimes, there are so many things you are aware of: arms, feet, hips, but if you can become relaxed, you will profit. You will reach a point where you get that feeling of locomotion, where everything gets fluid. You are gliding, easy."

The *Medical Tribune* recently reported that senior citizens do not exercise enough. By exercising, the article meant going to a gym for a full workout, exercising all the muscle groups. It is hard enough to get the average person to do an aerobic workout or to go swimming or biking. Less than 5% of us exercise daily. When you factor in all the diseases due to faulty diet and lack of exercise, you have disaster.

One exercise that is easy to do at home is sit-ups. Doing them properly will tighten your stomach and abdominal muscles. Place a pillow on top of your ankles and anchor the feet under a bed. In doing them, never put your hands behind your neck, because that will pull the neck and spine up and can throw your spine out of place. Instead, cross your arms over your chest. Only come up about nine inches, which will be enough for you to get complete expansion and compression. Exhale coming up and inhale going down.

Another simple exercise that can be done with equipment available in most gyms. It is the slow and rhythmic lifting of weights from a seated posture, doing the lift from 10 to 15 times. The general formula to go by is that if you want muscles that are big, bulky and have greater strength, then use a heavier weight and less repetitions. If you want muscles that are lean and fast, use lower weights and more reps. I would suggest 15 reps, 3 sets.

For strengthening the shoulders, upper chest and upper back, lift barbells of a comfortable weight, going from the arms hanging toward the waist till they are at shoulder height. As you move, don't crane your neck, but practice deep breathing, allowing deep releasing of oxygen.

Remember, an average gym will have about 20 pieces of equipment, but that does not mean you have to use all 20. If you tried to use them all, many of the exercises you would do would be redundant. You might be using a slightly different grip, but you would be working the same muscle group as on a different machine. You can work out on the slant board and any of the crunch machines, but the most important thing to keep in mind is to exercise everything: the hamstrings, calves, abdominals, upper chest, shoulders, arms and neck.

RELAXING AND COORDINATING THE MUSCLES

Feldenkrais

Where exercise strengthens and adds to muscle suppleness, sometimes, bad patterns of movement or chronic tensions have established problems in the joints or muscles. Feldenkrais is a practice that helps eliminate the problem of poor movement habits.

Sharon Oliensis, a guild certified practitioner, talks about her discipline. "Dr. Moishe Feldenkrais developed this method to relieve chronic muscle tension and stress. It uses very gentle movements. Either the student does them to him or herself, guided by the instructor, while lying on the floor, or the student lies on something like a massage table and the teacher uses a hands-on approach, taking the student through gentle movements so that he or she lets go of a chronic holding or stress pattern. This helps the student develop a greater sense of ease and flexibility so breathing and coordination improves."

Oliensis runs her hand lightly over the back of a clothed, standing male patient. She senses the curve of the spine and muscle development along the spine. Everyone's spine is different. As her hand moves up and down its length, the student directs his awareness to the point she is touching. Together, they make discoveries about its length and shape, as well as it sensitivities and insensitivities. One of the principles is to bring awareness to those parts of our body of which we were previously unaware, and develop the knowledge to alter old patterns. Then, she tests freedom of hip movement.

The patient lies on his back. "I lift his legs and press down through the soles of his feet to see how movement transfers up through his skeleton, through the pelvis, ribs and up to the top of his head. Then I can see and he can feel what is the pathway a movement most easily takes and where there are resistances to the movement. Based on that, combined with what he has told me, I can judge what to work on in any individual session. Part of the therapy is his body learning beneficial patterns, which comes of his learning to differentiate between parts of his body that are relaxed and parts which are still tense. Normally, the part that has been worked on will feel more in contact with the table, larger, wider, smoother. The side not worked with will feel as if rising off the table. The key for the nervous system is to learn a new way of behaving and recognize, simply enough, that one can feel this way or that way, relaxed or tense."

Yoga

Another means of keep the body young and the muscles flexible is to relax and strengthen it with yoga.

Mary Dunn, senior yoga teacher at the Iyengar Yoga Institute of Greater New York, says, yoga is a way to help alleviate the aches and pains and tensions that come from daily living as well as the general malaise and fatigue that may overtake a person.

When you come home from work with legs feeling tired and heavy, Dunn says, do a modified shoulder stand. With the back on the floor and a pillow under it, lift legs up and point them to the sky, bracing them against the wall. This will open up the chest and lungs, make the shoulder and the breath relaxed, so you can leave the tension of the day behind.

One of the methods of yoga is stretching. Most of our experience of stretching comes when we have to do some work, reaching for something on a shelf, for instance. Yet, if we were asked to replicate that reaching motion, we would feel constricted, because we were not stretching properly. We need to train the nervous system so as to bring consciousness into the body so all the joints are open. When we have opened all of them, we have stretched the nerves that accompany those muscles. When we relax, they relax, and since the nerves go back to the brain, it relaxes too.

ENERGY PRACTICES

Chakra Psychology

Aside from dealing with muscular tensions produced by our stressful environment, it is necessary to develop methods of channeling our energy, not letting it get dammed up and frozen the way our muscles can be when we do not know how to relax them. Indian and Chinese methods can play an important role.

An Indian practice, chakra psychology, is related to yoga and focuses on the energy we receive through breathing.

Shyam Bhatnagar of Sri Center International of New York City tells us there are seven chakras along the spine that influence our nervous system. It takes years to develop awareness of these nodes—six to seven years for the first.

Each of these chakras can teach a form of awareness:
- body awareness
- gender
- social identity
- consider ourselves lovers of the divine, people who love nature and mankind
  - the arts and creativity
- androgyny, resolving sexual dualities as well as being the center for meditation
- what reality is and what the underlying substratum is on which we superimpose our simplifying projections. At this last chakra can be found divine consciousness.

Bhatnagar tell us a number of practices, both enjoyable and beneficial, lead to a deepening experience of the chakras. First, synchronize breathing with the respiration of the cosmic bodies in heaven. We need to be aware of these bodies. The sun affects us most because it is our father. Without the sun, there would be no life on this planet. Second is the moon. These two heavenly bodies have a relationship and our body is constructed based on this relationship. To get in tune with this relationship, we need to do breathing exercises.

The right nostril is the solar or sun-dominated one, while the left is moon dominated. Conversely, the right brain hemisphere is lunar while the right is solar. When you are predominantly breathing with the left nostril, your right hemisphere will be more dominant. Breathing predominantly with the right nostril, you will find the left hemisphere in control. At any time, one of the nostrils will be dominant.

It may seem from casual observation that you are using both nostrils equally, Bhatnagar states, but there is a slight difference. There is a way to determine dominance. Place the thumb first under one then the other nostril. Breathe in, breathe out. Next time you do this, be aware of the temperature. Whichever side feels cooler is more open. If your digestion is not good, lie on the left side after and before eating, he advises. If you are in a situation in which you feel you cannot express your feelings, lie on the right side. When the right side is open, you will have more courage to express yourself. This is help you can get from the cosmic forces.

MEDITATION

A way to keep our senses alert and relaxed is through mindfulness meditation.

Beverly McGregor, Ph.D., a psychologist and founder, co-director of The Health Institute in Dallas, points out the value of mindfulness meditation. "It has to do with being aware of what is around us at every moment. In practice, we can learn to be calm and centered. When stressors come up, we can respond in a better way. We can be fully present in what is happening.

"You may be watching a sunset or seeing a lake. Suddenly a thought comes up—'I wish this other person were sharing this with me,' for instance. Suddenly we are thinking of something else, and not fully present with the lake."

Mindfulness meditation helps one to escape distracting and, hence, detracting thoughts that stop one from living in the moment.

ATTITUDES AND BELIEF SYSTEMS

The expression "our health care system" is a misnomer. It has never dealt with being healthy. You have to focus on keeping yourself healthy. Pasteur was only one half right. He recognized that there were germs and they played a role in illness. That's correct. But he was wrong when he said the germ would cause the disease. The milieu your body is in will cause the disease. Germs will alter depending on your body.

A funny thing I have wondered about is why so many people interested in health are sick. Some of the sickest individuals I have ever met are in the health movement. It is not all about a deficiency of nutrients. I have studied the healthiest individuals I could find. And afterwards, along with Dr. Martin Feldman and Dolores Perri, I developed a protocol for wellness that will optimize a person's overall life with, among other things, diet, supplements, exercise and positive life affirmations. Anyone who has followed this regimen has seen substantial, sometimes radical, improvement.

Life is not so simple that you can change one thing and see real improvement. For that, you have to change the whole field.

Number one is attitudinal change. With the wrong attitude, you will become sick. Negative attitude, meaninglessness, bad disposition, these always lead to disease. The disposition is the catalyst. You get breast cancer not only because of estrogen in the food, but because of attitude.

In poorer foreign countries, I will often meet people without the material wealth we have, but they have meaningfulness and purpose. They have balance. People in their 70s up to their 90s, loving and honoring life, not feeling angry or rejected.

A healthy person looks for a message in a crisis. Before he or she overreacts, he or she assesses the situation. Nothing is so bad it cannot be dealt with. Nothing you cannot survive. Look beyond the crisis toward solutions. You may not be able to change the crisis, but you can shift attitude and remain focused and balanced.

Meaninglessness exacerbates physical and psychological conditions. Stop beating up on yourself. Take the responsibility to love yourself. Most people are lovable if they let their real self show.

Bhatnagar puts it like this. "Some people seem to say, 'I don't like myself, but I want you to love me.' That's cheating. If a person starts to cheat on you, it's unfair. You have to love yourself first. Otherwise, there is dependency."

Stop making excuses. There is no need for any illness. But to say this, you must be willing to look into those dark places in your psyche that you have avoided or denied. Be willing to be consistently disciplined in your eating, in meditation. The moment that you are helpless—you pig out or you get angry—it is all for nothing. Then, it is gone. And how many games do you have to play before you realize you always lose?

Stan Huff, Ed.D., a licensed professional counselor, talks about changing yourself: "Visualization and imagery will help a person change some negative messages, escape old roles or the tyranny of negative experiences so as to replace these with a more positive set of roles and messages. A person can replace these counterproductive stories with more affirmative ones that fit better with who you deserve to be."

He explains that visualization is an active form of meditation that allows the patient to see images in the mind's eye that can influence the emotions and reduce stress. It gives the person new options and choices in ways to relate to the world.

You have to start honoring the little child within you. The child is the healer. I have never seen an adult who did not use this child as a vehicle for healing. A child has wonderment, acceptance, openness. Children do not reject you because you are black or white. They do not care. They love you for being you. I see these deadly serious people hanging out in doctors' offices. They are not using their inner child. No way is healing going to happen.

Quiet that mind. Find out how healthy you want to be. On a scale of 1 to 100, how healthy do you want to be?

Dolores Perri, R.D., a nutritionist, tells us, "Don't believe anyone who says you cannot do it. When I see people in their 80s running marathons, people cutting down their cholesterol without drugs, I know you can do it."

Put all the parts of wellness together. If you leave out one part because it is inconvenient, then you have problems. Put them together and you will reverse the aging process and be able to look forward to productive later years when you will be passionately alive.

INDEX